DATE DUE

NOV 4 1997			
MAR 3 0 1999			
MAY 2 8 2001			
AUG 2 9 2018			

Demco, Inc. 38-293

Evolution of Infectious Disease

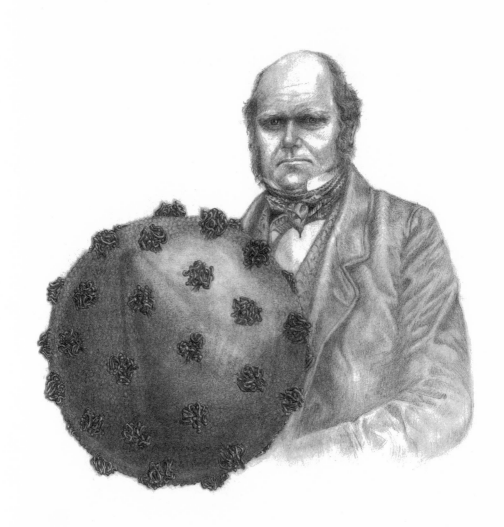

Evolution of Infectious Disease

Paul W. Ewald

Department of Biology
Amherst College

Oxford   New York
OXFORD UNIVERSITY PRESS

1994

Oxford University Press

Oxford New York Toronto
Delhi Bombay Calcutta Madras Karachi
Kuala Lumpur Singapore Hong Kong Tokyo
Nairobi Dar es Salaam Cape Town
Melbourne Auckland Madrid

and associated companies in
Berlin Ibadan

Copyright © 1994 by Paul W. Ewald

Published by Oxford University Press, Inc.,
198 Madison Avenue, New York, New York 10016-4314

Oxford is a registered trademark of Oxford University Press

Library of Congress Cataloging-in-Publication Data
Ewald, Paul W.
Evolution of infectious disease / by Paul W. Ewald
p. cm. Includes bibliographical references and index.
ISBN 0-19-506058-X
1. Host-parasite relationships. 2. Communicable diseases.
3. Evolution I. Title
[DNLM: 1 Communicable Diseases-etiology. 2. Evolution
3. Host-Parasite Relations. WC 100 E94e 1993]
RC112.E93 1993 616.9'0471-dc20 DNLM/DLC 92-48386

The frontispiece represents the merging of evolutionary biology, symbolized by Charles Darwin, with current knowledge about infectious processes, symbolized by the human immunodeficiency virus. The conical capsule inside the virus encloses the virus's genetic instructions. As discussed in Chapter 9, the projections from the virus's surface (called gp120) allow the virus to enter white blood cells by attaching to receptors (called CD4) on the surface of the cells, much like a hand grasps a doorknob to enter a house. *Illustration by Jennifer Nolan.*

5 7 9 8 6 4

Printed in the United States of America
on acid-free paper

Acknowledgments

When I was a graduate student, I, like most graduate students, spent time wondering what insights I might eventually have and where they would come from. And, like most students of ecology and evolution, my mind would wander to the classic, romantic stories in this field: Charles Darwin generating the principles of natural selection from his observations of finches in the Galapagos, or G. Evelyn Hutchinson gaining insights about the structure of ecological communities by peering into a pool full of aquatic insects in front of the little church of Santa Rosalia on the outskirts of Palermo, Sicily. Hutchinson entitled the paper that grew from his insights "Homage to Santa Rosalia." If I were to follow Hutchinson's lead, I would have to call this book "Homage to Manhattan, Kansas" because my impetus to apply evolutionary insights to the health sciences originated from a rather bad case of diarrhea that I acquired while I was conducting research near a little garbage dump on the outskirts of Manhattan, Kansas. Between the urgent dashes, I had long stretches of time to ponder the broader significance of my predicament. A chain of questions began forming. Should I treat the diarrhea or should I let it run its course? Why was this particular organism causing me more problems than the other organisms that I had encountered during my previous 23 years? And why was it that even though I was in extreme discomfort, it was no worse? Unlike other agents of diarrhea, this bug was not a threat to my life.

The ideas presented in this book have taken shape over the ensuing 16 years to answer this chain of questions and the additional questions that each answer generated. I am particularly grateful to those scientists who, early on, recognized the value of pursuing such questions and fostered my interest in doing so. Sievert A. Rohwer and Gordon H. Orians encouraged my early efforts to apply evolutionary principles to infectious disease and enlightened me about the relevance of evolutionary thinking whenever living things are the subjects of study. William D. Hamilton urged me to pursue these studies from our first meeting in 1978; he has also suggested that every evolutionary biologist should send me 50 dollars because the unification of evolutionary biology with the health sciences should help raise evolutionary biology's impoverished status in the minds of many outside the field. (If anyone is interested, that would be 70 dollars after adjusting for inflation.)

Many scientists contributed valuable ideas and perspectives during the middle and later stages of this work. Mary Jane West Eberhard helped me to recognize the value of comparative methods for fostering the integration of evolutionary biology and epidemiology, in part through her insights on Darwin's development of the principles of evolution. By never letting me off the hook during spirited exchanges, William G. Eberhard helped me to identify assumptions, weaknesses in arguments, and alternative hypotheses. David I. Ratner was always ready to provide mini-lectures on things molecular. My drawing together of information, ideas and arguments also benefitted from discussions with Richard D. Alexander, Roy M. Anderson, Tom Butynski, Geoffrey Cowley, Richard A. Goldsby, William B. Greenough, III, Jan Kalina, Jonathan Kingdon, Olga F. Linares, Elizabeth E. Lyons, Stephen S. Morse, Gerald Myers, Randolph Nesse, Gerald Schad, Robert Smutz, Andrew Spielman, James Strain, and George C. Williams. I thank Robert J. Biggar, Fernando Gracia, Moslem Udin Khan, Miguel Kourany, Leonardo J. Mata, Gerald Myers, Benjamin Schwartz, and H. Shimanuki for taking the time to clarify research findings and provide unpublished results. I note with appreciation the hundreds of scientists who have sent reprints and preprints of their work. William B. Greenough, III, Ethan J. Temeles, and George C. Williams provided numerous helpful comments on the manuscript, as did Nadine Alexander and Jennifer Nolan, who also expedited the final stages of manuscript preparation.

Many students have made contributions during discussions and by passing along relevant references. In particular, I thank Meg Abbot, Steve Bennett, Shagufta Bidiwala, Steve Boorstein, Beth Ellingwood, Tony Goldberg, Kathy Hanley, Marta Heilbrun, Kathleen McKibben, Karen Kiang, Lara Litchfield, Jennifer Nolan, Sarah Rubenstein, Jennifer Schubert, Bruno Walther, Kurt Weber, and Lowell Weiss. For help in obtaining articles and books I am grateful to Leeta Bailey, Margaret Groesbeck, Michael Kasper, Floyd S. Merritt, Susan Lisk, and Susan Edelberg of the Robert Frost Library at Amherst College, E. Tooke and P. Heddle of University of London's Book Depository, and the librarians at the London School of Hygiene and Tropical Medicine.

Many of the hypotheses presented in this book were developed and preliminary data were obtained while I was supported by the Michigan Society of Fellows and the Division of Biological Sciences at the University of Michigan from 1980 to 1983 and by an NSF/NATO postdoctoral fellowship at Imperial College during 1984 and 1985. Amherst College nurtured the research since 1983 by granting a Miner D. Crary Fellowship, a Trustees Faculty Fellowship, an Amherst College Faculty Research Award, sabbatical funding, and logistical support. The work was also aided by a fellowship from the Occupational Health Program at Harvard School of Public Health. The later stages of research and the final drawing together of ideas into this book were made possible by a George E. Burch Fellowship in Theoretic Medicine and Affiliated Sciences awarded by the Smithsonian Institution and hosted by the Smithsonian Tropical Research Institute.

My parents, Sara and Arno Ewald, fostered during early formative years a tendency to look from different perspectives and explore interests wherever they may lead. Christine Bayer Ewald has been both a source of support and a source of sources throughout my work on the evolution of disease.

Contents

Evolution of Infectious Disease

CHAPTER 1

Why This Book?

Given enough time a state of peaceful coexistence eventually becomes established between any host and parasite.

Rene Dubos (1965)

Disease usually represents the inconclusive negotiations for symbiosis...a biological misinterpretation of borders.

Lewis Thomas (1972)

The ideal of parasitism is actually commensalism.

Paul D. Hoeprich (1989)

A BREAK WITH TRADITION

Few ideas have been so ingrained in the literature of medicine and parasitology as the idea that parasites should evolve toward benign coexistence with their hosts. Few ideas in science have been so widely accepted with so little evidence. And few ideas are so at odds with the fundamental principles on which they are supposedly based, with such a great potential for missed opportunity.

The proponents of this idea rarely trace it to fundamental evolutionary principles; when they do they reveal a misunderstanding of the most basic evolutionary process: natural selection. One can pardon the early proponents. Theobald Smith (1934), Hans Zinsser (1935), and N. H. Swellengrebel (1940) were writing at a time when evolutionary biologists were just beginning to integrate natural selection with their newly found understanding of genetics (Fisher 1930, Haldane 1932). Even those writing on the subject through midcentury can be excused. Until William D. Hamilton (1964) and George C. Williams (1966) clarified the process of natural selection, even prominent biologists focusing on evolutionary processes were more than a bit confused (e.g., Wynne-Edwards 1962, Lorenz 1964). As the time since Hamilton and Williams's landmark writings has passed from years to decades, however, the perpetuation of this idea that parasites inexorably evolve to benignness has become distressing; it serves as an indicator of just how disconnected modern evolutionary biology is from modern health sciences. In recent years both theoretical and empirical studies have led to a rejection of obligate evolution to benignness (Levin & Pimentel 1981, Anderson & May 1982, Ewald 1983, 1988, 1991a, Levin 1983, May & Anderson 1983), yet it is still presented in well-respected journals and medical texts as the foundation upon which evolutionary arguments are built (e.g., Palmieri 1982, Doyle & Lee 1986, Hoeprich 1989, Snewin et al 1991, Waters et al 1991).

The confusion of prominent biologists and medical scientists alike can be traced to a misunderstanding about the levels at which natural selection acts. When advocates of obligate evolution to benignness write on the subject, they often phrase their arguments in terms of what is best for the parasite species or for most individuals within the species (Holmes & Bethel 1972, Palmieri 1982, Hoeprich 1989). Burnet and White (1972), for example, state, "For Nature, survival of the species is all that counts." Simon (1960) writes that "attenuated infection represents a state in which the most favorable conditions are provided for the greatest number of individuals over the longest period of time." But there is no reason to presume that natural selection favors what is best for the greatest number of individuals over the greatest amount of time. Natural selection favors characteristics that increase the passing on of the genes that code for the characteristics. If more rapid replication of a virus inside of a person leads to a greater passing on of the genes that code for that rapid replication, then replication rate will increase even if the more rapid growth of the virus population within a person causes the person to be severely ill, or leads to an overall decrease in the numbers of the virus among people, or hastens the eventual extinction of the virus.

Proponents of obligate evolution toward commensalism write about how inefficient parasites are if they reproduce so extensively that they leave behind millions of progeny in an ill or dead host, and how this inefficiency is a mark of poor adaptation of the parasite to its host (Swellengrebel 1940, Thomas 1972).

replication does not enhance transmission sufficiently, the more harmful fast replicators will be favored. Similarly, if the specifics of mutation, transmission, or pathogen reproduction increase the genetic variation of the parasites within a host, the slow replicators may be disadvantaged (Wilson 1980). Although many variations on the theme exist, these tradeoffs are fundamental to the application of natural selection to the evolution of host–parasite relationships. More generally, understanding these tradeoffs provides the key to understanding the evolutionary paths that our disease organisms have taken in the past and will take in the future. By studying these tradeoffs this book attempts to identify the circumstances that favor evolution toward any particular level of harmfulness, from extreme benignness to lethality.

Prior to the last quarter of the twentieth century, a scattered few scientists have disagreed with the conventional wisdom that adaptation should lead inexorably to benign states of coexistence. The malariologist G. R. Coatney and his colleagues (1971) expressed their reservations, writing that the "body of evidence is, in our view, somewhat less than convincing." The virologist C. H. Andrewes (1960) also distanced himself from the traditional view, although haltingly. While affirming his belief in the idea that efficient parasites are benign, he observed that when pathogens are transferred into new hosts, they may increase in virulence, and concluded that pathogens evolve toward an intermediate, "optimum" virulence to facilitate transmission. He illustrated this idea with the sneezes and coughs of respiratory diseases, which may facilitate transmission by distributing pathogens in the environment.

The strongest disagreement with the traditional viewpoint came from Ball (1943), who focused on a corollary of obligate evolution toward benignness: that particularly severe disease is an indication of a recent and imperfectly evolved association. He attacked this idea by showing the numerous exceptions, and concluded that if there is a tendency for parasites to evolve toward benignness, it is of no predictive value because knowledge about virulence does not provide knowledge about the duration of the association between host and parasite. Ball's criticisms, like the more guarded warnings of Andrewes (1960) and Coatney et al. (1971), were ignored largely, I think, because none of these authors provided a general alternative framework for understanding why different host–parasite associations have evolved different levels of virulence. Without the advancement of such a framework, the idea that host–parasite relationships should evolve to a state of benign balance was apparently too appealing to be rejected, in spite of the fact that there was no good evidence for it. Since the late 1970s this situation has changed. We can now see not only an alternative framework but also the beginning of two new disciplines that are emerging from the controversy: disciplines that synthesize our knowledge about treatment of disease, spread of disease, and evolution, from the submicroscopic realm of molecular biology to the superorganismal realms of ecology and evolutionary biology.

But the number of lost organisms is not the relevant number. We might as well say that maple trees are poorly adapted because 990 out of every 1000 helicopter-like seeds are doomed to an early death. The number relevant to natural selection is the number of genes passed into the succeeding generation. Would the genes coding for production of 1000 seeds be left in greater numbers than the genes coding for production of 100 seeds? The 1000-seed strategy may be vastly more wasteful in terms of seed death and tissue destruction, but if it ultimately yields more trees in succeeding generations, it will be more efficient in terms of evolutionary success. So too, a parasite that reproduces massively inside a host, leaving billions of pathogens to die after the final transmission event, will contribute more genes for that rapid reproduction into future generations than a parasite that by virtue of its lower rate of reproduction leaves fewer organisms stranded in the host but gets its descendants into fewer hosts.

Indeed, looking at the problem from this perspective, one might wonder whether the less harmful, slower reproducers could ever win. How could they pass on more copies of their instructions for slower reproduction in the midst of competition with the fast reproducers? The resolution to this problem lies in understanding the potential for pathogens inside of a host to be very similar genetically. The population of viruses inside of a person may number in the billions, a number generated by growth of the virus population from a few successful colonists. As a consequence of this growth, a particular genetic instruction in one virus stands a good chance of being in many if not most or even all of the other viruses inside the person. If a gene regulates the virus's replication at a low level and restricts the degree of tissue invasion, it may lose out in competition with any faster-reproducing competitors inside the person. But if the illness caused by the fast replicators severely curbs the prospects for transmission, then people who by chance become infected with slowly replicating colonists might transmit their pathogens to other people and thereby to future generations at a faster rate than those infected with the rapidly replicating colonists.

This argument is tricky because the advantages that the slower replicators achieve through slower reproduction are shared with any rapidly replicating cohabitants. The slow reproducers therefore tend to lose when they cohabit a person with fast reproducers. But because the population of pathogens in a person tends to grow from a few colonists, they may be genetically similar to one another; a slow replicator will often cohabit a person with other slow replicators, and fast replicators will often cohabit with fast replicators. The slow replicators will contribute more to succeeding generations when slow replication sufficiently enhances the chances for transmission to new hosts. [Those versed in the terminology of evolutionary biology will recognize that this process represents cooperation or altruism among the pathogens, which is generated by the inclusive fitness effects (Hamilton 1963, 1964) of slow replication; one can say that the slow replication evolves by kin selection (Maynard Smith 1964)]. When slow

EVOLUTIONARY EPIDEMIOLOGY AND DARWINIAN MEDICINE

Evolutionary biology is so firmly integrated with the rest of biology that it is not possible to mark a boundary between them. But modern medicine has been a peninsula. It is broadly and firmly connected with most regions of biology such as anatomy, physiology, biochemistry, molecular biology, and genetics, but has just a few thin bridges traversing the gulf to evolutionary biology. Knowledge about the evolution of antibiotic resistance is perhaps the best developed bridge between the disciplines. The discovery of the evolutionary basis for sickle cell anemia—protection against malaria—is another.

There are probably many reasons for the paucity of bridges. One stems from inadequate appreciation of the pervasiveness of evolutionary principles. From secondary school through medical school, the fundamental relevance of evolution to all of human life often has been ignored or even suppressed. Had it been different, the ideas presented in this book probably would have been addressed decades sooner, perhaps as early as a half-century ago, when evolutionary biologists were uniting the principles of genetics and natural selection. As will become clear in the pages that follow, the redress of these oversights may be a life-or-death matter for millions of people each year, and a quality-of-life matter for tens of millions more.

Realizing that scientists writing about the evolution of virulence have been incorrect throughout most of the last century is one thing; finding out what is correct is quite another. Application of evolutionary principles does not lead to the conclusion that all parasites evolve toward benignness. But can evolutionary principles help us understand why some parasites cause severe disease while others are nearly always extremely mild? This book is a dogged attempt to resolve this question and to understand the implications of this resolution for the future of the health sciences, in theory and in practice.

The question is at the heart of an emerging discipline: evolutionary epidemiology (Ewald 1988). Traditional epidemiology investigates the prevalence and spread of diseases within and among populations of hosts over ecological time scales. Epidemiology broadened the previous emphasis of health practitioners, which was on care of sick individuals, to a larger scale: the nature of disease processes among populations of individuals. Evolutionary epidemiology broadens the scale of inquiry still further to assess how the characteristics that traditional epidemiology has identified to be important—lethality, illness, transmission rates, prevalences of infection—change over time as hosts and parasites evolve in response to each other and to outside environments.

The integration of evolutionary biology with the health sciences is also spawning an overlapping discipline, termed Darwinian medicine, which takes an evolutionary approach to the entire spectrum of issues related to health and disease (Williams & Nesse 1991). Darwinian medicine and evolutionary epidemiology are complementary in several ways. Whereas evolutionary epidemiology focuses on the spread of diseases, Darwinian medicine focuses more on the individual patient. Darwinian medicine, for example, encompasses treatment of psychiatric disorders and physical trauma, and emphasizes the evolutionary molding of developmental processes and genetic diseases. Central to both disciplines is the action of natural selection, but because Darwinian medicine focuses more on individual patients, it gives more attention to human evolution. From the perspective of Darwinian medicine, senescence, for example, is an inevitable consequence of selection for traits that are beneficial during the early and middle years of a maximum life-span. These traits eventually take a toll during old age, but by the time this toll comes due in nature, the organism may have already died from other causes. Natural selection, therefore, favors the senescent developmental arrangement: Buy now, pay later. The immediate fitness benefit outweighs the cost of deferred payment because organisms tend to die young in nature: A 30-year-old man killed by a mastodon will never pay the price of a heart attack brought on by decades of atherosclerosis.

Defining epidemiology broadly to include nonhuman hosts, evolutionary epidemiology spans a broader spectrum of host–parasite relationships; it extends beyond medical settings to encompass parasitism in nature and agriculture involving both plant and animal hosts. The two disciplines overlap broadly, especially where the interpretation and treatment of human infectious diseases are concerned. Both disciplines emphasize that appropriate patient care requires an understanding of the evolutionary processes affecting the disease-causing organisms and the responses of the host to these organisms.

Because the evolution of human characteristics is relatively slow, evolutionary epidemiology and especially Darwinian medicine consider time spans that encompass the evolution of *Homo sapiens* and even our ancestral species in which relevant characteristics, like immunological defenses, may have evolved. Pathogens, in contrast, may evolve substantially over time periods of a few weeks. When considering infectious diseases from the pathogens' "point of view," a few decades of medical records may offer a potential for evolutionary change that is comparable to the entire time span of our genus *Homo*. The evolutionary process for pathogens is therefore best considered to be a process in progress. The pathogens are a moving target of our research. We and our activities are part of the environment that pushes this process down one course or another. The following pages emphasize evolutionary epidemiology. George Williams and Randy Nesse offer a complementary overview of Darwinian medicine (Williams & Nesse 1991).

In preparing this book, I have tried to eject specialized terms whenever possible. Technical terms are superb for transmitting complex ideas rapidly and concisely to colleagues, but they create viscous barriers to interested outsiders.

And if there is one thing that a synthesis of evolution and the health sciences needs, it is input from outsiders. People in the health sciences need the foundation of evolutionary principles as much as they need the foundations of molecular biology. Evolutionary biologists need to grasp the complex and specialized knowledge of immunology, molecular biology, and medical treatment if they are to provide evolutionary insights into medical problems. Because evolutionary changes in disease organisms depend on past, present, and future cultural environments, historians, sociologists, anthropologists, and psychologists need to be involved. Perhaps most importantly, if we want people outside of the health sciences to continue to foot the bill for expensive long-term research, and to make intelligent decisions about which bills to foot, the information must be accessible to those outside of science and academia.

Having said all of this, I must concede that there are some terms, like evolutionary fitness, ribonucleic acid (RNA) and virulence, with which I could not part. To help readers with these stragglers, I have provided a glossary at the end of the text. Some terms that I use will mean different things to different people. When I use these terms I shall try to be clear about the definition that I am using. When I use the term *parasite*, for example, I am referring to any organism that lives in or on another organism and causes harm to that organism. Theoretically, I define *harm* as a negative effect on a host's evolutionary fitness. *Evolutionary fitness*, in turn, is a measure of the individual's success at passing on its genes into future generations through its survival and reproduction. In practice, however, we can rarely measure this effect; moreover, effects of disease that might drastically reduce the fitness of humans living in nature may have no negative effects on fitness in our modern society. In practice, then, we can think of harm, crudely, as the presence of illness and increased chances of death that result from parasitism, keeping in mind the important caveat discussed in the next chapter: Many aspects of illness may actually be beneficial rather than harmful to the host. When I use the term *virulence*, I am referring to the degree of harm to the host caused by the parasite. I use *parasite virulence* when I am writing about the degree to which the parasite's characteristics impose negative effects on the host. The flip side is *host resistance*. When resistance is lowered, a disease may be more virulent, even though the parasite's inherent virulence is unchanged. Together these two components, parasite virulence and host resistance, determine how negatively the host will be affected.

My emphasis will be from the parasites' point of view rather than from the hosts'. It is not that I have any fondness for the smallpox virus or the cholera bacterium, or even our ubiquitous companion, the common cold virus, whose virulence is high enough to trigger special attention from parents and spouses, but mild enough to allow its victim to savor this care. No, I emphasize the parasites' point of view because the health sciences have strongly emphasized the humans' point of view. This concern for humans has led health scientists to investigate in striking detail how host characteristics influence virulence; indeed, tremendous progress has been made from this perspective. We are now learning how diet, exercise, stress, and genetic differences between people affect the severity of our illnesses. Every year, general principles are refined and applied to new situations. Throughout history, for example, there has been general awareness that physical fitness and a good diet make people better able to ward off disease. This general awareness has been gradually transformed into a finely woven understanding of countless threads of information. The threads may seem contradictory at first, but eventually we see that the apparent contradiction arises from the difference between our imagined pattern and the real pattern. Early on, health scientists discovered that our immune systems are more able to combat infection when we have an adequate intake of vitamins, protein, and other nutrients. More recently, the negative effects of overintake of these nutrients—particularly fats, sugars, salt, and cholesterol—have been clarified. When dietary fats are restricted, for example, heart disease is reduced and our immune systems operate more effectively. Still more recently, researchers have identified beneficial effects of what once would have been considered severely restricted amounts of food. When laboratory animals are fed just enough food to meet their needs, they have lower rates of cancer, longer life-spans, and improved immune responses. Dietary restriction may even improve abilities to fight off infectious diseases such as influenza (Effros et al. 1991), although it may have the opposite effect in some diarrheal diseases (Greenough & Bennett 1990).

Modern health sciences have been particularly perceptive and ingenious when discerning the how our bodies work in health and disease. Modern health sciences have not been particularly perceptive or ingenious when addressing the long-term reasons why our bodies and their pathogens act the way they do. This book will *not* recount the marvelous achievements in the former category, but, rather, will point out the inadequacies in the latter. My hope is that by recognizing these shortcomings and setting out to remedy them, we shall generate a more farsighted approach to infectious disease. The short-range approach of the past assesses what our medical policies can accomplish, given the current characteristics of our disease organisms. The long-range approach of the future adds an evolutionary dimension to this assessment. It asks how our medical, social, and political activities have changed and will change these relationships by changing the disease organisms themselves.

WHY STUDY THE EVOLUTION OF DISEASE?

Because the answer to this question will vary from person to person, I shall try to answer it only on a personal level. By spelling out the reasons why I think this problem is worthy of our attention, I hope that I may help the reader to customize his or her own answer to the question.

One reason I want to understand the evolution of parasitism stems from the pervasiveness of the parasitic mode of life: Most of the species on our planet are parasites (Price 1980). We cannot understand nature and our place in nature without understanding parasites. But I, like most humans, am anthropocentric. As much as I value other species, I value human life more. Although I have tried to divorce my values from my assessments of the evolutionary processes that occur between host and parasite, the subject matter itself cannot escape being a reflection of these values. As a consequence, I tend to focus on the parasites that cause humans the most suffering and death. If we understand why diseases cause this suffering and death, we have a better chance of alleviating these effects.

Besides these general reasons for learning about the evolution of disease, there are some practical personal reasons. Each of us will have many encounters with infectious diseases. When they occur we need to decide on a best course of action. Should we treat our symptoms or should we let them run their course? Determination of the appropriate treatment requires application of evolutionary thinking. Yet modern medicine has been largely inattentive to this application. Until this inattentiveness is remedied, the patient and doctor together must take up the slack. In the absence of hard data, this process will inevitably be sloppy, but a sloppy, educated guess is better than a random guess. A framework for making these guesses and for structuring future research is outlined in the next chapter.

At a larger scale, policymakers must be cognizant of evolution to determine how to fund medical research and interventions for improving health. This need has always been pressing for people in poorer countries who have never had a respite from widespread death due to infectious diseases. It was less pressing for people in richer countries during the middle decades of this century. In the fourth edition of *Natural History of Infectious Disease*, Burnet and White (1972) stated, "Young people today have had almost no experience of serious infectious disease. The classical pestilences, smallpox, plague, typhus and cholera have been banished effectively for a hundred years or more and in the last half century the standard childhood infections have progressively lost their power to kill." AIDS has changed this rosy outlook for the wealthy countries and has further burdened the labored progress of less wealthy countries toward this goal. A general theory for the evolution of disease should be able to explain more than the decline of the classical pestilences and standard childhood infections. It should also be able to explain why this new pestilence has arisen, how it may evolve in the future if we continue our present policies, and what we can do to change this future evolutionary course.

At various places in this book I hold up Burnet and White's book to what may seem like wrathful scrutiny. Actually, I admire their book for its attempt to integrate epidemiology with ecology and evolution, but I contrast my ideas with theirs for several reasons. First, their book is one of the most lucid and thoughtful of the many books and articles written on the ecology and evolution of disease. Among medically oriented people, it has become the standard analysis of infectious disease from an ecological and evolutionary perspective. I think, however, that rigorous applications of ecological and evolutionary principles will often lead to rejection of their conclusions.

I also wish to make these contrasts because people in the health sciences often seem to evaluate my arguments like lightning and then tell me to read Burnet and White, who already wrote the book on the subject. By showing explicitly how application of current evolutionary thinking differs from "the book on the subject," I hope that I shall cause a pause in readers who might otherwise view this book as merely supplemental to previous books that interpret disease as a temporary state of imbalance in an otherwise balanced Nature.

When the apparent imbalances arise, they may be caused by old pathogens in new places or by altered pathogens. Old pathogens in new places present no problem for traditional arguments. Their high virulence can be explained by insufficient time for accommodation between host and parasite. The altered pathogen is what draws out the murkiness in traditional arguments.

An article from a news magazine of science offers an illustration (Weiss 1989a). Encapsulating views from leading thinkers in epidemiology and disease history, the article analyzes whether devastating epidemics might arise in the future. But nowhere in the expert testimonies is there any consideration of an evolutionary mechanism. The speculations on future epidemics are instead made by analogy with past epidemics. The article begins, for example, by describing a six-month influenza epidemic that resulted in the deaths of more than 17 million chickens in Pennsylvania, and then quotes a well-respected virologist as saying that the world's human population is like Pennsylvania's chicken population; that is, large numbers of humans are vulnerable to an explosive and lethal epidemic, just as the large numbers of chickens in Pennsylvania in 1983 were vulnerable. The implicit assumption of this argument is that large numbers of hosts are vulnerable to highly lethal epidemics as long as the right mutation comes along. New plagues are ascribed to mutation without considering whether the harmful or the benign variants within the population of mutants will be more successful. The traditional approach considers the first step in the evolutionary process (that heritable genetic variation is created), but not the second step—the sieve of natural selection. Researchers have thus concluded that severely lethal epidemics will occur in the future, but their focus on mutation leaves them with no foundation for predicting which kinds of parasites will be the progenitors of the lethal outbreaks, how bad the lethal outbreaks will be, or how we can reduce the lethality of the outbreaks that do occur by suppressing the evolution of increased virulence.

To be sure, the 1983 chicken epidemic had its human counterpart—a pandemic of influenza that began toward the end of 1918 and killed about 20 million people before it subsided about a year later. But why did the highly virulent rather than the less virulent influenza variants spread through our species in 1918 (and the Pennsylvanian chickens for that matter)? Conversely, why have all of the other influenza epidemics since then been so much less lethal? I think that we can begin to provide reasonable answers to these kinds of questions by integrating the fundamental principles of evolutionary biology with our knowledge of epidemiology. Most of what I have to say in this book is an attempt to do just that.

More generally, I am trying to use this book to reach people in the health sciences who are interested in looking beyond the currently prescribed boundaries of their fields. But I am also writing to reach biologists with an interest in the health sciences, and anyone else who shares an enthusiasm for learning why we are the way we are. I want people to see that evolution is not just something we should learn about to make us more broadly educated. It is that, but it is also going on around us all the time and is having deeply relevant effects—effects that could determine whether we and our loved ones will live or die. And no organisms are evolving faster with more pressing consequences than are the parasites among us: from the parasites of our agricultural resources, to the vectors of our lethal diseases, to the protozoa, bacteria and viruses that will kill millions of us this year. If we want to understand and manage our world better, we had better try to understand the evolution of infectious disease.

CHAPTER 2

Symptomatic Treatment
(Or How to Bind
The Origin of Species to
The Physician's Desk Reference)

EVOLUTIONARY FUNCTIONS OF SYMPTOMS

"You're just treating the symptoms." This admonition derives from the idea that problems are the effects of underlying causes, and to resolve a problem fully one must nullify the underlying cause. Applying the idea to infectious diseases, a twentieth-century physician might say that treating the symptoms of a disease may provide some comfort to the patient, but it is generally of little consequence to the future course of the problem at hand.

A physician with a firm grasp of evolutionary principles would disagree. The consequence of treating a symptom depends on the reasons why the symptom has evolved. One who argues "You're just treating the symptoms" is tacitly assuming that symptoms are side effects of an infection. An evolutionarily astute observer recognizes that symptoms might be just side effects, but they might represent adaptations that benefit the host or the parasite. For easy reference, I shall call the former a *defense* by the host and the latter a *manipulation* of the host (Ewald

1980), and I shall use *symptom* broadly to encompass both objective signs of disease and subjective manifestations.

Host defenses can be behavioral, morphological, physiological, or biochemical; they can provide repair to host tissues, barriers to invasion, protection from toxins, destruction of parasites, or inhibition of parasite multiplication. Manipulations by parasites alter the host's behavior or physiology to help convert host tissues into parasite growth and reproduction or to facilitate transmission to new hosts. The route through which manipulations benefit the parasite may be circuitous, if, for example, the alteration involves counterdefenses that permit evasion or neutralization of host defenses. [Williams and Nesse (1991) provide a similar breakdown, and Hart (1990) provides a framework for understanding the spectrum of behavioral defenses.]

The decision to treat or not to treat a symptom should depend on whether the symptom is a defense, manipulation, or side effect. If a symptom is a defense against the invading organism, symptomatic treatment may decrease the ability of the host to overcome the disease. On the other hand, if a symptom is a manipulation of the host by the parasite, symptomatic treatment may help the host recover or help control the spread of the disease to other hosts.

DEFENSIVE SYMPTOMS AND FEVER

Virtually all symptoms of infectious diseases can be explained hypothetically as a defense, but fever is the most frequently cited example. What to do about fever has been a source of controversy throughout history. In Greek writing, it was seen as part of the disease, the state of imbalance among the "humours." In more recent centuries, expert advice about fever depended more on the expert consulted than on the current state of evidence. Over the past two decades the controversy has continued, but the focus of the controversy has shifted to experimental evidence instead of "expert" opinion. For this shift we can thank Matthew Kluger, who had the insight to choose as his study subject the desert iguana (*Dipsosaurus dorsalis*). Prior to Kluger's insight, people were focusing on animals that generated their body heat internally. To reduce fever, an experimenter would have to do some fairly major messing about with an animal's physiology. Consider, for example, use of aspirin. When fever is reduced with aspirin, so are pain, the inflammatory response, and other processes that could help the animal defend itself against parasites. If such aspirin treatment worsened disease, one would not know whether this exacerbation resulted from reduced fever or the sabotaging of other activities that were helping to control the infection. Realizing that desert iguanas keep their body temperatures constant and warm by shuttling between warm and cool microhabitats, Kluger suspected that they might run fevers by moving to even warmer microhabitats when they are infected. When he infected the iguanas with a bacterium called *Aeromonas hydrophila*, he found that they did run a fever. He then conducted the critical experiment, which showed that infections became more severe when iguanas were kept at the lower temperatures preferred by uninfected iguanas (Kluger et al. 1975).

But just because a symptom is a defense against one kind of parasite does not mean that it is an effective defense against a different species or even a genetically different parasite of the same species. In fact, there are good theoretical reasons for presuming that fever will not always function as a defense. Most obviously, some pathogens will be more resistant than others to febrile temperatures. Because the turning off of a febrile response to these pathogens would require prolonged host evolution in response to the particular pathogen, there very well might be insufficient time for such a response. But even if there is sufficient time, hosts may have limited options. Shutting down the febrile response to one kind of pathogen might also turn off the response to other pathogens that trigger fever by the same mechanism. This restriction of host options could allow pathogens to manipulate the system in their own favor.

Consider a pathogen that is not suppressed by fever. Because metabolic processes generally speed up with temperature, such a pathogen could conceivably benefit from the high temperatures, producing more progeny in a given period of time. The host would have limited options for dealing with this threat. Turning off the fever response to this pathogen could cause the host to suffer more harm from other pathogens which would no longer be suppressed. Given enough time, we might expect the host to evolve a mechanism for distinguishing between fever-resistant and fever-susceptible pathogens, but time is on the side of the pathogens, which have a greater potential for rapid evolution. Growth of laboratory strains of the polio virus, for example, is typically inhibited by febrile temperatures, but if the virus is grown in the lab at febrile temperatures, it rapidly evolves an improved ability to withstand them (Lwoff 1959).

Evolutionary logic provides clues about where to look for pathogens that benefit from fever. The proportion of infections that trigger fever varies greatly among the different pathogen species. Like pathogens grown in the lab under high temperatures, pathogens that virtually always trigger fevers would be under strong selective pressure to develop abilities to reproduce under febrile conditions. If there are pathogens that benefit from fever, those uniformly associated with fever would therefore be prime candidates.

Another part of the spectrum may encompass pathogens that are neither suppressed nor enhanced by fever. If the host can differentially respond to such pathogens, then one would not expect them to trigger fever because such fevers would harm the host.

A survey of the existing information on fever does reveal a great variety of outcomes. One of the agents of lizard malaria, *Plasmodium mexicanum*, grows just as well at febrile temperatures as it does at normal temperatures; accordingly, it does not trigger fever in one of its primary hosts, the western fence lizard (Schall 1990). Whether this lizard generates a fever in response to any parasite, however, is unknown.

Grasshoppers and their parasites not only illustrate this point but also show how resolution of these ambiguities may have important consequences for agriculture. During their population explosions, grasshoppers may parasitize bumper crops, transforming them into stubble in a matter of days. Yet, the grasshoppers, too, may be ravaged by parasites. Especially lethal are *Nosema* protozoa and *Entomophaga* fungi–two groups of sit-and-wait parasites (see Chapter 4) that reproduce massively inside of grasshoppers, often killing them within a week or two.

One of these pest species of grasshoppers, *Melanoplus sanquinipes*, runs a behavioral fever when infected with *Nosema acridophagus* (Boorstein & Ewald 1887). Grasshoppers kept at these febrile temperatures survived longer and gained weight more rapidly than when they were kept at the temperatures preferred by uninfected hoppers (Boorstein & Ewald 1887); however, a closely related parasite, *Nosema locustae*, did not trigger a fever in the same species of grasshopper (Hanley 1989).

Such variations in febrile responses have consequences for the usefulness of parasites for biological control programs. If *Nosema* are used in biological control programs, their effectiveness would depend on which species is used and the temperature ranges available to the hoppers in nature. On hot sunny days, the *M. sanquinipes* would be able to combat infections with *N. acridophagus* by running high fevers, and little if any control of the hopper populations by the parasite would be expected. During cool cloudy days, control would be feasible. Historical data are consistent with this idea: In northern latitudes, outbreaks of *Melanoplus* and other grasshopper species tend to occur during hot, sunny years (Edwards 1960, Gage & Mukerji 1977).

Even when a symptomatic defense *is* triggered by each of two closely related parasites, the parasites may be different in their susceptibility to the defense. Grasshoppers infected with a U.S. strain of the fungus *Entomophaga grylli* sunned themselves, generating a fever of 100°F, which destroyed the fungus. But an Australian variety of this fungus was resistant to such a fever (Anonymous 1989a, Carruthers et al. 1992).

Fever in mammals is associated with a variety of immunological changes that could either enhance or inhibit effective control of pathogens (Lorin 1987). Because of these associations and the internal heat production of mammals, the evidence for and against a defensive role for mammalian fever seems to be especially difficult to interpret. When rabbits and mice are kept in warm environments, they have higher body temperatures and are better able to survive life-threatening infections (Lwoff 1959). But these experiments do not separate any negative effects of high temperature on the virus from correlates of the higher body temperature. Mammals kept in cold environments may die more often

some limited reproduction, but researchers have not assessed the effects of aspirin because aspirin did not have an effect in the influenza B model (Sanchez-Lanier et al. 1991).

In ferrets, repeated cycles of influenza reproduction occur and aspirin increases symptoms of Reye's syndrome (Deshmukh 1985). When ibuprofen is substituted for aspirin, ferrets still die from the treatment. Their illness shows some similarities to Reye's syndrome but does not involve the type of liver abnormalities that are typical of Reye's syndrome (Mukhopadhyay et al. 1992). The compounding effect of ibuprofen on influenza infection is consistent with the inflammatory sabotage hypothesis, but the difference between the effects of aspirin and ibuprofen indicates that the negative effects of treatment involve other complications, perhaps attributable to differences between the particular biochemical processes affected by these drugs. How these effects are related to Reye's syndrome in humans is unclear, but they certainly do justify keeping a lookout for any associations between antiinflammatory drugs like ibuprofen and Reye's syndrome. These effects, and the evolutionary logic presented above, suggest that to be on the safe side, it is best to avoid antiinflammatory drugs during viral infections, at least until additional studies are completed. The more general conclusion is that proper treatment of symptoms depends on the evolutionary functions of the symptoms that are influenced by the treatment. This conclusion adds another facet to current considerations, which typically distinguish between antifebrile drugs primarily on the basis of toxicities and biochemical rates of activity (Lorin 1987).

The impact of these decisions on an average individual may be relatively slight. About 20,000 influenza infections will occur for every case of Reye's syndrome attributable to influenza (Keating 1987). But the large numbers of people affected by general policies may translate into thousands of Reye's syndrome cases each decade. These numbers certainly warrant more thorough investigations of these issues and more cautious use of symptomatic treatment until these investigations are carried out.

MANIPULATIVE SYMPTOMS AND CHOLERA

Some pathogens of humans have apparently evolved to manipulate us for their own benefit. Consider the predicament of the bacterium that causes cholera: *Vibrio cholerae*. A group of *V. cholerae* swallowed by a person are faced with a daunting ordeal. First the invaders encounter the stomach's acid bath which decimates them. For *V. cholerae* it is like the hot oil and pitch that was dumped on raiders of medieval castles, but with worse odds. The stomach acid kills nearly a million raiding *V. cholerae* for each one that makes it through (Hornick et al. 1971). Those breaching this barrier then face another formidable task: to compete with a population of other bacteria, which are generally well adapted for surviving in the gut and may have mechanisms for killing or suppressing invaders (Cooperstock 1987). Unless the normal flora of the gut is experimentally decimated by antibiotics, the probability of infection is low for most would-be invaders (Bonhoff et al. 1964). But here is where *V. cholerae* has an advantage. It uses its propeller-like tail and its analogue to our sense of smell to seek out the crevices in the lining of the small intestine. Upon adherence to the intestinal lining, it releases a toxin that causes biochemical changes in the intestinal cells, which in turn cause a massive flux of water and solutes into the intestinal cavity (Miller et al. 1989). The alkaline, salty flood favors the growth of *V. cholerae* over competing bacteria and washes the competitors out of the intestines. Within hours of the onset of severe cholera, stools are transformed into a turbid effluent, each liter of which may be dominated by over 100 billion *V. cholerae* (Gorbach et al. 1970). A comparably talented invader of a castle would, upon reaching the top of the wall, be able to lower the drawbridge and grab onto the castle walls tightly while commanding a flood to wash out the residents through the open gate, leaving the castle to be controlled by the invader and any other wall-clinging comrades. These invaders would plunder the castles riches and its resources to procreate, sending perhaps a trillion progeny out the gate to invade others (Finkelstein 1973). The castle and its contents may be thoroughly ravaged, but as long as the total number of invaders is increased or maintained, this strategy will remain through time.

Microbiologists working with *V. cholerae* have independently arrived at similar explanations (without the medieval metaphors) for the function of cholera toxin (Barua 1970, Gorbach et al. 1970 Finkelstein 1973, McNicol & Doetsch 1983). One unappreciated aspect, however, is the complexity of the evolutionary processes involved. The explanation implies that any *V. cholerae* that "cheated" on the others by producing less toxin after a successful invasion would have a competitive advantage. Toxins favor the spread of *V. cholerae* over pathogen species that cannot withstand the flood inside the intestine, but toxin is expensive to produce: Strains that manufacture little or no toxin typically outproduce those that manufacture more toxin when both are on growth media where the proposed benefits of toxin cannot be realized (Basu et al. 1966, Baselski et al. 1979, Hamood et al. 1986). Once a group of *V. cholerae* is established in the intestinal tract, individuals within the group that secrete less toxin can channel the resources they have saved into survival and reproduction.

This argument proposes that the production of cholera toxin is maintained through a kind of group selection (*sensu* Wilson 1980): Only those groups of invading *V. cholerae* that make it into the intestine with at least some toxin producers are expected to infect the intestine successfully. Indeed groups containing only mutants that do not produce toxin are inept at establishing infections; their numbers decline strongly within a few hours after introduction (Baselski et al. 1978, 1979, Sigel et al. 1980). Similarly, ingested groups of cholera bacteria are more likely to initiate infection if they collectively produce substantial toxin (Sigel et al. 1980).

For most pathogens such conflicting selective pressures are probably unimportant because the small amount of environmental mixing makes the pathogens in a person closely related. Conflicts of interest within the group of pathogens inside a host are therefore small, much like the small conflicts of interest among the cells in our body. But because *V. cholerae* are often transmitted by water, the *V. cholerae* infecting a local population of humans undergo frequent mixing. The infecting dose should therefore tend to be a genetically heterogeneous sample of the *V. cholerae* found in the local human population. And it is under such conditions of frequent mixing and separation into small groups that natural selection should favor characteristics that contribute to group success (Wilson 1980).

If this argument is correct, the *V. cholerae* organisms that produce less toxin should tend to displace those that produce large amounts of toxin as the infection progresses within an individual host. Consequently, the toxin production should be greater among the *V. cholerae* present early during an infection than among those present later during the infection, particularly when the colonizing groups produced toxin abundantly. Because infant mice are excellent indicators of the potential of *V. cholerae* strains to produce disease in humans (Sigel et al. 1980), experimental data from mice can be used to evaluate this prediction. Isolates made early during infection with classical strains of *V. cholerae* elicited more fluid accumulation—a primary manifestation of toxin production—than isolates made two to four days later (Sigel et al. 1980). Interestingly, this trend is opposite to that expected by the researchers who gathered the data (Sigel et al. 1980), apparently because they were considering the problem in terms of the necessity of virulence factors for successful infections rather than the change in selective pressures that occurs as group colonization progresses to within-group competition. The trend toward decreased toxin production during an infection did not occur among the el tor strains (Sigel et al. 1980), which tend to produce less toxin than classical strains (Huq et al. 1983, Turnbull et al. 1985). High levels of toxin production appear to help groups get established but become a liability once establishment occurs. Similar reductions in toxin production occur in other bacteria that generate diarrhea by releasing toxins (Cooperstock 1987).

Given these tradeoffs, one might expect *V. cholerae* to evolve the ability to finely tune their toxin production. They do in fact do so. Toxin production is turned on along with several other changes useful for a takeover by *V. cholerae*, in response to cues peculiar to life in the intestinal tract (Miller et al. 1989). But even though production of toxin is regulated facultatively by a complex control system, toxin production is turned on to different levels in different *V. cholerae*. The classical *V. cholerae*, for example, typically have copies of toxin genes in different sites in the chromosome; this arrangement generates high levels of toxin production. The el tor types have only one such control site (Moseley & Falkow 1980, Kaper et al. 1981). Within this site, however, different el tor strains may repeat the instructions to different degrees, resulting in different amounts of toxin production. Although these levels of toxin production are generally lower than those of classical *V. cholerae*, passing el tor strains through mice can cause them to evolve increased toxin production. Further evidence for genetic variation in virulence comes from transferring or neutralizing the genes that control toxin production; such alterations can change toxin production by a few fold to about 10 fold (A. A. Khan et al. 1985, Hamood et al. 1986).

The secretory activity, which is triggered by the toxin and causes the diarrhea, does not seem to be defensive. Infected people are harmed because too much of their body fluids are lost through the diarrhea. If this indirect effect of the toxin could be blocked, the risk of death could be eliminated. Indeed, compensating for the fluid loss by drinking a rehydration solution does eliminate nearly all death from cholera (Hirschhorn & Greenough 1991).

If the secretory response to cholera toxin is a manipulation, we might expect natural selection to favor host defenses against this manipulation. Such defenses may be absent, however, because secretory responses may be defenses against other toxins, which are widespread in nature. The secretory aspect of diarrheal responses probably helps dilute and eliminate such toxins before they damage tissues or cellular machinery. Once the secretory response serves as a defense against some toxins, it may be very difficult to evolve insensitivity to the cholera toxin because the benefits of reduced sensitivity to cholera toxin may be outweighed by increased vulnerability to other toxins.

These considerations suggest that the diarrhea caused by *V. cholerae* is best explained as a manipulation of the host to facilitate transmission of the bacteria. This conclusion has a bearing on treatment. Symptomatic treatment that reduces diarrhea should help the infected person and help control the spread of *V. cholerae*. Treatment with aspirin, indomethacin, or other antisecretory drugs, for example, may be able to break the biochemical chain of events that causes the efflux of fluids (Finck & Katz 1972, Jacoby & Marshall 1972, Holmgren 1981, Petersen & Ochoa 1989, van Loon et al. 1992). In so doing, such compounds may reduce the spread of the most virulent bacteria while protecting the patient from dehydration and providing symptomatic relief.

One of the major efforts at symptomatic treatment is to replenish fluid loss largely by encouraging the drinking of a sugar and salt solution called *oral rehydration therapy*. This kind of treatment has the potential to increase rather than decrease the release of *V. cholerae*. A patient who survives diarrhea through this therapy may release more pathogens than one who dies early during the infectious period; moreover, among surviving patients, standard oral rehydration therapy does not reduce the duration or amount of diarrhea (Hirschhorn & Greenough 1991). Coupling rehydration treatment with a drug or other substance that reduces secretion, however, could benefit the ill person and reduce the transmission from the ill person at the same time. Researchers may have found just such an ingredient: starch (Hirschhorn & Greenough 1991). Rice starch, for example, appears to reduce the duration of diarrhea and stool output by reducing the flux of fluids into the intestine (Rahman et al. 1991). Measurements are needed to determine whether these reductions are associated with a reduction in the total number of organisms released during each infection. If so, this kind of symptomatic treatment could simultaneously help the patient and control the spread of *V. cholerae.*

Diarrheal and febrile illnesses are also often associated with anorexia, a loss of appetite. Theoretically this anorexia, like the diarrhea and fever, could be a defense if the host were reducing food intake to starve out the pathogen. Alternatively, it could be a manipulation if the alteration of the host food intake reduced the host's ability to muster an immunological or physiological defense against the pathogen. Finally, it could be a side effect benefiting neither the host nor the pathogen. Data on supportive care indicate that at least for some diarrheal diseases, the first of these three hypotheses can be rejected. Feeding the patient throughout the infection reduces the severity and duration of disease (Greenough & Bennett 1990). For these diseases, the manipulation hypothesis and the side effect hypothesis are still valid. If the anorexia is a manipulation, feeding the patient will not only improve the patient's sense of well being, but it will also reduce the spread of the disease. If this dual benefit occurs increased investment in this intervention would be warranted.

An evolutionary assessment of the biochemical mechanisms of disease sometimes reveals that chemical causes of disease may not be what they appear to be. Edmund LeGrand (1990ab) has come to this conclusion about lipopolysaccharides. These part-fat, part-sugar compounds protrude from the membranes of many bacteria, trigger fever, blood clotting, anorexia, and inflammation, and are therefore generally presumed to be damaging toxins. Several facts suggest, to the contrary, that these lipopolysaccharides facilitate our ability to recognize and destroy bacterial invaders. As LeGrand emphasizes, each of the responses to lipopolysaccharides may offer protection against bacterial invasion. These responses could be damaging if they were uncontrolled, but lipopolysaccharides also trigger production of chemicals that keep these symptoms in check. Lipopolysaccharides are probably not a bacterial tool for invading or manipulating the host because they are common to all species, whether parasitic or not, within one of the basic subdivisions of bacteria. Rather, these compounds appear to be an essential component of the bacterial cell membrane, an Achilles heel that our bodies make good use of.

SIMULTANEOUS MANIPULATION AND DEFENSE

The preceding descriptions show how complicated adaptive interpretations of symptoms may be. But there is another major complication: A symptom may benefit both the host and the pathogen infecting it at the same time.

Shigella is the primary bacterial cause of dysentery—bloody diarrhea brought about by invasion of the cells lining the intestine. The invasiveness of *Shigella* raises the possibility that the diarrhea it induces could be a defense as well as a manipulation. In this case diarrhea could benefit the patient by washing out the *Shigella* to reduce the contact time between the bacteria and the intestinal lining. The reduced contact should reduce destruction of intestinal tissue as well as the invasion of other tissues. This diarrheal defense hypothesis has been tested by experimentally administering diphenyloxalate hydrochloride with atropine. This drug, sold under the trade name Lomotil, decreases diarrhea by reducing the motility of the gut. If the gut motility is washing away the dangerous *Shigella*, this symptomatic treatment should harm the host. That is just what happened. Treated patients were still sick when the untreated patients had recovered (DuPont & Hornick 1973).

But the diarrhea also may benefit the *Shigella* by facilitating transmission. To envision this benefit, I encourage you to conduct a simple experiment that I have run repeatedly. The next time you visit an institutional toilet, sacrifice a few feet of the paper roll, placing it evenly on the sitting surface. Then flush. Notice the numerous droplets that appear on the paper. Then think of the millions of bacteria in each milliliter of fecal material. If the person before you had a fluid case of diarrhea, a billion bacteria may have been evenly distributed in the basin, just before the flush before last. At flush-time thousands of bacteria may have been catapulted onto the seat, and ingestion of less than 200 can cause disease (DuPont et al. 1972). How careful were you to avoid touching the toilet seat with your hands or to avoid touching the parts of you that touched the seat? You may smugly think that you have outsmarted the bacteria by washing your hands carefully before you left, but you had to touch the faucet *after* you washed your hands. Think about the previous visitor. Before the fingers of that visitor touched the faucet, they were on the other side of porous toilet paper—hardly a comforting thought, especially considering the quality of institutional toilet paper.

In spite of the potential importance of curbing lavatory transmission for improving the quality of life, few scientific studies of the phenomenon have been published. Admittedly, it is not the most glamorous research environment. Yet, a dedicated English scientist, R. I. Hutchinson, did complete a scientific study in four institutional lavatories and in a private home during outbreaks of diarrhea caused by *Shigella sonnei* (Hutchinson 1956). She recovered *S. sonnei* from about one-third of the toilet seat samples, and showed experimentally that diarrheal stools contaminated the toilet seats whereas solid stools did not. About half of the children in nursery schools handled the toilet seat while sitting on it;

about one-third of these children then touched their faces or mouths before washing their hands. Contamination of fingers occurred through all five tested types of toilet paper when stools were fluid and through four of the five types when stools were solid. *Shigella sonnei* survived under lavatory conditions for a few days when exposed to low humidity, high temperatures, and indirect sunlight, but survived for weeks when exposed to high humidities, low temperatures, and little indirect sunlight. Accordingly, outbreaks of this organism occurred during the winter months, when the latter conditions were common in lavatories.

The diarrhea caused by *Shigella* infections is therefore best interpreted as being beneficial to both the host and the parasite. Such jointly beneficial symptoms should be common because they are relatively stable evolutionarily. Symptoms that are solely manipulative but not defensive should exert selective pressure on the hosts to evade the manipulation. Symptoms that are solely defensive should exert selective pressure on the parasites to overcome the defense. When the symptom aids both parasite and infected host, these pressures diminish. The losers are those who become infected as a result of the diarrhea. But their loss does not influence the evolutionary game played by the parasite and the host from which they were infected (unless the recipients are relatives of the infected people).

Their loss however, is relevant to policymaking. When a symptom benefits both host and parasite, symptomatic treatment may be a difficult and sensitive social issue. Neutralization of the symptom would be harming the patient but helping to control the spread of disease. The difficult decisions about treatment would have to weigh the expected harm to the patient due to treatment against the expected benefits to others who might otherwise contract the disease. When infected people are less capable of practicing hygienic measures, the tradeoff shifts toward symptomatic treatment. When infected people are isolated from others, the tradeoff shifts toward withholding of treatment.

These decisions also must consider the degree to which the diseases can be controlled by measures other than symptomatic treatment. Even though defensive symptoms may on balance help the patient, they may be associated with some costs; fever, for example, may cause tissue damage, and diarrhea may result in loss of valuable salts and nutrients. If neutralization of defensive symptoms is accompanied by effective antibiotic treatment, then the pathogen could be eliminated without paying these costs. So long as the overall effects of the antibiotic are more beneficial than the overall effects of the defensive symptom, antibiotic treatment is favored. One problem is that we do not yet know enough about the costs of symptomatic treatment. Another problem is that pathogens evolve antibiotic resistance, which reduces the value of antibiotics as a substitute for defensive symptoms or compels an increase in the dosages and hence the costs (i.e., the side effects of the antibiotic) imposed on patients in order to provide the same level of protection. The lack of emphasis on functions of symptoms has led to the present lack of knowledge about these functions, which in turn forces physicians and patients alike to try to make treatment decisions without an adequate knowledge of the compromises that will result from the decisions.

The available information about diarrhea exemplifies the need to analyze every parasite–host combination as a separate case rather than making sweeping generalizations about symptomatic treatment. Even when consideration is restricted to a given symptom associated with a given pathogen, it may be detrimental to treat the symptom with one drug but acceptable to treat it with another. As mentioned above, treatment of diarrhea by suppression of gut motility in *Shigella* infections worsened infections. Treatment of diarrhea with bismuth subsalicylate (the active ingredient sold under the trade name Pepto-Bismol), however, caused no discernible negative effects (DuPont et al. 1977). This difference between symptomatic treatments may be attributed to the coating and antibacterial actions of bismuth preparations, which may replace the defensive action of the diarrhea (Goldenberg et al. 1975, Domenico et al. 1991, Gump et al. 1992). But another part of the difference reflects a more fundamental principle. A particular symptom may be comprised of separable components. *Shigella*-induced diarrhea results from high motility of gut contents and increased secretions of the cells that line the intestinal tract. Suppressing *Shigella* diarrhea by countering the increased motility seems to sabotage a symptomatic defense, but reducing fluid flux into the intestine by using bismuth subsalicylate does not worsen the prognosis (Ericsson et al. 1986). In *Shigella* infections, fluid secretion may therefore be a manipulation of host physiology for transmission, as in cholera. Reducing secretory activity by symptomatic treatment may harm the pathogen by reducing the fluidity of stools necessary for effective transmission. The dehydration, however, is probably a side effect that is harmful for both host and *Shigella*—and for *V. cholerae* for that matter. It may harm the pathogen by reducing the chances that the person will be physically able to transmit the pathogen (e.g., if the person dies or is severely incapacitated) and may harm the person by lowering the volume and solute concentrations of body tissues.

The preceding discussion has focused on diarrhea, but similar arguments could be made for most symptoms. Coughs, for instance, by expelling pathogens from the respiratory tract probably help transmit pathogens to susceptibles, but they also may help protect the person from further damage by the pathogen. The difficulties in assessing the latter possibility are analogous to those mentioned above for fever. In hospitals, for example, patients treated with barbiturates develop pneumonia more frequently and more rapidly (Eberhardt et al. 1992). This effect may result from the barbiturate's suppression of coughs, or it might result from the barbiturate's suppression of white blood cell migration, or both (Eberhardt et al. 1992).

SYMPTOMS OF NONINFECTIOUS DISEASES

When illness is not caused by an infectious agent interpretations are simpler. If the disease is not caused by an organism, the symptom cannot be a manipulation by an organism. In these situations the overall effect of symptomatic treatment is more likely to be negative because a defensive function is, by default, more likely. Less obviously, recognition of the defensive function may improve the attention given to people whose symptoms are less pronounced.

Margie Profet has provided two of the best illustrations. Any father or mother can testify that parenthood has its downsides, but mothers experience them first. Nausea, vomiting, and an aversion to many foods often begin within a month after conception. Taking an evolutionary approach to the problem, Profet (1988, 1992) evaluated the possibility that these symptoms could represent a defense that protects the growing fetus from toxins in the environment. The growing fetus is especially vulnerable to toxins because the cells in its body give rise to many critical tissues during development. If a toxin causes a mutation in the cell of an adult, the cell generally can be sacrificed with little harm. If a toxin causes a mutation in a cell of an embryo or a young fetus, that change may be passed on to many millions of cells in the developing fetus, and cause severe abnormalities along the way. Profet showed first that the foods triggering nausea tend to contain compounds that can cause mutations. She then analyzed the benefits of this nausea by comparing miscarriages. Women who experienced little or no pregnancy sickness had miscarriages about twice as frequently as those whose pregnancy sickness was severe enough to cause vomiting (Profet 1992). By recognizing that nausea may be a symptomatic defense and that this defense is meager in some women, health practitioners should be able to improve their counseling. Instructing women to ignore or suppress nausea may be destructive. An evolutionarily astute practitioner would inform the patient about the probable protective function of these sensations and advise avoidance of foods that contain the most culpable compounds.

Profet (1991) has similarly applied evolutionary thinking to another pervasive reaction that is generally considered to be an unhelpful side effect: the allergic response. Given the complexity of its components and control, we need to assess why the allergic response has evolved and is maintained in so many species. Although allergies can sometimes be life-threatening, they may be defensive in general because a very small proportion of the allergic response machinery seriously impairs or kills its host. Allergies are triggered by immunoglobulin E (IgE), a class of antibodies that has had no other clearly identified function. Realizing that IgE triggers allergic responses after it binds to potentially carcinogenic chemicals, Profet argued that allergic responses could help expel these chemicals (e.g., by sneezing them out), or slow them down and sequester them once they are in the body (by triggering the inflammatory response).

In accordance with this argument, people with different intensities of allergy also have different risks of developing cancer. But predicting the relationships between cancer and allergy is very complex. More intense allergies could result from a greater inherent ability to invoke allergic defenses, in which case one would expect fewer cancers among people exhibiting strong allergic responses. Alternatively, intense allergies should occur more strongly in people with greater exposure to dangerous chemicals. The greater exposure in turn could result from a greater level of allergy-causing compounds in their environment or from a reduced ability of the body to neutralize these compounds with safer detoxification mechanisms. In this situation, one would expect more cancer among people exhibiting stronger allergic defenses.

Over 20 different studies have assessed whether allergies are associated with cancer. The majority show fewer cases of cancer in allergy-prone people, a few show more cases of cancer, and a few show no association (Profet 1991). The tendency to find associations between allergy and cancer bolsters the idea that allergies are a defensive response. If a large proportion of the studies had found no association, the hypothesis would have been weakened. But only a few studies found no association. In these studies the two causes of stronger allergies mentioned above may be offsetting each other: Some people may have strong allergic responses and a *high* risk of cancer because they are exposed to *high levels* of cancer-causing compounds; others may have strong allergic responses and a *low* risk of cancer because their strong allergic defenses are protecting them more effectively against *any particular level* of cancer-causing compounds.

How should and how will these insights affect treatment policy? To envision an answer to this question, imagine that an extraterrestrial student of transportation came to observe a typical American city in 1940. It carefully studies police cars, fire engines, passenger cars, and trucks, and readily understands that these machines have different functions in the society. But it sees that some of the factories make vehicles that do not serve any obvious function and tend to generate explosions, which sometimes hurt people. The alien decides that although people work hard to build them, these machines have no essential value. Perhaps they provide some minor entertainment when they are used for unclear purposes in secluded areas. The alien, in its beneficence, decides to alter these machines so that the explosions provide a spectacular display but cannot hurt anyone—and without functional American tanks, Hitler won the war.

I expect that many allergy researchers will not take kindly to these ideas. After all, the logical deduction is that the central thrust of research on allergy may have been misguided. Current funding of allergy research is fostering development of innovative approaches to make nonfunctional the branch of the immunological system that is responsible for allergies. One approach, for example, aims to nullify IgE activity by saturating the body with receptors that bind to IgE. Once bound, the IgE can no longer bind to white blood cells to set in motion allergic responses. Disabling the allergic response, instead of helping people, might therefore make them vulnerable to a greater threat, such as death from cancer. The attitude of many researchers working in this area is perhaps very much like that of our beneficent alien. Noting that mice without deficient allergic responses show no apparent immunological deficiency, an NIH researcher summed up a commonly held view: "Maybe these cells are involved in some immunological defense, but maybe not so critically that if you inhibited that receptor [involved in the allergic response,] you'd have any real problem" (Weiss 1989b). Maybe the researchers are not looking at the right time and in the right place. If the alien looked at tanks only in America, it would not have witnessed their value in Europe during the World War II. Neutralization of the allergic components of the immune system may not lead to immediate immunological vulnerability, but may lead to increased rates of cancer and other mutation-induced diseases years later.

Given the economic considerations and vested interests, Profet's paper probably will be controversial, without having an immediate effect on the status quo of allergy research and clinical practice. If widespread suppression of allergic responses does continue, it will provide the opportunity to draw together an additional test. The firm evolutionary foundation of her hypothesis and its potential consequences, if true, warrant investment in long-term studies of people to find out whether those who suppress their allergies with medications have higher cancer rates.

If Profet's ideas are correct, a great deal of additional research will be needed to answer questions critical to appropriate treatment. How much of the variation in allergic reaction is a response to a varying threat from the allergy-causing compounds as opposed to differences among people in their inherent sensitivities? Which intense responses are overreactions? Clearly, if a person dies from anaphylactic shock, the cost of the allergic response was greater than any life-saving benefits that might have accrued. What is needed is the ability to predict the damage from treatment relative to the damage from lack of treatment.

At the beginning of this section I mentioned that interpretations are simplified when diseases are not caused by parasites because the manipulation hypothesis is often not viable. But some allergic responses could be a manipulation, or a manipulation and a defense simultaneously. Bee stings provide an illustration. The venom injected by bees could conceivably have no harmful effects aside from the negative effects of the allergic response. If so, the allergic response is strictly a manipulation, and suppression of the response should be beneficial. But what if the venom does have direct harmful effects? Let us say that the venom causes some tissue destruction. In this case, the allergic response is still a manipulation: The bee has evolved the venom to manipulate its victim's behavior, that is, to deter it from harming the colony of bees. But by using a toxic compound, the bee's threat is real and the allergic response may carry a benefit. The question to be asked is a specific version of the general question that must be asked for all allergic responses: At what point does the negative effect of the allergic response outweigh the negative effect the venom would have if the allergic response were suppressed?

Many of the common allergic responses could be manipulations. Allergic responses to secondary compounds in plant tissues could be manipulations of vertebrates to reduce trampling or eating of the plant. The allergic response to dust mites and their products could cause people to withdraw from dusty areas; or sneezes might rescue dust mites from nasal tar-pits. The general evolutionary theory of allergic responses offers a clear framework for identifying and resolving such questions.

THE NULL HYPOTHESIS: SYMPTOMS AS SIDE EFFECTS

At the beginning of this chapter I mentioned that symptoms might be neither defenses against the host nor manipulations by the parasite, but rather side effects—consequences of infection that benefit neither host nor parasite. In spite of the tendency by many to presume that treatment of symptoms is inconsequential, the evidence for symptoms being side effects is more scanty than the evidence for symptoms being defenses or manipulations.

The least ambiguous example of a side effect is death. Death is too drastic a measure to be considered a defense except in the most extreme circumstances, one of which is described in Chapter 4. Similarly, death rarely benefits the pathogen unless the death facilitates transmission, as it might if transmission occurs by a scavenging cannibalism or predation (see Chapter 4).

The lack of support for the side effect explanation should not be surprising. In scientific jargon it is a *null hypothesis*. Acceptance of the null hypothesis requires rejection of the working hypotheses, which are in this case the defense and manipulation hypotheses. The limited testing of the working hypotheses means that acceptance of the null hypothesis is at present justifiable in very few circumstances; and it is precisely this null hypothesis that is needed to justify the reproach "You're just treating the symptoms."

CHAPTER 3

Vectors, Vertical Transmission, and the Evolution of Virulence

---

THE VIRULENCE OF VECTORBORNE PARASITES

Hypothetical tradeoffs

Why has falciparum malaria been so lethal and the common cold so mild? The first step toward an answer is to identify the tradeoffs associated with different levels of virulence. Consider first a parasite that depends on the mobility of the host for transmission. Rhinoviruses, for example, cause the common cold by reproducing inside the cells that line our nasal passages. The viruses are shed from these cells into nasal secretions, which trickle out through a runny nose or blast out in droplets during a sneeze. The trickle may be blocked with a finger, which then may contact fingers of others during a hand shake or by way of a borrowed pencil. When these contacted fingers then contact the noses to which they belong, or when these noses inhale the droplets from a sneeze, some lucky rhinoviruses may be planted onto fertile ground. Whichever of the two routes occurs, host mobility is critical. If the virus reproduced so extensively that the person was too ill to leave home, the thousands of rhinoviruses released from the nose that day would be destined to die from exposure to the elements. A few might eke by, perhaps by infecting a caring spouse, but such transmission could hardly be considered a great success, especially if the spouse became immobilized. For rhinovirus, a person's mobility enhances the prospects for transmission.

Accordingly, the reproduction of rhinovirus within our noses is highly restricted. It is limited to a small proportion of the many cells lining our nasal passages. A few cells will be infected in a spot, yet their neighbors will be infection-free. Off in the distance, many cells away, the pattern repeats itself, and so on throughout the nasal lining (Dearruda et al. 1991). When viewed under the microscope, infected cells do not show obvious damage (Winther et al. 1990). As a result of this highly restricted reproduction, rhinovirus infections are about the most benign of human infections; no death attributable to rhinovirus has been reported (Benenson 1990).

But what if a virus is transmitted by, say, a mosquito? If a mosquito-borne virus reproduces so extensively that the host is immobilized from the illness, the parasite obtains the fitness benefits from the reproduction while paying little if any costs. So long as the vector can reach the ill person, it can transport the pathogens from the immobilized infected host to susceptibles. In fact, experiments with rabbits and mice indicate that transmission to mosquitoes is facilitated by illness, because ill hosts are less able to keep mosquitoes from biting (Waage & Nondo 1982, Day & Edman 1983, Day et al. 1983). Although ethical considerations limit comparable studies using humans, the limited data suggest a similar effect; when people keep their arms still, mosquitoes have longer feeding bouts (Lenahan & Boreham 1976). The immobilization associated with extensive reproduction inside the host therefore may be beneficial rather than costly to the parasite. What's more, if a parasite is vectorborne, extensive multiplication and spread throughout the body provides a benefit. Virulent vectorborne pathogens tend to reach higher densities in the blood and in cell culture than milder pathogens, and mosquitoes tend to be infected more frequently when they ingest more pathogens (Coatney et al. 1971, Reisberg 1980, Hardy et al. 1983, DeFoliart et al. 1987, Morens et al. 1991). Extensive multiplication and spread within a vertebrate host should therefore increase the probability that a biting vector will become infected. Without systemic spread, a vector would have to bite close to the site of the bite that infected the host. In sum, vectorborne parasites that reproduce extensively in the vertebrate host should win big: They get great fitness benefits and pay little fitness costs.

Vectors and the lethality of human diseases

This hypothesis provides a readily testable prediction. Parasites transmitted by biting, terrestrial arthropods should be especially virulent in humans or other vertebrate hosts. I tested this prediction using the viruses, bacteria, and protozoa that regularly infect humans. In applying this prediction to humans, I assume that pathogens have been evolutionarily molded by transmission through humans. The test therefore excludes pathogens that are transmitted rarely or never from infected humans to other humans. On this basis it also excludes pathogens that reproduce extensively in external environments such as soil or water and those that tend to cause diseases only in unnatural situations such as in association with wounds and medical procedures. The test excludes pathogens that live in our gastrointestinal tracts because they may rely on food in the tract instead of relying solely on host tissues; moreover, as discussed in the next chapter, some of these diarrheal pathogens are transmitted by analogues of arthropod vectors that may influence their virulence.

Categorization of most pathogens as vectorborne or nonvectorborne is relatively straightforward. One exception is the agent of plague, *Yersinia pestis*. Because this bacterium is transmitted by both fleas and respiratory secretions, I excluded it from the analysis.

Categorization of virulence is more complicated because the intensity of particular symptoms is not necessarily a reliable indicator of the severity of the infection. Sometimes an intense symptom, such as a high fever, might indicate that the pathogen is being dealt with effectively (see Chapter 2). In contrast, if someone dies from an infection, it is fairly safe to say that the infection was virulent. I therefore used as an indicator of virulence the number of deaths that occur for every 100 untreated infections (i.e., percent mortality; for other details, see Ewald 1983).

By using death as an indicator of virulence, I am not considering death to be beneficial to the pathogen. Rather, I view death as an occasional side effect that is nearly always costly to both parasite and host (see Chapter 2). Pathogens that exploit hosts more extensively should tend to cause death more frequently, but may still do so at a low frequency. Even these more lethal pathogens, however, may incur relatively little cost from host death when infection triggers a potent immune response that eliminates the parasite from surviving hosts. From the pathogen's point of view, a dead host and an immune host are not much different.

The results of this test, shown in Figure 3.1, reveal that vectorborne pathogens of humans are more severe than nonvectorborne pathogens. This tendency for vectorborne pathogens to be severe is robust. It occurs, for example, if pathogens are grouped according to genus. Consideration of immobilization among those pathogens in the less severe categories would, if anything, strengthen the association between virulence and vectorborne transmission; while most nonvectorborne pathogens in the less severe categories generally are not debilitating, most of the vectorborne pathogens are regularly debilitating. Chikungunya and dengue viruses, for example, cause death in less than one out of 100 infections. The name chikungunya originates from a Swahili word meaning "that which bends up" (Halstead 1981); victims feel such excruciating pain in their limb joints that they lie on their backs with their arms and legs bent above them. Similarly, dengue is known as break-bone fever; it makes bones feel as if they are breaking (Halstead 1980).

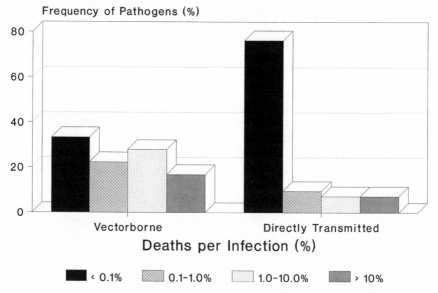

FIG. 3.1 Mortality associated with untreated infections transmitted by arthropod vectors compared with those transmitted directly from person to person. The lethality of vectorborne diseases is significantly greater than that of directly transmitted pathogens. ($p < 0.01$; ordered chi-square test).

Levin and Svanborg Edén (1990) devalued the association between lethality and vectorborne transmission, arguing that vectorborne diseases are more frequent in the tropics where mortality is greater for reasons other than the inherent virulence of the parasites. But if only temperate zone vectorborne pathogens are included, the average mortality of arthropodborne pathogens in Figure 3.1 does not decrease. They also argued that arthropodborne parasites might be more severe simply because the bites of arthropods introduce such parasites through the skin, the body's first line of defense. But this argument ignored a second test, which included only pathogens that are inoculated through the skin. This test is described in the following section.

Adaptive severity or restricted adaptation?

The theory supported by Figure 3.1 presumes that the greater virulence of vectorborne pathogens results from their adaptation to humans. In spite of the dramatic difference in lethality between vectorborne and nonvectorborne parasites of humans, this difference has not been addressed in the medical literature. Interestingly, an historian did offer an explanation for the high virulence that occurs among some vectorborne pathogens. W. H. McNeill (1976) based his explanation on the conventional premise: that evolutionary adaptation of parasites to their hosts pushes the relationship toward benignness. He then proposed that a parasite is not capable of evolving to a benign equilibrium in both the arthropod vector and the vertebrate host; thus, according to his *restricted adaptation hypothesis*, evolution to benignness is restricted to one of the two hosts. McNeill reasonably proposed that evolution to benignness occurs in the vector rather than the vertebrate host because a healthy vector is more important for transmission than, say, a healthy human.

The restricted adaptation hypothesis and the *adaptive severity hypothesis* that I proposed above can be distinguished by assessing how the severity of infection changes in parasite populations that have experienced different opportunities for adaptation to humans. According to the adaptive severity hypothesis, parasites that cycle primarily between humans and vectors will be more virulent in humans than will parasites that cycle primarily between nonhuman vertebrates and vectors. The restricted adaptation hypothesis does not yield this prediction.

This difference between these hypotheses stems from the tendencies for human immune systems to be able to control nearly all organisms that have not had a history of adaptation to humans. As an illustration, consider malaria parasites that use a monkey species as their primary vertebrate host. These parasites should have adaptations that are specialized for both monkey and mosquito environments. If some were introduced into a human, they would encounter a biochemical environment that differed from the monkey environment to which they had adapted. A human immune system, on the other hand, must be able to neutralize a continual barrage of novel and familiar organisms if the person is to survive. The human, therefore, should have the advantage when fighting against parasites that are adapted to nonhuman hosts. The result should be a relatively benign encounter. If the parasite were then repeatedly passed from person to mosquito to person, the variants that most effectively evaded the human arsenal and grew on the human soup of nutrients would tend to be preferentially transmitted to mosquitoes and hence to successive human hosts. Because the adaptive severity hypothesis presumes that extensive reproduction in humans does not jeopardize transmission, the more rapidly reproducing descendants should get the benefits of reproduction at little cost. Their virulence therefore should be greater than that of the pathogens originally introduced into the human from the monkey.

What one predicts from the restricted adaptation hypothesis depends on whether any evolution toward benignness is possible in the vertebrate host. If at least some evolution toward benignness is possible, then the restricted adaptation hypothesis predicts that the more a pathogen cycles between humans and vectors, the less virulent it will become in humans. If no evolution toward benignness is possible in the vertebrate host, then one would expect the virulence in humans to remain unchanged.

The information needed to test these predictions was gathered inadvertently over the past century and recorded in the epidemiological literature. This information permits comparisons of vectorborne pathogens that are closely related to one another but differ in the degree to which they have cycled in humans. Thirteen such comparisons can be made. In all but one, the greater the cycling in humans, the more severe is the disease in humans (Ewald 1983). The available evidence therefore supports the adaptive severity hypothesis rather than restricted adaptation hypothesis.

The exception involves sleeping sickness: the less virulent Gambian form has cycled in humans more than the more virulent Rhodesian form. This exception illustrates how the prevailing view can shape what scientists see. Until the 1980s, obligate evolution to benignness was the prevailing view. Accordingly, the milder nature of Gambian sleeping sickness was offered repeatedly as evidence that parasites generally evolve toward benignness as they adapt to humans (e.g., Herbert & Parratt 1979). The general lesson is clear. The biomedical literature is so rich, and host–parasite relationships are so variable, that one can find an example that is consistent with almost any hypothesis. Host–parasite relationships must be sampled without bias to test the general validity of hypotheses, rather than selected to support a particular hypothesis.

These tests draw attention to the need for more finely tuned investigations to gather more precise data from different populations and for running experimental tests using laboratory animals. Experimental tests are feasible because parasites can evolve substantially over time periods of months.

Evidence of this feasibility comes from medicinal use of a malaria organism called *Plasmodium knowlesi*, during the first half of this century. Like most malaria parasites naturally found in monkeys, *P. knowlesi* causes relatively mild malaria in humans when first transferred from monkeys. About 1000 parasites occur in each cubic millimeter of blood, one-tenth the number typically occurring in the three most mild species of human malaria (Coatney et al. 1971, Ewald 1983). Because fever seems to suppress the organism that causes syphilis, and *P. knowlesi* generates fever, *P. knowlesi* was inoculated into patients with neurosyphilis before effective antisyphilis drugs were available. It was then transferred from patient to patient with a syringe and a needle—in effect, a technological mosquito. After 170 such transfers, the malaria had become as dangerous as the neurosyphilis. Densities of the malaria parasite had risen to 500,000 per cubic millimeter and the disease had become life-threatening. Experimental mosquito-borne transmission yielded similar results, although the small number of transfers makes the trends equivocal (Contacos et al. 1962, Chin et al. 1968).

The insufficient time hypothesis

Historical changes and typhus. Writers proposing that diseases as a rule evolve toward benignness have made heavy use of certain historical examples of organisms that once were frequently lethal but now rarely kill. The list typically includes the agents causing diphtheria, whooping cough, and measles. But these writers have overlooked a pattern in the historical changes in death rates from particular disease agents. The diseases that have declined in virulence over time are typically nonvectorborne. The pathogens that are transmitted by arthropod vectors may have been reduced or eradicated in certain areas, but where they exist they have continued to cause severe disease. Human malaria, for example, can be traced back to the earliest civilizations (Garnham 1977, Krotoski 1985).

Burnet and White (1972) provide a detailed account of what I shall call the *insufficient time hypothesis* to explain the evolution of virulence. They introduce this hypothesis using rickettsial diseases like typhus as illustrations. They then draw the following conclusion: "These stories of human intrusion into rickettsial ecosystems illustrate the frequent finding that many of the most lethal infections of man are ecologically infections of other vertebrates—or of insects—which reach man only by accident . . . . One might even argue that all highly lethal infections of man, classical smallpox for instance, are caused by agents which have only recently (in a biological sense) become human diseases."

Well, let us take a closer look at typhus. Drawing upon Hans Zinsser's (1935) conjectures, Burnet and White (1972) imply that epidemic typhus probably originated in Europe in the sixteenth century. They state, "No clear evidence of typhus fever is found prior to this period" (p. 147). But their assessment neglects to mention an alternative explanation. Typhus may have been described first during the 16th century because the insightful Italian physician Girolamo Fracastoro was alive then (see chapter 10). One of Fracastoro's achievements was the description of different diseases as different entities, and one of the entities he clearly described was typhus. Using the poorer earlier descriptions, other authorities trace typhus to earlier centuries. In fact, the edition of *Zinsser's Microbiology*, published in the same year as Burnet and White's book, traces typhus back twice as far, to a monastery in Salerno in 1083 (Smith 1972). The poor quality of clinical descriptions prior to the sixteenth century make the absence of clear documentation extremely weak evidence for the absence of the disease. Such absence is especially weak for typhus, which was not clearly clinically differentiated from typhoid fever until the early nineteenth century (Smith 1972).

Noting the high virulence of the typhus rickettsia for lice and the transmission of rodent typhus to humans, Burnet and White (1972), like Hans Zinsser (1935) before them, concluded that "the typical louse-spread typhus is a modern development." But we now know that high virulence tells us little if anything about the previous duration of the relationship. Epidemic typhus may be a recently evolved disease. Alternatively, the high virulence in the louse might result from a combination of some unique aspects of louseborne transmission. First, lice cannot transmit the typhus rickettsia *vertically*, that is, from parent to offspring (Saah & Hornick 1979). Because some of the low virulence of vectorborne pathogens in their vectors can be attributed to vertical transmission, one would not expect infections in lice to be as benign as vertically transmitted, vectorborne pathogens usually are in their vectors (see the section INFECTIONS IN THE VECTORS, in this chapter, below).

Second, lice lack the primary line of defense found in vectors such as fleas: the protective sheath lining their intestinal tract. A given level of pathogen multiplication might therefore have a more virulent effect in lice than in fleas. Accordingly flea-borne typhus is lethal in lice.

Third, lice tend to abandon ship when the ship generates a fever. Fevers of 102–6°F generally occur 5 to 21 days after an infected louse bites (Smith 1972), and typically continue until death or recovery a week or two later (Saah & Hornick 1979). The louse is capable of transmitting infection four to six days after the ingestion of rickettsiae. Even though the infection may kill the louse within one to three weeks (Saah & Hornick 1979), the louse's aversion to febrile hosts means that it will not stay on a typhus victim for long. If densities of uninfected humans are high, an infected louse is almost certain to move from a febrile host to at least one other host before its demise. Under such conditions even a doomed louse may transmit typhus as effectively as a mosquito transmits malaria.

Burnet and White go on to say, "There are some slight differences between the rickettsiae that produce the 'rat type' typhus and those of 'louse type' infections, but they are no more than the differences between local races of the same species" (p. 147). In fact, the mortality in humans caused by the "louse type" typhus is about ten times greater than that caused by the "rat type" (Snyder 1975, Ewald 1983), and biochemical comparisons suggest that the typhus rickettsia transmitted by lice is neither a "local race" of the rat type nor a "modern development." Myers and Wisseman (1980) hybridized genes from the different types of rickettsiae to one another—the greater the percentage of hybridization, the greater the evolutionary similarity of the types. The hybridization of all louse types was 100%, but the hybridization of louse and rat types was only 70–7%. To get a feel for the significance of this difference, consider the hybridization of an entirely different genus of rickettsial organism. *Rochamlimaea quintana* is a louse-borne rickettsia that caused debilitating but nonlethal epidemics of trench fever among infantrymen in World War I. Its hybridization to either of the typhus rickettsiae ranged from 25% to 33% (Myers & Wisseman 1980). These percentages indicate that the agents of louse typhus and rat typhus are best considered different species that diverged from each other far longer ago than was suggested by Zinsser, and Burnet and White.

Falciparum malaria: insufficient time or adaptive severity. Causing nearly 300 million new cases of malaria each year, the four species of *Plasmodium* generate more death and illness than any other vectorborne parasite of humans (Hoffman et al. 1992). The insufficient time hypothesis has recently been invoked to explain why one of these species, *Plasmodium falciparum*, is more lethal than the others. *P. falciparum* is more closely related to the bird plasmodia than are the other primate plasmodia (Waters et al. 1991), although it is still unclear whether the jump was from birds to humans or humans to birds (Brooks & McLennan 1992). The discoverers of this close relationship proposed that this avian origin explains why falciparum malaria is so much more severe than other human malarias. Presuming that parasitism evolves toward commensalism, they suggested that *P. falciparum* may have had as little as 10,000 years to evolve in humans, and that this relatively recent origin may explain why *P. falciparum* is particularly severe (Waters et al. 1991, and T. F. McCutchen, quoted by Rennie 1992). But 10,000 years is a long time!

Compared with the other *Plasmodium* species, *P. falciparum* has a faster reproductive rate, and a shorter period between infection and symptoms (Reisberg 1980). *P. falciparum* may infect up to 60% of the red blood cells in a person, whereas the other species generally infect less than 2% (Reisberg 1980). How much time does *P. falciparum* need to evolve a lower rate of reproduction? As mentioned above, *P. knowlesi* evolved increased rates of reproduction within a few years. If a reduction in reproductive rate were favored by natural selection, *P. falciparum* should be particularly able to do so rapidly. It has a great potential for generating the variability necessary for evolutionary change because different lineages recombine their genes sexually with short generation times (Walliker et al. 1987, Ranford-Cartwright et al. 1991). Accordingly, isolates of *P. falciparum* reveal a great amount of genetic variation, even when geographically restricted (Babiker et al. 1991, Mercereau-Puijalon et al. 1991ab).

Ten thousand years *is* a long time for evolution of a protozoal parasite like *P. falciparum*. Moreover, the other human malarias may have had little more time and perhaps even less time to evolve in humans. The evolutionary tree presented by Waters et al. (1991) shows that the other human plasmodia are about as closely related to some plasmodia that infect monkeys as *P. falciparum* is to the avian plasmodia. But each of these other species of human plasmodia appear to be less closely related to the simian plasmodia that Waters and his colleagues studied than to other simian plasmodia (Coatney et al. 1971, Ewald 1983, Cogswell et al. 1991, Gilks 1991). Interpretations about relative durations of evolution in humans might have been quite different if the tree had included these simian plasmodia and *P. reichnowi*, a species isolated from chimpanzees that is similar to *P. falciparum* (Garnham 1977).

Seasonality and vectorborne virulence

If the inadequate time hypothesis is not valid, why does *P. falciparum* induce more severe disease than the other human plasmodia? I suggest that a *virulence niche hypothesis* is more parsimonious than the inadequate time hypothesis. *P.*

falciparum's high rates of reproduction would be most beneficial when large numbers of susceptibles exist and when mosquitoes are available year round. Mathematical models indicate that *P. falciparum* can spread through a susceptible population far more rapidly than can the other human plasmodia, even though *P. falciparum* kills a higher proportion of those it infects. Moreover, frequent, continuous transmission should promote simultaneous infections with genetically different parasites, and simultaneous infection should promote increased virulence. The variant that reproduces faster to higher densities should have the competitive advantage. Not only does it use the body's resources preemptively, but also any immunity it triggers may suppress the more slowly reproducing competitors. Accordingly, simultaneous infections are ubiquitous in the heartland of *P. falciparum* (Conway et al. 1991).

But if mosquitoes are lacking for prolonged periods, *P. falciparum*'s strategy may be less successful than the strategies used by the three more mild plasmodia, which can survive inside of a person for a longer period of time (Garnham 1977). Two of them, *P. ovale* and *P. vivax*, can remain latent in people and then reawaken years later in numbers that can readily infect mosquitoes; the third, *P. malariae*, can remain infectious for several decades (Coatney 1976, Garnham 1977). In *P. vivax*, in some plasmodia that infect monkeys, and probably in *P. ovale*, this capability to cause renewed infection after years of latency is attributable to a special form of the parasite called a *hypnozoite* (sleeping animalcule), which lies dormant during the years between attacks (Krotoski 1985, Cogswell et al. 1991). Some strains of *P. vivax* also have a delayed incubation period; people become infected during the summer, but come down with malaria the following spring (Garnham 1977). The prolonged infectiousness of the three milder *Plasmodium* species must give them an advantage when mosquitoes or susceptible humans are temporarily unavailable. Under such conditions, *P. falciparum* should diminish more quickly than the three milder species.

These arguments suggest that *P. falciparum* has evolved to fill an ecological niche that is different from those filled by the other three species. The geographic distributions accord with this idea. *Plasmodium falciparum* tends to maintain itself only where mosquitoes and susceptible humans are present for a relatively large proportion of the year; for example, historically, it comprised a progressively smaller proportion of the transmitted plasmodia with increasing latitude (Bruce-Chwatt & de Zulueta 1980). Further support for this idea comes from variation in the timing of relapses within *P. vivax*. Isolates from areas with relatively continuous opportunities for infection have a reduced tendency for prolonged latency and relapse (Manson-Bahr & Apted 1982). A strain of *P. vivax* that originated in New Guinea, for example, did not show a sequence of dormancy and relapse (Coatney 1976). Strains from Venezuela, Nicaragua and El Salvador often cause short latencies and relapses within a few months, whereas strains from the temperate zones regularly show long delays before the initial disease and before relapses: A North Korean strain shows such long latencies that it was named *P. vivax hibernans* (Coatney et al. 1950, Coatney 1976, Shute et al. 1976, Garnham 1977, Krotoski 1985). These differences apparently result from the differences among the strains in their relative production of hypnozoites (Krotoski 1985).

A similar argument probably explains the intermediate virulence of trypanosomes transmitted between newts by leeches. The highly seasonal biting behavior of the leech favors those trypansomes whose reproduction is sufficiently restricted to permit survival within the newts throughout most of the year (Gill & Mock 1985). The argument also may help explain the intermediate virulence of many other seasonally restricted vectorborne parasites, such as *Plasmodium mexicana*, which causes lizard malaria (Schall 1990), and the *Plasmodium*-like *Leucocytozoon*, which sometimes kills ducks (Garnham 1977). In nature, the densities of latent and activated *Leucocytozoon* in ducks are typically low and the infections are mild (Desser et al. 1968). The severity of *Leucocytozoon* may undergo an evolutionary transformation, however, when the natural episodic potential for transmission is replaced by more continuous opportunities associated with domestication. The highest mortalities, which can approach 100%, occur in duck farms when new ducks are continually introduced (Siegmund & Fraser 1973).

Myxomatosis: time and virulence

Advocates of obligate evolution toward benignness frequently refer to Frank Fenner's study of myxomatosis (Burnet & White 1972, Wallace 1972, McNeill 1976, Essex and Kanki 1988, Pela & Platt 1989, Ampel 1991). The myxomatosis virus is naturally transmitted by mosquitoes between South American rabbits. It was introduced into Australia in middle of this century to control a burgeoning population of a different rabbit species, which had been stripping Australian rangeland since the latter half of the nineteenth century. When the virus was first introduced into Australia it killed nearly all the rabbits that it infected. Over the ensuing years, its lethality declined markedly because of increased resistance among the rabbits and reduced virulence of the virus (Fenner & Myers 1978).

Although scientists often refer to the myxomatosis experience as a model of evolution toward benignness, the rabbits might tell a different story. The mortality occurring in rabbits *after* the evolutionary decreases in the virus' virulence and the increases in rabbit resistance was comparable to the mortality of most virulent vectorborne diseases of humans; it was, for example, higher than the mortality associated with *Plasmodium falciparum* and the yellow fever virus. Perhaps more importantly, the trend toward decreased virulence documented during the first decade of the study has not continued. In fact, the inherent virulence of the virus may have increased during the subsequent decades. This reversal is consistent with current theory, which views the problem as an arms race between the virus's virulence and the rabbit's resistance (Dwyer et al. 1990).

Those who use this decline in rabbit mortality to bolster arguments about diseases eventually evolving to benignness, often emphasize that myxomatosis is benign in South American *Sylvilagus* rabbits. But this conclusion is based on sketchy evidence. For one thing, data from natural populations can be terribly biased. A severe illness in wild rabbits is not likely to last long. A sick rabbit will die from infection, recover, or be eaten by predators within a few days; moreover, once the infection is pervasive in the rabbit population, the infections should tend to occur in very young rabbits because young rabbits are most susceptible immunologically. The chance of seeing a wild rabbit ill with a moderately severe pathogen would therefore be vanishingly small unless the rabbit population is very dense and the pathogen has only recently entered the population (in which case the ratio of currently infected to previously infected rabbits could be high).

Falciparum malaria offers an illustration. If one travels to an area with endemic falciparum malaria, inhabitants at any given instant will typically show substantial immunity and few severe symptoms, even when the protozoan can be isolated from their blood. Authors arguing in favor of obligate evolution to benignness have suggested that these findings support the idea that coevolution leads ultimately to a benign state of balance between host and parasite (Swellengrebel 1940). But a closer look at infection across age groups leads to a different conclusion. Data from one of the most extensive field studies of malaria, the Garki Project, showed that virtually all Nigerian babies become infected with falciparum malaria during their first year of life, and many of them die (Molineaux & Gramiccia 1980). Epidemiologists who came into an area and made a snapshot study of the relationship between postnatal villagers and malaria therefore missed the conflict. A photographer coming into a war-torn country months after a major battle may photograph injuries, scars, and rubble but little of the death that results from combat. How wrong it would be to conclude from the pictures that warfare is not lethal.

INFECTIONS IN THE VECTORS

The notion that pathogens evolve to benignness in vectors has been similarly perpetuated on precarious footing. According to Burnet and White (1972), for example, the rickettsiae that cause Rocky Mountain spotted fever "establish a harmless infection which persists through the life of the tick." At about the same time that their book was published, Burgdorfer and Brinton (1975) were conducting the controlled experiments needed to arrive at the correct answer. They found that this pathogen reduced the ability of ticks to lay eggs and sometimes killed them.

Evolutionary principles suggest that pathogens should be relatively benign in their vector hosts. A mosquito-borne *Plasmodium*, for example, may pay a great price if it reproduces so extensively in the mosquito that it makes the insect ill. A delirious mosquito may be inept at reaching a susceptible host and avoiding swats if it gets there. The benefits of extensive reproduction in the vector should also be relatively low. Because vectors are smaller than vertebrate hosts, extensive exploitation of vector tissues would yield a smaller amplification of parasite numbers than extensive exploitation of vertebrate tissues. Also, because the number of bites made by a mosquito is generally far less than the number of mosquitoes biting a human, the potential for spread from a mosquito to different humans is less than that from a human to different mosquitoes. These considerations indicate that vectorborne parasites should specialize on their vertebrate hosts as resource bases for amplifying their numbers and on their vector hosts as agents of dispersal. The result should be severe disease in the vertebrates and benign infections in the vectors.

The first half of this chapter confirmed the expected severity in vertebrate hosts, but did not address the second issue. Are infections in vectors relatively benign? Yes. Viruses transmitted between vertebrates by mosquitoes, for example, may suppress egg production or development but almost never kill their hosts (Ewald & Schubert 1989); viruses that infect mosquitoes but are not transmitted between vertebrates by the mosquitoes, regularly kill the mosquitoes before they reach adulthood (Ewald & Schubert 1989).

There is, however, an alternative explanation for the mildness of vectorborne parasites in their vectors. Many of these parasites can be transmitted from mother to offspring, and such vertical transmission should favor evolution toward benignness. A pathogen that decreases the reproductive success of its host reduces its potential for transmission to the host's offspring. This extra cost of virulence should increasingly favor benignness as the potential for vertical transmission increases (Fine 1975, Ewald 1987a).

This theoretical virulence-reducing effect of vertical transmission has been demonstrated by a series of experiments using viruses that infect bacteria. As the potential for horizontal transmission is reduced, the viruses becomes more benign (Bull et al. 1991). When possibilities for horizontal transmission are eliminated altogether, the viruses rapidly lose their genes for horizontal transmission and destructive infection (Bull & Molyneux 1992). The reproductive success of the infected bacteria increases accordingly. Within weeks the bacteria begin growing at rates comparable to uninfected bacteria (Bull & Molyneux 1992). In a similar experiment, an association between a plasmid and its bacterial host evolved to a mutualistic association (Bouma & Lenski 1988), in accordance with evolutionary predictions (Ewald 1987a).

The importance of vertical transmission has also been affirmed by evidence from nematodes that parasitize fig wasps. The nematode species often harm the wasps severely, but those that tend to be transmitted vertically have mild effects on the fitness of their wasp hosts (Herre 1993). This result is noteworthy because the associations between nematodes and fig wasps appear to be very ancient, and nematodes have a great potential for rapid adaptation to their insects hosts (Herre 1993, Jaenike 1993).

These studies underscore the need to account for the influences of both vertical and vectorborne transmission on evolution of benignness in vector hosts. The association between vertical transmission and benignness can be evaluated independently of vectorborne transmission by restricting analysis to parasites of mosquitoes that are not part of a mosquito–vertebrate transmission cycle. Protozoal parasites offer the richest data base. The protozoal parasites that are more frequently vertically transmitted rarely cause the death of female mosquitoes. Parasites that are rarely or never vertically transmitted from infected females, on the other hand, nearly always cause substantial death of females (Ewald & Schubert 1989).

Clearly, vertical transmission of vectorborne parasites must be taken into account. Indeed, among viruses that use mosquitoes as vectors, the more vertically transmitted the virus the more benign it is (Ewald & Schubert 1989). But these vectorborne viruses are much less lethal to their mosquitoes than either the nonvectorborne, vertically transmitted viruses, or the nonvectorborne protozoa mentioned above (Ewald & Schubert 1989).

Studies of damage to mosquito cells and tissues reveal a similar difference. Mosquito cells typically shed vectorborne viruses at low rates with little if any overt cell damage; and the damage is least among vectorborne viruses that are frequently vertically transmitted. Nonvectorborne viruses, in contrast, typically reproduce extensively, destroying mosquito cells and tissues in the process (Ewald & Schubert 1989).

The literature on mosquito-borne viruses therefore reveals that vectorborne transmission is associated with benignness in vectors, independently of vertical transmission. In fact, viral reproduction often may be so restricted that large numbers of mosquito-borne viruses may not have enough viruses in their salivary glands to deliver an infectious bite. The viruses may never even make it from the mosquito's digestive tract to the salivary glands. Apparently, then, selection for benignness in vectors has led to a problem for the parasites that is opposite to the problem they experience in vertebrates. The variation in pathogen characteristics and host resistance causes some pathogen lineages to die with their vertebrate hosts because selection for high levels of reproduction sometimes led to host death; they were too severe. Analogous noise in the system has led other lineages to die in their vectors because they underproduced the numbers of progeny or disease-causing substances necessary for transmission; they were too benign.

The relative benignness of vectorborne parasites in their vector hosts does not mean that their associations will evolve toward commensalism or mutualism. The same kinds of tradeoffs that occur in vertebrate hosts should determine the degree of virulence toward which the vector–parasite relationship will evolve. The costs and benefits of benignness in vectors may change from day to day or even second to second.   If evolution can generate flexible parasite strategies that are responsive to these changing costs and benefits, then we might see indications of moderate virulence at very specific times in otherwise benign relationships.

As an illustration, consider the sequence of events associated with transmission by mosquitoes. As a mosquito bites an infected person, the parasites in the person and the mosquito have the same short-range objective: Both benefit if the mosquito drinks a large meal and escapes. The pathogen benefits itself if it helps the mosquito to reach this objective. And pathogens may do just that. The illness in the vertebrate might be one such example, especially in malaria because the vast numbers of parasites will never be transformed into stages that can survive in mosquitoes. The illness caused by their large numbers might benefit their genes by facilitating bites by mosquitoes. Less speculative, perhaps are the changes in blood viscosity generated by infection (Rossignol et al. 1985). The mosquito drinks its fill of this thinner blood and leaves the infected person more quickly, reducing the chance of being killed or deterred before it obtains a full meal. The mosquito then digests the blood meal; the parasites reproduce, and make their way to the salivary glands or other structures to await "deplaning." When the mosquito is flying toward a susceptible person, the interests of the mosquito and its parasitic passengers coincide. But shortly after landing, conflicts of interest arise.

For both mosquito and parasite, dining is perilous. If the mosquito hesitates, feeds too long, or steps on the wrong hair, its world may suddenly become two-dimensional. It is flatland as well for any parasites left in the mosquito. A foraging mosquito benefits by getting a large blood meal in a small amount of time. Too long a visit increases the risk of immediate death. Too small a meal reduces her potential for making eggs, and may necessitate another dangerous visit.

The parasites in the mosquito, however, have a different balance sheet. If an infected mosquito stays too long, the price is dear for the parasite, but not as dear as for the mosquito; only the parasites that did not travel down the mosquito's hypodermic tongue are left to die with the mosquito, but even these doomed parasites will have been partially successful insofar as some of their kin made the passage. More generally, the parasites benefit by successfully infecting as many new hosts as possible. Hindering the mosquito's feeding may provide parasites with a twofold benefit. It may increase the probing time, thereby increasing the chance that the visit will yield an infection. It may also decrease the amount of blood obtained in the meal, thereby increasing the number of additional visits that the mosquito will make before she dies.

Just such disharmonies occur among protozoal parasites and their vectors. Mosquitoes, for example, regularly bite and apparently transmit malarial parasites to more than one person during a single fill-up (Conway & McBride 1991). This multiple transmission apparently results from a pathological alteration of the mosquito's salivary gland by the protozoan, which reduces the amount of blood that can be safely siphoned from alert victims (Conway & McBride 1991). The protozoan that causes sleeping sickness has a similarly strained relationship with its vector, the tsetse fly. Infected tsetse flies spend more time probing because of damage to their salivary glands (Sivinski 1984). From the parasite's point of view, human behavior is part of the transmission arrangement: Incapacitation of ill people facilitates transfer of large doses to the mosquito, and the capacitation of uninfected people increases the number of people to which mosquitoes transmit infection.

The arguments presented above indicate that vectorborne transmission leads to relatively benign parasitism in the vector and severe parasitism of the vertebrate hosts. This pattern of virulence allows the parasite to use the vector for transport to new hosts, and the vertebrate host as a resource base.

CONTROL OF VECTORBORNE DISEASES

Genetic control

One prong of the current attack on vectorborne diseases has been to generate mosquito populations that are genetically resistant to vectorborne pathogens (Collins et al. 1986, Miller & Mitchell 1991). The hope is to create and propagate mosquito strains that can block the pathogens' ability to reach the saliva. But if this intervention proves successful, the success is likely to be short-lived, being nullified by the selection pressure that the intervention will place on the pathogens. The potential for the pathogens to overcome the engineered resistance may be great because the pathogens transmitted by the remaining unengineered mosquitoes will provide a continuing pool of pathogens under great evolutionary pressure to break into the engineered mosquito population. Accordingly, this evolutionary breakthrough may be delayed if the release of the genetically engineered population occurs in conjunction with a decimation of the natural mosquito population to reduce the evolutionary potential of the pathogen population. Pathogens with little genetic variability should take longer to break through the engineered defenses, as should pathogens that tend to use other species of mosquitoes and other species of vertebrates.

These considerations suggest that some success may be gained from current attempts to genetically engineer resistance to yellow fever virus in the major urban vector of the virus *Aedes aegypti*. The yellow fever virus does not have an extraordinarily high mutation rate; it often cycles in mammals other than humans and uses mosquitoes other than *Aedes aegypti*. But the approach offers virtually no hope for control of more destructive foes like falciparum malaria, because *P. falciparum*'s sexual reproduction will probably rapidly generate the genetic variability necessary to break through engineered defenses.

To be successful a large proportion of the mosquito population must be resistant, but as soon as the population of resistant mosquitoes becomes large, the selective pressure on the pathogens to overcome the resistance increases. Maintaining such defenses would be more feasible if the parasite had a strong negative effect on infected vectors, which could tip the competitive advantage in favor of resistant mosquitoes. But, as mentioned above, vectorborne parasites typically evolve toward benignness in their mosquito hosts. Resistant mosquitoes therefore should tend to have little competitive advantage over susceptible mosquitoes. Natural populations provide evidence for this concern. Some individual mosquitoes in nature are able to subdue malarial parasites by encapsulating them. Yet these resistant mosquitoes have not displaced susceptible mosquitoes in natural populations.

Chemical control

Malaria has been a severe pathogen of humans throughout history, and has shown no signs of evolving toward benignness. Because the malaria organism can reproduce sexually during its transmission cycle, it has a great potential for evolving around barriers that we place in its way. This potential is well illustrated by its responses to antimalarial drugs.

The use of quinine can be traced back to the mid-seventeenth century, when the Incas discovered the effectiveness of quina quina bark. During the empire building and warfare of the 1930s and 1940s the pressing need for antimalarial drugs led to the synthesis of a diverse family of quinine-type drugs. Confronted with Japanese monopolization of quinine-producing areas in Java, the Western nations developed synthetic drugs like chloroquine. During the 1960s, plasmodia resistant to chloroquine had emerged, and today the most severe form of malaria is resistant to chloroquine throughout large regions of Africa, Southeast Asia, and South America.

One of the mechanisms of resistance apparently involves an enhancement of a biochemical pump for expelling the drug. If drug-sensitive malaria are leaky boats doomed to sink because their bilge pumps cannot pump out the drug at a sufficient rate, the resistant strains are leaky boats that remain afloat because they have many more of these pumps. Having multiple copies of the genetic instructions for these pumps, these strains can make enough pumps to keep the drug at nonlethal levels inside the cell. Generating this mechanism of drug resistance is apparently not a great evolutionary challenge. Mammalian cancer cells have evolved similar pumps for ejecting anticancer drugs, and *P. falciparum* has evolved two different sets of pump instructions (Wilson et al. 1989).

The increasing resistance of *P. falciparum* to most of the widely used antimalarials has necessitated the use of drugs with more damaging, even life-threatening side effects (Peters 1987, Björkman & Phillips-Howard 1991). It has also spurred the search for other families of antimalarials. One compound found by this search is the active ingredient in an herbal treatment of malaria that was used in China about a century before the Incas were using quinine (Klayman 1989). Like quinine, the active ingredient has provided the basis for a family of synthetic drugs that hold promise for treatment of malaria—that is, until the treated malaria organisms begin to develop resistance to them as well. The first signs of resistance to this family of antimalarial compounds have already been documented (Doury et al. 1992, Oduola et al. 1992). Similar signs of resistance across the entire armamentarium of antimalarial drugs has led researchers to conclude that the future will offer an ongoing succession of new antimalarial drugs and new resistance to the drugs (Peters 1987).

Given the limitations of antimalarial drugs, researchers have long tried to apply to malaria the principles of vaccination used so successfully against some bacteria and viruses. Indeed the limited options available have led policymakers to focus on vaccines as the most hopeful long-term solution (Turner-Lowe 1991). The continuing attempts will undoubtedly eventually yield some sort of malaria vaccine. But *P. falciparum*'s potential for varying its external proteins (Certa et al. 1987, Lockyer et al. 1989, Hughes 1992) and its past success at evolving around antimalarial compounds suggest that such a vaccine would provide a short-term rather than a long-term solution.

Evolutionary control

Although evolutionary considerations darken the outlook for long-term control by vaccination and antimalarial drugs, the evolutionary principles outlined in this chapter offer hope for approaches that will simultaneously provide short-term and long-term control. Theory predicting that vectorborne diseases should be more virulent than nonvectorborne disease is based on the idea that vectors can transmit the pathogens from immobilized hosts. This ability has undoubtedly been true for most of our evolutionary history with vectorborne pathogens. But if we can intervene so that pathogens no longer could be transmitted from immobilized hosts, we may tip the competitive balance in favor of the more benign variants.

Making houses and hospitals mosquito-proof would be the most feasible way to accomplish this goal for mosquito-borne pathogens like malaria. Recent studies in Sri Lanka, for example, showed that people living in houses with incomplete mud or palm walls and thatched roofs had both malaria and indoor mosquitoes twice as frequently as people living in houses with complete brick and plaster walls and tile roofs (Gamagemendis et al. 1991). Making the better built houses even more mosquito-proof, with screens on all houses, for example, should further decrease exposure to vectorborne diseases. In Thailand, residents of houses with full screening and doors that opened outward suffered dengue at one-fifth the rate of people living in unscreened houses (Ko et al. 1992). But perhaps more importantly, if these improvements were made on a broad scale, malaria variants that affected people adversely enough to necessitate bedrest would achieve virtually no propagation during incapacitating illness. So long as their increased virulence was at least partly due to heritable genetic differences, the population of vectorborne pathogens would evolve toward benignness. The protective immunity generated by a mild *P. falciparum* strain against distantly related lethal strains (Fandeur et al. 1992) indicates that this forcing of *P. falciparum* to evolve reduced virulence would be enhanced by immunological resistance. Because this immunity appears to be more long-lived than previously thought (Deloron & Chougnet 1992), mild strains of *P. falciparum* circulating in a human population have the potential to act like a vaccine against more virulent strains.

Widespread housing improvement may thus provide a benefit not just for the owners of the improved houses but potentially to all within reach of the malaria transmitted from the region.   The most obvious benefit should be a stronger reduction in the frequency of *falciparum* malaria than in the frequencies of the milder *vivax*, *malariae* and *ovale* malarias, but indicators of virulence should show a reduction in the virulent strains within species as well, particularly within *P. falciparum*. This effect contrasts starkly with the tendencies for *P. falciparum* to swamp milder strains as it becomes resistant to antimalarial drugs in areas with long mosquito seasons (Peters 1987). In Minas Gerias, Brazil, during the early 1960s, for example, malaria caused by *P. falciparum* was one-tenth as common as malaria caused by *P. vivax*. By the late 1960s, the proportions were reversed (Peters 1987).

The association between long quiescent periods of *P. vivax* infections and seasonal exposure to vectors (see above) illustrates the responsiveness of plasmodia to different opportunities for transmission. The screening intervention would offer a new twist on transmission opportunities by creating a continual disfavoring rather than a temporary disfavoring of the more rapidly reproducing plasmodia; any plasmodia that reproduced so extensively that they incapacitated their host would suffer, whether this burst of reproduction occurred early or after a period of latency. Such screening should also decrease the virulence of other diseases, like dengue, whose vectors would otherwise invade houses.

The need to consider these long-term evolutionary options is heightened by the failings of past campaigns. At midcentury, the goal of long-term cohabitation with a milder pathogen would have been unacceptable. The goal then was local and eventually global eradication. Now that vectorborne parasites have been educating us for over 30 years, goals are more modest. In malarial campaigns, for example, hopes for eradication have been replaced by hopes for suppression, which have now been replaced by hopes for controlling the spread of malaria in the face of increasing drug resistance (Peters 1987, Brown 1992).

One of the brightest success stories is yellow fever. Yet even with yellow fever, the sense of triumph at midcentury has given way to the realization that the present efforts will at best restrict yellow fever to regional flare-ups (Monath 1991). The recent resurgence of *Aedes aegypti* in areas vulnerable to yellow fever epidemics (Miller & Mitchell 1991) may make even this limited goal a rosy scenario. More yellow fever was reported to the World Health Organization from 1988 through 1990 than at any time since 1948; about 200,000 cases now occur annually (Anonymous 1992). Resistance to insecticides is one reason for this resurgence. *Aedes aegypti* has become more effective at transmitting yellow fever and dengue in the presence of control efforts because it has evolved such resistance (Weiss 1990). These considerations are sobering because yellow fever is one of the most controllable of vectorborne adversaries. *Plasmodium falciparum* is showing no signs of being tamed by vaccines or antimalarial drugs in spite of decades of effort.

Protection from mosquito bite is currently considered to be a valuable prong in a multipronged approach to reduce transmission (Turner-Lowe 1991). Of the options available within this prong, mosquito-proof housing should impose the strongest evolutionary suppression of virulence. Bed nets reduce illness and death from malaria (Bermejo & Veeken 1992) and might similarly cause an evolutionary suppression of virulence if they were used comprehensively by all sick individuals. But the motivation to use nets and repellents is strongest for uninfected individuals who are trying to avoid infection. Infected individuals have relatively less to gain from their use, and, if they are ill, may be less able to use them fastidiously. Ill people do not have to remember to use their own mosquito-proof house, or be motivated to do so.

The evolutionary effectiveness of vector-proof housing will undoubtedly depend on the particulars of the pathogen, the vector, and the local human community. In some cases the effectiveness may be altered by the presence of other interventions. When *falciparum* malaria is untreated, the forms of the parasites that can infect mosquitoes, called gametocytes, appear in the blood during severe illness (see Figure 286 in Kitchen 1942); gametocytes that appear after severe illness subsides tend to infect mosquitoes poorly, probably because the host's activated immune response inhibits transmission (Sinden 1991). When *falciparum* malaria is treated, however, the gametocytes tend to appear after illness subsides (see Chapter 14, Figure 14 in Garnham 1966). These considerations suggest that mosquito-proof housing will be most effective in areas where treatment is ineffective, for example, where *P. falciparum* is resistant to antimalarial drugs, or distribution of the drugs is not feasible.

We shall not know whether making houses mosquito-proof will cause a strong evolutionary shift toward benignness until we try this intervention on a large scale—one that encompasses an entire interbreeding population of pathogens. If it does not work, what have we lost? We shall have spent some money to provide people with a better standard of living: They will have better homes, fewer insects in their homes, and thus fewer vectorborne infections. If it does work, we shall have provided an extra bonus for these residents, visitors to the area, and others who incur economic and health costs from vectorborne diseases: Vectorborne pathogens will become milder, causing less suffering and lower financial expenditures for treatment and for short-term control measures. Mosquitoes can evolve resistance to DDT, and *Plasmodium falciparum* can evolve resistance to chloroquine. Let them "try" to evolve resistance to mosquito-proof houses. Their most viable evolutionary option is to make their human hosts less sick, and that is our goal as well.

Phrased more generally, this approach proposes that we can artificially raise the fitness costs that pathogens incur from harming the host. When these costs are so raised, natural selection should favor pathogen variants that do not immobilize the host and thus do not incur these costs. In theory, the same approach could be used to drive directly transmitted pathogens to have even milder effects than they now have. If our policies in schools and the work-place required students and employees to work at home if they felt even mildly ill, the pathogens that caused such illness would tend to be purged from circulation. The net result should be an evolutionary reduction in the inherent harmfulness of directly transmitted infections. Given the current socioeconomic pressures of our society, I doubt that our policies could presently be changed sufficiently to facilitate this transition. I am more optimistic about the future. As information technology improves, employees and students will be more able to conduct their work at home and verify the completion of this work to employers and teachers. When this occurs the socioeconomic costs of working at home will drop, allowing us to raise the fitness costs incurred by illness-causing pathogens, and cause these directly transmitted organisms to become even more mild than they are.

CHAPTER 4

How to Be Severe Without Vectors

USING PREDATORS IN PLACE OF VECTORS

Vectorborne transmission is a special case of a broader phenomenon. If we replace the word "vector" with "consumer" and "host" with "consumee," we can apply the same principles to "carnivorous transmission" (Ewald 1987a). When parasites are transmitted from prey to predator through the act of predation, increased use of the prey's tissues should result in exceptionally low fitness costs to the parasite because parasites inside of weakened, less mobile prey can still be transmitted effectively to the predator. The selection for virulence in the consumee should be even more extreme when parasites are transmitted to scavengers by scavenging; in this case, death of the consumee can benefit the parasite by facilitating transmission.

Consider the tapeworm, *Echinococcus granulosus*, which is transmitted from ungulates like sheep, to wolves. The parasite is debilitating and sometimes even lethal in sheep, which certainly must make the sheep easier for the wolves to capture. But the parasite typically causes no overt symptoms in wolves, which disperse them in their feces. Sheep complete the cycle when they inadvertently consume the parasites while grazing. Humans enter into the cycle when they accidentally ingest wolf fecal material, for example, when they handle wolf carcasses during wolf hunts and then touch their mouths with their fecally contaminated hands. The parasites thus enter people during the part of their cycle when they normally would be entering sheep; accordingly, the parasites initiate the severe stage of their life cycle. The result is hydatid disease in which a massive, debilitating and often lethal cyst grows in the person's liver.

Evolutionarily, the wolf in the wolf–sheep cycle is like a giant mosquito. Because of its large size it kills the sheep in the process of becoming infested. But a dead sheep cannot become infested, so, unlike the mosquito, the wolf does not transmit the parasite to sheep by bite. Rather, wolves transfer the parasites to the environment where the sheep will eventually ingest them.

This association of severe disease in the prey host and mild disease in the predator is not a special case. One need open only a few parasitology texts (e.g., Olson 1974) to see that the association occurs in nearly all parasites whose life cycles require transmission from a prey host to a predatory host by predation.

USING A STAGE OF LIFE IN PLACE OF A VECTOR

Some parasites can be thought of as chimeras: part vector and part internal parasite. In such cases the internal parasite can cause severe damage, immobilization, and even death of the host, so long as it can break out of the host and move to new hosts on its own. This description may conjure up an image from the movie "Alien," in which a developing parasite erupts from John Hurt's abdomen as part of its life cycle. Although I found this scene disturbing, it did make me appreciate not being an aphid. Most of us are familiar with these small green or brown insects that live in groups, suck sugar-laden juices from plants, and become a gooey handful of insect mush when we accidently grab their branches. Few, however, are familiar with *Aphelinus jacundus*, a wasp about the size of a pinhead. When a female wasp finds an appropriate aphid, she lays an egg in it and then departs. A few weeks later, the aphid becomes lethargic and eventually stops moving. A bulge forms in its abdomen which then rips, and a wasp nearly the size of the aphid emerges. When the wasp is flying between hosts, it transports its eggs to new hosts, much as a mosquito transports the parasites of malaria. After the egg hatches, the larval wasp incurs little if any cost from extensive use of the aphid's tissues, so long as the wasp can transform itself into its "vector stage" to leave a dead or dying aphid.

This most extreme price paid by wasp-infested aphids has apparently led to a most extreme defense. In Chapter 2, I mentioned that we can generally presume death to be too drastic to be a defense against parasitism. Not so with at least one aphid parasitized by a wasp. The pea aphid, *Acyrthosiphon pisum*, is lethally parasitized by a wasp called *Aphidius ervi*. Because the pea aphid reproduces asexually, the members of a local group can be about as closely related as identical twins. When one is attacked by *Aphidius ervi* it apparently commits suicide. It saves its sisters from its own fate by dropping off the plant onto the hot dry ground where it usually dies before the larval wasp has developed sufficiently to emerge. When the ground is not hot, parasitized aphids are no more likely to drop than unparasitized aphids (McAllister & Roitberg 1987). The dropping into a lethally hot microenvironment therefore appears to be a suicidal act that protects the other unparasitized hosts (as it was, incidentally, at the end of third movie in the "Alien" series).

Although the relationship between a parasite's mobility outside of its host and its virulence has not been systematically studied, the vast majority of lethal insect parasites have a highly mobile stage (Askew 1971). The severity of such highly adapted parasites is contradictory to the conventional belief in evolution toward commensalism. Advocates of the conventional view did a semantic sidestep to deal with this contradiction. They set these lethal parasites apart from "true" parasites, calling them *parasitoids*, or parasitic predators. However, the mortality inflicted by these mobile parasites ranges relatively continuously from 100% to the much lower mortality typical of vectorborne parasites. Considering that their lethality is explainable by the same evolutionary forces that lead to severity among "true" parasites, it is more parsimonious to view parasitoids as parasites possessing characteristics that favor evolution toward one end of the continuum that spans from intense mutualism to lethal parasitism (Ewald 1987a).

Why are humans spared from such destructive guests? We are infested with a few parasites that use a similar strategy. When botflies encounter wounds they may lay eggs from which maggots grow. They are disgusting, but generally not life-threatening. Their relative mildness in us can be attributed to their small size relative to us, and to our ability to limit the numbers of eggs laid by swatting or shooing flies. In smaller, more helpless vertebrates such as bird nestlings, these parasitic flies can be as damaging as *Aphelinus jacundus* is in aphids. But even in large vertebrates such parasites can be relatively severe if the host does not have effective means of avoiding them. Deer, for example, suffer from flies that lay eggs in their noses. The maggots hatch, eat, and grow during their migration to the deer's lungs. The tissue damage maims and sometimes even kills infested deer.

This argument about body size and virulence can be expanded to provide a clearer view of the entire spectrum of consumer relationships from mutualism through parasitism to predation. When consumers approach the size of their host, their options for living in or on the host—that is, for being parasitic—narrow. A lion would be better off if it could get all of the nutrients it needs to survive and reproduce competitively without killing the zebra upon which it feeds. A dead zebra may provide more food than the lion can eat; furthermore, the lion's predatory activities continue to eliminate the most vulnerable individuals, often making future attacks more difficult. How much more leisurely the lion's life would be if it could move to a very vulnerable zebra to take a few bites and return again and again as hunger arises. The death of the zebra is not in itself useful to the lion, just as the death of a human from falciparum malaria is not useful to the protozoa that cause the malaria. The death is a side effect of an intensity of dining that facilitates the consumer's survival and reproduction. The lion benefits from a relatively great use of zebra tissue because it is big relative to the zebra, and it is mobile; when a zebra dies, the lion can move to other zebra to get some more zebra tissue.

It takes some imagination to picture what it is like to be living at a scale so small that consumers are midway between typical predators and parasites. We do not, for example, find mites directly threatening the lives of humans. At worst they might transmit an infectious disease or cause the intense itching and eczema that we call scabies. For smaller animals the situation may be more serious. Honeybees die from infestations of the mite, *Acarapis woodi*, which crawl into the bee's breathing tubes and drastically reduce their air intake (Hart 1989, Cowen 1991). Imagine dozens of spiders crawling through your nose and into your lungs to feast on your lung tissue, eventually killing you by clogging your breathing passages. Mosquitoes are a bother to us, but when they feed on a mouse they are the size of a vampire bat. Swallow bugs can be responsible for about half of all deaths among nesting cliff swallows. A single nest may contain up to 2500 bugs (Brown & Brown 1990). If a group of 2500 vampire bats attacked and killed a person by feeding on him, would we call the bats parasites or predators? The larger the parasite becomes relative to the host, the more predator-like it becomes because its options for being anything but a predator narrow.

When consumers become small relative to their consumees, additional options present themselves. The individual parasite can dine on its host without causing death; if it is small enough, it may not even cause any detectable harm. Tiny parasites therefore have an option that the lion does not have; they can take a few very tiny "mouthfuls." But the possibility of this option does not mean that it is the option favored by natural selection. Tiny consumers also have the option of reproducing in or on the host. And because populations can grow geometrically, tiny parasites can, through reproduction, use up resources more like a predator than like a freeloader. The tiny consumers can take vast numbers of tiny mouthfuls after they have undergone vast amounts of multiplication inside of the host. This multiplication is little different from growth of body size: The cells of the unicellular parasites are simply separated from one another. In this context, the *Plasmodium falciparum* inside a person collectively have a relatively large body size: They can infect nearly half of a person's red blood cells. The evolutionary approach to virulence emphasizes that the collective body size of parasites—and the harm they cause—will often depend on readily identifiable characteristics of the relationship: transmission from sick or dead hosts, vertical transmission, and the mobility of parasites outside of the host.

LETHAL PARASITISM AND MANIPULATION OF HOSTS

Lethal parasitism opens new evolutionary avenues for host manipulation. If the host is going to die anyhow, there is little long-term price to pay from making the host do things that hurt the host but help the parasite. A wasp called *Aphidius nigripes* does just that when it parasitizes the potato aphid, *Macrosiphum euphorbiae* (Brodeur & McNeil 1989). Like the immature *Aphelinus jacundus* and *Aphidius ervi*, immature *Aphidius nigripes* eat away at the insides of the aphid until the aphid is little more than a casing, from which the adult wasp erupts. But before the aphid dies, the larval wasp often enters a dormant state, which is presumably an adaptation for passing through inhospitable times of year. But entering dormancy is particularly risky for *Aphid. nigripes*. Over such a long period of time, its aphid host might be eaten by predators or killed by exposure to the physical environment; moreover, the wasp can be lethally parasitized by another wasp, called *Asaphes vulgaris*. Dormant *Aphid. nigripes* would presumably be better off if its aphid host sat quietly in a safe place. And this is just what the aphid does; when parasitized by dormant *Aphid. nigripes*, it moves into curled leaves or other protected sites where it eventually dies. In these sheltered sites, *Aphid. nigripes* has a lower chance of falling victim to *Asaph. vulgaris* (Brodeur & McNeil 1989). The wasp has manipulated the last act of its aphid host for its own protection before doing in the aphid.

The greater survival of *Aphid. nigripes* in the protected sites suggests that the change in the aphid's behavior is a precise manipulation rather than a haphazard destruction of normal behavior. So does one other piece of information. When *Aphid. nigripes* does not go into a dormant state, the aphid's behavior is altered but in a different way: The aphids crawl into exposed positions. Parasitism per se therefore does not lead to movement toward protected sites.

The lethality associated with consumee-to-consumer transmission has also raised evolutionary options for bizarre forms of manipulation. The classic example involves *Dicrocoelium dendriticum*, a trematode worm that moves from its ant host to its sheep host when the sheep eats the ant. Some of the *D. dendriticum* in the ant facilitate this transmission by migrating to the ant's brain, where they short-circuit the ant's behavior. The rewired ant crawls up a blade of grass, clamps down on the grass with its jaws, and waits to be consumed by "predatory" sheep. After entering the sheep, the trematode releases its progeny among the sheep feces, which ants ingest to start the cycle over again. Variations on this theme are ubiquitous among the parasites transmitted from prey to predator by predation. Under laboratory conditions, the tapeworm *Echinococcus multilocularus* often kills the field mice it inhabits, but before doing so, it causes them to become obese. In nature, the sluggish mice become easy and apparently rich targets for foxes, the other host in the worm's life cycle. The trematode *Leucochloridium pardoxum* is transmitted to birds when they eat infested snails. This parasite does not just slow down the snail; it transforms the snail's antennae from narrow hairpins to bulging, colorful caterpillars, which seem to make the snails irresistible to the birds that *L. paradoxum* must enter to complete its life cycle.

In a symposium on behavioral manipulation of hosts by parasites, N. A. Croll asked one of the leading researchers in this area, J. C. Holmes, whether predatory hosts, like the birds that consume *L. paradoxum*, are idiots (Holmes & Bethel 1972). Why do they not evolve the ability to alter their behavior to avoid consuming the parasitized prey? Holmes answered, "Definitive hosts are not idiots . . . . The system involves a tradeoff with acquisition of parasites being traded for easier capture of prey." He noted that for his study systems parasitism imposes little tissue damage in the predators. So far so good. But then he added, "It must be emphasized that it is the population's energy balance that is involved; individual hosts could occasionally lose out." The framework proposed in this book offers a more comprehensive answer that is consistent with evolutionary processes. These systems are stable in general because the predators are used like vectors; parasites cause them little harm because the parasites need them for dispersal to new prey hosts, like malaria parasites need mosquitoes. Whether the population of predators benefits or suffers is not the issue. Rather, the issue is whether the predators that choose to eat parasitized prey benefit from doing so. The predators benefit so long as the fitness costs they incur from being parasitized are less than the benefits they get from easier capture of prey. This argument points to a key test for assessing whether the predators are or are not idiots. If the accessibility of, say, snails that are not parasitized by *Leucochloridium* is increased, then the birds, if clever enough, will begin choosing unparasitized snails when the density of these snails becomes so great that the loss in fitness from passing up parasitized snails is less than the loss in fitness from becoming parasitized.

USING THE MOBILITY OF SUSCEPTIBLES IN PLACE OF A VECTOR

Sit-and-wait transmission and virulence

Vectorborne transmission explains why the agents of malaria, yellow fever, typhus, and sleeping sickness are severe whereas most of the nonvectorborne pathogens are more mild. But a great deal of variation among nonvectorborne pathogens remains to be explained. Kuru is one of the most lethal nonvectorborne diseases. Its extreme lethality is explained by a quirk of its life cycle: Death facilitates transmission because transmission occurs when individuals killed by the disease are eaten by other people. This mode of transmission is unique (thankfully) among the pathogens summarized in Figure 3.2. Explaining kuru's lethality therefore still leaves us asking questions about the remaining pathogens. Why, for example, are smallpox and tuberculosis so much more severe than the other nonvectorborne diseases?

One possible answer can be termed the sit-and-wait hypothesis. A pathogen can be transmitted from an immobilized host to a susceptible host in two ways. It can be transported there, by something that is mobile, like a mosquito. Or, it can sit and wait for a susceptible individual to come to it. Its success at sitting and waiting depends on its ability to survive in the external environment. Like vectorborne pathogens, sit-and-wait pathogens could gain the benefits of multiplication inside of hosts while paying little cost through immobilization of the host. Sit-and-wait parasites should therefore be especially virulent.

After generating the sit-and-wait hypothesis to explain the often high virulence of pathogens infecting insects (Ewald 1987b), I wondered whether the sit-and-wait strategy might explain some of the variation in lethality among nonvectorborne pathogens of humans. If so, pathogens that can survive longer in the external environment should be more lethal. Bruno Walther and I have just finished a test that confirms this prediction among respiratory tract pathogens of humans. Nonvectorborne pathogens typically survive for hours to a few days in the external environment and kill about one to ten out of every 100,000 people who are infected. But the species that survive for weeks to years tend to cause death more frequently. Leading the pack is the smallpox virus which kills one in ten and can survive for more than a decade outside of the host. The agents of tuberculosis and diphtheria can survive for months and are correspondingly severe. The remaining pathogens tend to survive for periods of hours to days and tend to cause lethality less frequently. So, sit-and-wait transmission explains why the agents of smallpox and tuberculosis are so severe.

An analogous test has not yet been conducted on insect pathogens, but indications are that the sit-and-wait hypothesis applies to them as well. Some of the nuclear polyhedrosis viruses that infect insects make the smallpox virus look relatively benign. They can kill nearly all that they infect, and can survive for many years in the external environment. One problem with the sit-and-wait strategy is that the pathogen has to sit and wait in the right spot. At least one of the nuclear polyhedrosis viruses times its lethality to facilitate its entrance into new hosts. It blocks the hormone that allows larvae to molt into adults (O'Reilly & Miller 1989). The larval insect therefore dies in larval microhabitat, where succeeding generations of susceptible larvae will be present.

The sit-and-wait strategy should work especially well when living sites for the hosts are limited and protected. If sites are limited they will tend to be visited by new hosts soon after the last host has been killed. If these sites are protected from light, desiccation, and extreme temperatures, sit-and-wait transmission should be facilitated by prolonged survival outside of the host. In this regard, it is not surprising that honeybees are victims of particularly voracious sit-and-wait parasites. When honeybee larvae are infected with the bacterium *Bacillus larvae*, they face virtually certain death (Morse & Nowogrodzki 1990). Because its spores can easily survive over 50 years in the external environment (H. Shimanuki, personal communication), *B. larvae* has a large window of time during which sites of destroyed colonies can be sources of infection. Being resistant to infection, the adult bees can transmit the spores on their body surfaces. *Bacillus larvae* can therefore move to new colonies directly through contact between adult bees or indirectly through flowers, or it can infect new colonies that are established at the contaminated site. Another route of transmission is by way of beekeepers who spread the bacterium by moving honey, pollen, or brood combs between colonies (Shimanuki 1990). Whatever the route, the extreme durability of *B. larvae* allows effective transmission even though infected larvae are consumed before they are ever mobile.

The sit-and-wait hypothesis may also be applicable to vertebrate agriculture. Bovine spongiform encephalopathy is a rather gruesome example of sit-and-wait transmission. Fear of acquiring human cases of this "mad cow disease" has led to the destruction of over 18,000 cattle in England, where an outbreak was identified in 1986 (Cherfas 1990). Like kuru, this disease causes neurological damage and death, after which it is transmitted by consumption of infected brain tissue. It appears to have been introduced into cattle by the use of infected sheep brains as a feed supplement. (In sheep the pathogen is apparently the cause of a similar disease called scrapie.) In the absence of feed contamination, the pathogen seems to be perpetuated by gradual dissemination from dead animals. It can survive for years in the soil, ready to infect and kill grazers that inadvertently eat food contaminated by the remains of an infected animal (Weiss 1991).

Sit-and-wait transmission and our future

At first glance, the sit-and-wait hypothesis might seem to be largely of historical relevance to human disease. Smallpox has been eradicated. Diphtheria has plummeted wherever widespread vaccination has been enacted. Tuberculosis had been receding steadily during the latter half of this century as standards of nutrition and housing improved and effective antibiotics came into use. The AIDS pandemic has contributed to a reversal of this progress. HIV cannot bring back smallpox from extinction, but it is now helping to bring back tuberculosis in countries like the United States and is exacerbating the longstanding tuberculosis problem in poorer countries. The downward trend in the incidence of tuberculosis stopped in rich and poor countries alike during the mid-1980s as the AIDS pandemic took hold (Sudre et al. 1992). With its yearly death toll of about 3 million, *Mycobacterium tuberculosis* now ends more human life than any other species of pathogen, and this annual toll is expected to rise (World Health Organization 1992).

HIV and *M. tuberculosis* enhance each other's dangerousness. With its intrinsically high virulence, *M. tuberculosis* tends to accelerate progression of HIV infections to AIDS (Hill et al. 1991). The damage to the immune system caused by HIV accelerates the development and contagiousness of tuberculosis and diminishes the effectiveness of tuberculosis tests (Stead & Lofgren 1991, Heckbert et al. 1992, Johnson et al. 1992, van der Werf et al. 1992). These interactions decrease the chances of detecting *M. tuberculosis* infections before they progress to dangerous stages, and appear to have an amplifying effect on the spread of the tuberculosis epidemic in hospitals, prisons, and shelters for the homeless (Daley et al. 1992, Dooley et al. 1992ab, Pearson et al. 1992).

Because *M. tuberculosis* can cause dangerous, contagious infections even among people with intact immune systems, the amplification of *M. tuberculosis* by the AIDS pandemic may have a serious impact on people who have very low risk for HIV infection. The elderly are particularly vulnerable to *M. tuberculosis*. In Arkansas, for example, *M. tuberculosis* infections were nearly twice as common among people who had lived in nursing homes for about 2.5 years than among people beginning their residence in the nursing homes (Stead et al. 1985). Each year about one out of every 25 residents became infected. The danger in hospitals serving AIDS epicenters like New York City has been even greater. Highly contagious tuberculosis patients often remain in crowded hospital settings for prolonged periods before appropriate infection control procedures can be instituted (Centers for Disease Control 1991). In such settings large proportions of hospital personnel have become infected, sometimes fatally (Centers for Disease Control 1991, Dooley et al. 1992b). HIV-infected hospital personnel are particularly vulnerable not only because they are more likely to die from *M. tuberculosis* infections, but also because they are disproportionately exposed: HIV-infected personnel often volunteer to care for AIDS patients (Castro et al. 1992).

Compounding the problem is the increasing resistance of *M. tuberculosis* to the antibiotics that have proved so successful in past decades. This resistance reduces the chances for recovery, and thereby increases the extent to which infected people may act as sources of infection for others (Beck-Sagué et al. 1992). Resistant bacteria are particularly widespread in some urban areas like New York City and in developing countries, and new replacement drugs are not in the offing (Centers for Disease Control 1991, Davidson & Le 1992, Dooley et al. 1992a, Edlin et al. 1992). In countries with meager resources for health care and high rates of infection, *Mycobacterium tuberculosis,* whether sensitive to antibiotics or not, will soon be enhancing its reputation as a major killer (Fitzgerald et al. 1991).

The spread of tuberculosis in concert with AIDS is particularly ominous in Africa, where one out of three people is infected with *M. tuberculosis* (Sudre et al. 1992). AIDS is the leading killer, for example, in the Ivory Coast, being responsible for one in six deaths. Tuberculosis has increased substantially since the mid-1980s to become the third leading cause of death in Abidjan (DeCock et al. 1991). The spread of tuberculosis in concert with AIDS has occurred in other African countries as well as in North and South America and Europe; tuberculosis may occur in from one of 50 AIDS patients in some groups to more than half in others (Hughes & Corrah 1990, FitzGerald et al. 1991, Nauclér et al. 1991, Ong & Mandal 1991). In Africa, over a quarter million cases of HIV-associated tuberculosis occurred in 1990 (Sudre et al. 1992). With one-third of the world's population infected with *M. tuberculosis* and with HIV still spreading, we can be certain that the problem of HIV-induced tuberculosis will get worse. The theory presented here indicates that, ultimately, sit-and-wait transmission deserves much of the blame for this problem and more generally for the millions of deaths from tuberculosis that will occur this year and each upcoming year into the foreseeable future.

CHAPTER 5

When Water Moves like a Mosquito

WATERBORNE TRANSMISSION AND VIRULENCE

If I were to ask a person on the street to name the world's most dreaded afflictions, few in economically prosperous countries would say diarrhea. Yet diarrheal diseases have levied one of the greatest death tolls since the middle of this century, being primary causes of from 4 to 20 million deaths annually, mostly among young children (Hardy 1956, Puffer & Serrano 1973, Rohde & Northrup 1976, Rowland et al. 1977, Walsh & Warren 1979, Snyder & Merson 1982, Gibbons 1992). And they probably have been no less culpable for at least the past few centuries.

Clearly, diarrheal diseases are a major health problem. But only in recent years have biologists been able to explain why some diarrhea-causing organisms have evolved to cause extremely severe diseases, like cholera and typhoid fever, whereas others cause just a few urgent dashes per day.

One of the explanations recognizes a similarity between the wings of mosquitoes and the ways humans use water. Like pathogens transmitted by mosquitoes, waterborne pathogens can reap lucrative profits from transforming us into pathogen production machines. A person immobilized with a severe case of diarrhea will release pathogens into bedding and clothing, which will tend to be washed; or fecal material may be discarded by attendants directly into toilets, sewers, or other conduits of water. When the water contaminated with such fecal material mixes with unprotected drinking water, hundreds of susceptible people can become infected by the pathogens released from a single immobilized host.

This process has been documented repeatedly over the past two centuries when water supplies have been inadequately protected (Snow 1855/1966, Prescott & Horwood 1935, Seal & Banerjea 1949, Pollitzer 1959, Robertson & Pollitzer 1939, Levine et al. 1976).

Recognizing the analogy between this kind of transmission and transmission by arthropod vectors, like mosquitoes, I refer to this process as *transmission by a cultural vector*.   Specifically, I define *cultural vector* to be a set of characteristics that allow transmission from immobilized hosts to susceptibles when at least one of the characteristics is some aspect of human culture (Ewald 1988). I use the term "culture" in the broadest sense to encompass any aspect or product of human activity that is passed on nongenetically from person to person. A cultural vector can transport (1) the pathogen from the infected individual to susceptibles, (2) the infected individual to susceptibles, or (3) susceptibles to infecteds.

In the case of waterborne transmission, the cultural vector includes the materials tainted by the immobilized host, the person removing the feces and tainted materials, any sewage system transporting the contaminated water to drinking water supplies, any noncultural variables contributing to contamination of the drinking water (e.g., moving bodies of water such as streams), and any persons and equipment delivering the contaminated drinking water to susceptible people. Because the potential pool of susceptibles is often extremely large for waterborne pathogens, pathogens may gain tremendous fitness benefits from increased use of host resources for their own propagation.

In contrast, when transmission occurs by person-to-person contact, immobilization may severely reduce the number of susceptibles that can be infected; moreover, the probability of infecting a contacted susceptible should plateau rapidly as reproduction of directly transmitted pathogens increases because they are not diluted. Person-to-person transmission should therefore favor less virulent variants than waterborne transmission. This cultural vector hypothesis therefore predicts that the virulence of diarrheal pathogens should be positively associated with their tendencies for waterborne transmission. A review of the relevant literature confirmed this prediction (Table 5.1).

Levin and Svanborg Edén (1990) provided an alternative explanation of this association. They suggested that the ingestion of pathogens in water might increase the infective doses, thereby causing more severe disease. This suggestion can be rejected, however, because waterborne outbreaks of the severe pathogens are not more lethal than nonwaterborne outbreaks of the same pathogens (Ewald 1991a). Nor can this strong positive correlation between waterborne transmission and mortality be explained by possible correlates of these two variables, such as fly-borne transmission, historical period, or desiccation resistance (Ewald 1991a). The available evidence therefore supports the idea that waterborne transmission causes an evolutionary increase in virulence.

TABLE 5.1   Waterborne Transmission and Lethality of Diarrheal Diseases

Pathogen	Mortality (%)	Waterborne (%)
Vibrio cholerae, classical biotype	15.2	83.3
Shigella dysenteriae, type 1	7.5	80.0
Salmonella typhi	6.2	74.0
Vibrio cholerae, el tor biotype	1.42	50.0
Shigella flexneri	1.35	48.3
Shigella sonnei	0.45	27.8
Enterotoxigenic Escherichia coli	<0.1	20.0
Campylobacter jejuni	<0.1	10.7
Nontyphoid Salmonella	<0.1	1.6

Note: These results represent all pathogenic bacteria of the gastrointestinal tract that are regularly transmitted between humans in community settings and for which both waterborne transmission and mortality could be adequately quantified. Mortality percentages refer to the number of deaths that would occur in the absence of effective treatment for every 100 infections. Waterborne percentages refers to the average number of outbreaks involving waterborne transmission for every 100 outbreaks reported in the literature with an identified mode of transmission. Mortality is significantly correlated with the degree of waterborne transmission ($p < 0.01$, Spearman rank test). References, selection procedures, and calculations are presented by Ewald (1991a).

GEOGRAPHIC PATTERNS

The evolutionary linkage of virulence to waterborne transmission presumes that pathogens can evolve their current states of virulence over time periods of centuries to millennia. This assumption can be evaluated by looking at the time scales over which pathogens can evolve key characteristics critical for their survival in response to cultural changes. The medical literature provides only one intensely studied example of such a characteristic: antibiotic resistance. Pathogens can evolve antibiotic resistance on a time scale of weeks to months (Ewald 1988).

If waterborne transmission favors highly virulent pathogens during even remotely similar time scales, introduction of uncontaminated drinking water should result in an evolutionary reduction in virulence. Evaluating this prediction involves use of the public health records, much as a paleontologist uses a fossil record. Ideally, one would like to have genetically distinct competing conspecific pathogens whose frequencies are traceable before, during, and after the introduction of pure drinking water—that is, since the mid-nineteenth century in industrialized countries. Unfortunately, the lack of detailed identification of variants within species until the early decades of the twentieth century hinders this goal, but two approaches are feasible.

1. Because closely related bacterial species (i.e., those belonging to the same genus) have been identified throughout the century, changes in their prevalences can be monitored. Competition among species within a genus should be weaker than competition within a species; nevertheless, the serological, nutritional, and ecological similarities of species within a genus should make the prediction applicable, though the trends are likely to be looser than in comparisons within species.

2. Frequencies of intraspecific variants can be quantified over part of this period. The general prediction outlined above is still valid for the past 50 to 60 years because water purification generally spans several decades and is still incomplete in many countries.

Comparisons within genera do show a correlation between purification of water supplies and a shift from severe to benign species. Massive improvements in water purification occurred in the United States, for example, during the first quarter of this century (Gay 1918). By the 1930s, the most deadly dysentery bacterium, *Shigella dysenteriae* type 1, was being replaced by the moderately severe *Shigella flexneri* (Hardy et al. 1940, DuPont 1979). Water purification improved steadily into the middle of this century (Gorman & Wolman 1939, Craun & McCabe 1973), when *S. flexneri* became replaced by the more benign *Shigella sonnei* (Centers for Disease Control, Shigella Surveillance Reports, 1968–83).

Salmonella show a similar trend. The most deadly *Salmonella* (*S. typhi*) decreased while the more benign *Salmonella* species increased in absolute frequency (Gay 1918, Wolman & Gorman 1931, Stebbins 1940, National Academy of Sciences 1969, Centers for Disease Control, *Salmonella* Surveillance Reports 1968-1978).

The timing of such transitions across geographic areas should be correlated with the timing of improvements in water supply. Geographic areas with later purification can be considered "controls" for the prior purification in "experimental" areas. The actual trends are consistent with this prediction; for example, water supplies in the United Kingdom were purified decades before purification in the United States (Burnet 1869, Fuertes 1897, Robins 1946). The transitions from the deadly *S. dysenteriae* type 1 to moderately virulent *S. flexneri* to the relatively benign *S. sonnei* occurred about three decades later in the United States than in the United Kingdom (Fraser & Smith 1930, Bøjlen 1934, Hurst & Knott 1936, Bowes 1938, Felsen 1945, Hutchinson 1956, Gillies 1968). The United States in turn purified its water supply about a quarter century before the initial improvements in Poland, and *S. dysenteriae* replaced *S. flexneri* about a quarter century earlier than in Poland. Japan and Western Europe purified their water supplies at about the same time as the United States and experienced replacements of *S. dysenteriae* with *S. flexneri*, and *S. flexneri* with *S. sonnei* synchronously with the United States (Futaki 1926, Acton & Knowles 1928, Shiga 1936, Manson-Bahr 1944, Felsen 1945, Aoki 1968, Szturm-Rubenstein 1968, van Oye et al. 1968, Takeda 1983). Most of China did not experience these improvements in water supply and did not show this pattern of replacement. *S. dysenteriae* was still common in China 40 years after it had disappeared from Japan and the United States (Aoki 1968). But the water supplies of Hong Kong and Shanghai were improved early in the century, just shortly after Japan and the United States were making major progress in water purification. Accordingly, the *S. dysenteriae* had virtually vanished from Shanghai and Hong Kong shortly after disappearing in the United States and Japan (Aoki 1968, Shu-Cheng 1983). An analogous difference occurred between New York City and rural New York during the first half of this century, when water purification in the city was many years ahead of that in the rural areas (Stebbins 1940).

Although India has made substantial improvements in water supply in some areas, availability of pure water has been comparable to that in most of China, and so has the composition the *Shigella*: *S. dysenteriae* and *S. flexneri* have been common throughout the century and show no signs of giving way to *S. sonnei* (Heffernan 1914, Manifold 1928, Wats et al. 1928, Manson-Bahr 1944, Little & Bornshin 1930, Boyd 1940, Panda & Gupta 1964, Sharma et al. 1967, Feldman et al. 1970, Sakazaki et al. 1971, Rajasekaran et al. 1977, Kaliyugaperumal 1978, Paniker et al. 1978, Khan et al. 1979, Macaden et al. 1980, Arora et al. 1982, Agarwal et al. 1984, Macaden & Bhat 1985, 1986, Santhanakrishnan et al. 1987). Water quality in Bangladesh is generally worse than in India and the prevalence of *S. sonnei* remains slightly lower (Khan & Mosley 1968, Huq 1979, Stoll et al. 1982, Huq et al. 1983, Tacket et al. 1984, M. U. Khan et al. 1985).

Guatemala has one of the most contaminated water supplies in the Americas and was the source of the last major epidemic of *S. dysenteriae* in the Americas (Mata et al. 1966, 1970). This epidemic spread northward unabated until it arrived in the United States, where it disintegrated, presumably because it could not be maintained without waterborne transmission. Its transmission was studied in a barrio in Los Angeles on a person-by-person basis (Weissman et al. 1974). In this environment with its uncontaminated water supplies, every 10 infections, on average, gave rise to only four new infections. Within a few of these declining rounds of transmission, the organism died out. The situation to the south of Guatemala was similar. The organism was blocked in Costa Rica, where water supplies were relatively pure (L. J. Mata, personal communication). The prevalences of *S. sonnei* relative to *S. flexneri* to the south of Guatemala were also similar to those in other countries with early water purification. In urban centers in Costa Rica and Panama, both water purification and the increased prevalence of *S. sonnei* occurred by midcentury (M. Kourany, personal communication, L. J. Mata personal communication, Moore et al. 1965, 1966, Kourany & Vásquez 1969, Kourany et al. 1971).

The uniformity of these trends is remarkable, especially when one considers all of the other factors that could influence the composition of *Shigella* species. It is also remarkable because it suggests that the different species are negatively affecting one another. The shift from *S. flexneri* to *S. sonnei* in the United States, for example, was not associated with a decline in the overall frequencies of *Shigella* infection (Centers for Disease Control, *Shigella* Surveillance Reports, 1968–83, Reller et al. 1970). Such competition probably occurs largely through acquired immunity. The dysentery-producing *Shigella* species share a collection of components that are associated with basic processes such as infection of cells. Because these components are similar in structure, immunity generated against those found on one species of *Shigella* can also neutralize other *Shigella* species. This kind of cross-immunity should certainly have some inhibitory effect, but current evidence indicates this between-species immunity is substantially weaker than within-species immunity: Vaccines generated from a *Shigella* species protected against disease by other species only in some instances (Meitert et al. 1984, Wang 1984, Formal et al. 1991).

Regardless of the details about the interactions among the different species, the geographic patterns and their changes through time shows that water purification is associated with changes in the composition of *Shigella* species. As water is purified, the composition shifts in favor of the milder *Shigella*.

Similar changes have occurred among *Vibrio cholerae*, the bacteria that cause cholera. The relatively mild el tor type largely replaced the more virulent classical type throughout the world during the 1960s and 1970s. This displacement is often characterized as a sudden and relentless wave spreading across the Pacific Islands and southern Asia. Although this characterization may be valid on a broad geographic scale, it tends to overlook small-scale variations that provide clues to the reasons for the broader trends. The countries that were first invaded by the el tor *V. cholerae* generally had made improvements in purification of drinking water. Calcutta, India, for example, had established substantial access to unpolluted water supplies at least a decade before the major improvements in Dhaka, Bangladesh, which began during the mid-1970s but were only partially effective (Ghosh & Rao 1965, M. U. Khan, W. B. Greenough III, personal communications). The transition from classical to el tor occurred in Calcutta by 1964 (De et al. 1965, 1969). Although el tor was present in Bangladesh at that time, displacement of classical by el tor in Dhaka began about a decade later, and was incomplete (Khan et al. 1984a). Relative to surrounding countries, Bangladesh still has less access to pure water and it is the only country in which classical *V. cholerae* persists endemically (Siddique et al. 1991, 1992).

The cultural vectors hypothesis answers one other question that has troubled epidemiologists. Why did the tidal wave of el tor spread around the world, displacing classical *V. cholerae* during the 1960s? El tor *V. cholerae* was first identified in 1906 among pilgrims to Mecca who fell ill in the El Tor quarantine station on the Saudi Arabian coast of the Red Sea (De 1961). Why did el tor *V. cholerae* make so little headway in competition with classical *V. cholerae* for a half-century and then almost completely displace it within a decade? The cultural vectors hypothesis suggests that the extensive water purification projects in South Asia during the middle decades of the twentieth century tilted the competitive balance in favor of the milder el tor.

Applying this cultural vectors hypothesis to *V. cholerae* is complex because the relationships between virulence, host immunity, and competitive advantages are complex. *V. cholerae* causes cholera through the release of a toxin that apparently expels competitors by flushing them out of the intestine (Chapter 2). The classical *V. cholerae* generally produces more toxin than the less virulent el tor type (Turnbull et al. 1985). The greater the amount of toxin, the more voluminous the diarrhea (Petritsch et al 1992). The more extensive toxin production of classical *V. cholerae* should therefore lead to more rapid expulsion of competitors and eventually more *V. cholerae* flowing out of the intestinal tract.

Measurements suggest that this increase in productivity can be enormous. The density of *V. cholerae* in the outflow from symptomatic infections can be about 100 or even 1000 times greater than that from very mild or asymptomatic infections (Pollitzer 1959, Dizon 1965, Dizon et al. 1967, De et al. 1969). Similarly, the densities flowing from cholera cases are about ten times greater than the densities from relatively mild cases of choleraic diarrhea (De et al. 1969). A typical classical infection, then, can be expected on average to shed pathogens in the environment at a greater rate than does a typical el tor infection. The variation in virulence within each type of *V. cholerae* infection provides additional evidence that productivity of *V. cholerae* is linked to virulence rather than to some other characteristic of these two types. When a particularly virulent el tor strain was compared with a milder classical strain, the outcome was reversed: The el tor strain invaded with fewer organisms, caused worse disease, and produced more progeny in purer culture than did the classical strain (Lycke et al. 1986).

The goal of improving water supplies in Bangladesh has been severely hampered by financial limitations and a burgeoning population; consequently, a large proportion of the population still consumes fecally contaminated water (M. U. Khan, W. B. Greenough, III, personal communications). Around 1980, classical *V. cholerae* resurged in Bangladesh. This resurgence made clear the inadequacy of the tidal wave model of el tor expansion, but left epidemiologists at a loss for an explanation (Monsur 1983, Samadi et al. 1983, Edelman & Pierce 1984).

The general displacement of classical *V. cholerae* by el tor has been explained in terms of el tor's competitive superiority when co-occurring in culture media, its greater duration of excretion from infected hosts, and its greater ability to survive on surfaces and in nightsoil (Glass et al. 1982, Huq et al. 1983). But these arguments do not consider the broader set of pros and cons that result from rapid toxin production. When the entire transmission cycle is considered in areas where waterborne transmission is prevalent, classical *V. cholerae* may achieve competitive superiority over el tor even if el tor is superior in the absence of waterborne transmission. The price the classical type may have paid for this superiority is slow growth in competition with other *V. cholerae*: Profuse toxin production requires resources that could otherwise be funneled into reproduction.

The arguments relying on competitive superiority in the external environment also ignored the timing question. Why did severe *V. cholerae* apparently dominate benign forms for centuries, only to be rapidly replaced a quarter century ago? A stronger competitive ability of el tor outside the intestinal environment would surely favor coexistence, but it cannot explain the temporary displacement of the el tor biotype that has recently occurred in Bangladesh. Invoking this hypothesis, Huq et al. (1983) noted that the resurgent classical *V. cholerae* were able to compete with el tor in culture media better than the old classical strain. Yet, the resurgent classical *V. cholerae* still grew more poorly than el tor; the ratio of classical to el tor had dropped by 90% after 24 hours.

If el tor replaced the classical type because of water purification, why did the classical type resurge in Bangladesh? The cultural vectors hypothesis can explain this resurgence if transient immunity is taken into account. El tor and classical *V. cholerae* cross-react serologically; intense infections with one type provide substantial immunity against the other (Felsenfeld 1963, Lycke et al. 1986). Vaccination studies indicate that this cross-protection is partly a consequence of immunity to cholera toxin: The effectiveness of vaccines is improved by including portions of the toxin (Sack et al. 1991), which is virtually the same in the classical and el tor types of *V. cholerae*. These vaccines appear to protect against both types for several years before the immunity begins to wane. The cross-protection therefore indicates that one type of *V. cholerae* will inhibit the other for years through the immune system, even though the chances of simultaneous infection are small. The differences in the makeup of the two types, however, indicate that the immune-mediated suppression by one type will be stronger against its own type than against the other type. It is this stronger within-type suppression that could lead to oscillating relative abundances of the two types in Bangladesh. When immunity to el tor *V. cholerae* was low, the moderate improvements in the use of pure water that occurred during the mid-1970s may have favored el tor over classical *V. cholerae*, but as the immunity to the el tor type increased and the immunity to the classical type diminished, the lack of substantial improvement in water supply may have led to a resurgence of classical *V. cholerae*. Indeed, one characteristic of cholera epidemics in the past was a cyclic waning as recovery from disease increased the population's overall immunity, and then a waxing after susceptibles were added through new births and age-related declines in immunity (Pollitzer 1959).

When viewed from the perspective of the cultural vectors hypothesis, this cycling of classical *V. cholerae* helps explain another aspect of the el tor pandemic. Classical cholera pandemics typically wreaked havoc for a few years and then receded, but the most recent el tor pandemic has shown a greater tendency to persist in invaded areas (Glass et al. 1992). This difference can be explained by the classical type's reliance on waterborne transmission. When it invades a new area it spreads explosively, rapidly generating a large population of survivors, who are temporarily immune. Having exhausted the local supply of susceptibles, the pandemic recedes from the region. El tor *V. cholerae*, with its greater reliance on non-waterborne routes of transmission, should tend to have a less explosive spread that is less limited to populations with contaminated water. By the time the more slowly spreading el tor *V. cholerae* infects a substantial proportion of a population, the immunity of those infected at the outset may begin to diminish. This declining immunity along with introduction of susceptibles by birth and immigration, apparently allows the el tor type to persist in regions where the classical type could not.

These explanations yield predictions for the upcoming decades. If Bangladeshi water supplies are improved, the classical *V. cholerae* will either decline with progressively smaller future resurgences or will evolve to produce toxin at a lower, el tor-like rate. If water supplies deteriorate, *V. cholerae* will revert to more virulent states reminiscent of the past. If neither improvement nor deterioration occurs, severe and benign strains will cycle indefinitely into the future. Similarly, if a region has purer water than Bangladesh, it will experience less or no resurgence of the highly virulent *V. cholerae* of the classical type or of new mutant types. If a region has water supplies that are more contaminated than Bangladesh or comparably contaminated, then we can expect periodic resurgences of highly virulent *V. cholerae*. Just such an epidemic apparently began in India and Bangladesh during 1992 and 1993 (Albert et al. 1993, Ramamurthy et al. 1993). The agent is a third type of *V. cholerae*, which can produce more toxin than most of the *V. cholerae* that have been isolated in the past (W. B. Greenough III, personal communication). The theoretical framework developed above predicts that any lineages of this new type that enter and persist in regions with pure water will evolve lower levels of toxin production.

Similarly, if relatively mild *V. cholerae* spreads into new geographic areas with poor water supplies, its virulence should increase. The rapid population growth in Lima, Peru, during the last two decades dramatically outpaced the city's ability to deal with fecal contamination of the largely unchlorinated water supplies (Anderson 1991). When el tor *V. cholerae* arrived there near the beginning of 1991, apparently from the bilge water of a Chinese freighter, it was spread largely by water, causing about 300,000 cases of cholera in Peru (Epstein 1992, Glass et al. 1992). The overall death rate per case suggests that this invading *V. cholerae* was relatively mild. If the ideas about waterborne transmission mentioned above are correct, the extensive waterborne transmission during the first few months of the epidemic should have increased the virulence of the organisms. This idea has not been rigorously tested, but the available data are consistent with it. When the epidemic moved from the urban into the rural areas, nearly 5% of the cases resulted in death. In the coastal areas, where the epidemic began, the death rate was less than 1% (Epstein 1992). Measurement of toxin production of the *V. cholerae* isolated during the first six months of the Peruvian epidemic would help determine whether this difference in mortality resulted from increased virulence of the organism or poorer treatment in rural areas.

One could formulate posthoc explanations for the concordance of water purification and the historical changes in the prevalence of diarrheal pathogens by searching for cultural differences for each comparison. But I am aware of no general alternative explanation for these trends. Indeed, epidemiologists have repeatedly identified the large-scale replacement of classical *V. cholerae* by el tor *V. cholerae* as a fundamental unresolved problem (Glass et al. 1982, Monsur 1983, Samadi et al. 1983, Edelman & Pierce 1984).

The cultural vectors hypothesis also helps explain some apparent anomalies. As the more benign el tor biotype was beginning to increase in prevalence, Mackenzie (1965) observed that the increasing availability of pure water "has not diminished noticeably the incidence of sporadic cholera in endemic areas, though fulminating epidemics of cholera with high fatality rates are, generally speaking, less frequently encountered." He suggested that infections were more severe because waterborne transmission leads to high densities of ingested *V. cholerae*, but a given type of *V. cholerae* does not seem to be more lethal when it is acquired from water (Ewald 1991a). Mackenzie's observation may have resulted from an evolutionary change in the genetic makeup of *V. cholerae* populations. Such trends are just what is expected from the cultural vectors hypothesis: Reduction in the pervasiveness of waterborne transmission should have a stronger controlling effect on the most virulent strains, increasing the proportion of the less virulent strains.

The associations between waterborne transmission and severity of diarrheal diseases show how evolutionary principles may offer insight into the evolution of virulence. Because such comparisons are nonmanipulative, however, they do not control for potentially relevant correlates of waterborne transmission, such as general hygienic standards. The results therefore emphasize the need for two kinds of studies. The first involves comparative analyses of such correlates and pathogen prevalences for the three genera that include largely waterborne pathogens: *Vibrio*, *Shigella*, and *Salmonella*. The second kind of study involves monitoring of virulence genes in experimental areas scheduled for water purification and simultaneous monitoring in matched control areas, both before and after the purification.

THE ORIGIN OF CHOLERA

If the preceding framework for understanding the evolution of virulence is of general relevance, we should be able to explain why and when highly virulent diseases have evolved during human history. The rates of evolutionary change implied by this conclusion seem reasonable if one considers the rapid rates of evolution documented in response to some cultural characteristics; for example, during the first five months of an epidemic of *V. cholerae* in Tanzania, resistance of isolates to tetracycline changed from 0% to 76% (Mhalu et al. 1979). Such rapid evolution suggests that high levels of virulence may have evolved over time scales of weeks to decades after the presence of cultural conditions favoring increased virulence.

With regard to waterborne transmission one would expect, therefore, the evolution of increased virulence to date back to the earliest civilizations in which fecally contaminated water supplies became available to large populations of city dwellers. The Harappan civilization, which existed from 3000 to 1800 B.C. in Pakistan and India, is to my knowledge the earliest civilization in which extensive waterborne transmission could be expected.

Inhabitants of Harappan cities obtained water from public wells in streets or private wells within the densely packed houses. The rims of these open wells were typically within a few inches of the surface of the road or the floor of a house (Mackay 1931). Open wells of this type are notorious for spreading waterborne diseases when they lie within a network of leaky drainage lines, especially when flooding distributes surface contamination and allows backflow from drainage lines. The Harappan cities had a such a wastewater network surrounding these the open wells. The network consisted of brick-lined drain pipes that were typically a few inches to two feet below the surface of each street. Wastewater would pass into soak pits (approximately 100 cubic feet in volume) within which it would gradually seep into the ground. This drainage system formed a network enveloping the open wells, with drain openings often situated near well openings (Mackay 1931, Gokhale 1959).

The outside wall of houses had an opening or two through which wastewater flowed into either the road drainage system, a pit, or a large pot (Mackay 1931, Wheeler 1968). Wastewater from the pots would seep into the ground through holes in the bottom of the pot. Pots without holes apparently functioned to receive wastewater, and were carried into the street drainage system or allowed to overflow (Mackay 1931, Marshall 1931).

The water supplies in this system must have been extraordinarily prone to contamination, especially when flooding occurred. In fact, an early researcher (Mackay 1931) proposed that these drainage systems would not ordinarily be used for excrement because excrement would have clogged drains and contaminated the nearby wells. But several findings indicate that transport of excrement cannot be dismissed on these grounds: Excavations revealed latrines connected directly to the drainage system, wooden mesh screens along the drains for separating solid from liquid waste, and refuse heaps left in the streets by sanitary squads who periodically cleaned this drainage system through manholes in the streets (Marshall 1931, Wheeler 1966, 1968, Rao 1973).

After maintaining some of the finest cities in the world for centuries, the residents abandoned them at the beginning of the second millennium B.C. (Ghosh 1982). This deurbanization has attracted much attention from scholars over the past half-century. Hypotheses based on warfare, earthquakes, deforestation, climatic changes, and reduced trade have been advanced, but most can be dismissed on the basis of available evidence (Dales 1964, Ghosh 1982), and none is sufficient to explain the deurbanization of all the major cities within a century or so. Researchers have resorted to vague arguments about "fatigue of an overgrown culture" (Ghosh 1982). Perhaps the most widely held last resort involves some sort of ecological destruction. But this explanation is unsatisfying because one must propose that different cities hundreds of miles apart met their demise within a relatively short time span from different kinds of ecological disasters—for example, waterlogging in one area; desiccation in another; and deforestation, salinization, and erosion in still others (Ghosh 1982). The only firm conclusion that can be drawn from the literature is a general one: Some aspect or aspects of urban life became less attractive or more repulsive during the last few centuries of this civilization.

What could cause people who had so prized urban civilization to abandon it so pervasively? The concept of cultural vectors offers a new hypothesis that is not only consistent with the available information, but, I believe, more parsimonious than any previous explanation: The technological advancements of the Harappan culture favored the evolution of cholera or some similarly devastating waterborne disease.

Historically, when cholera has been transmitted by sewer-contaminated water, it has spread explosively and killed a large proportion of infected individuals within days of the first symptoms (Snow 1855/1966, Ewald 1991a). It wouldn't take a statistician to notice hundreds of city dwellers dying sudden deaths and the paucity of such mortality in rural areas. Given the hysteria that typically surrounds such epidemics and the tendencies to interpret pestilence as an omen or divine wrath, one could easily imagine wholesale emigration from a city, no matter how much a center of culture it was.

Once such a virulent pathogen evolved, the highest density of people infected with the pathogen should occur in the cities with the most extensive contamination of wells. The older, larger cities should meet this condition more frequently than the younger, smaller settlements; the older drains and wells would have been more prone to cross-connections, and larger cities would have been most able to maintain a steady rate of infections and deaths repelling potential inhabitants. The extensive flooding that occurred in some of the Harappan cities during the decades of deurbanization (Wheeler 1968) would have enhanced the chances of waterborne transmission and hence the maintenance of virulent pathogens.

Different cities probably would have had epidemics at different times, depending on the presence of virulent strains, movement between cities, and the connections between sewers and wells within cities; consequently, one city might deurbanize at one time, and another months, years or decades later. Those returning to the cities would still be confronting water supplies contaminated by sewage. One would therefore expect periodic outbreaks of waterborne disease, repelling people who could make a decent living elsewhere, leaving the city to squatters. The makeshift construction during the deurbanization supports this scenario.

The disintegration of commercial trade during this period is also consistent with the cultural vectors hypothesis. Commercial trade might suffer indirectly if the infrastructure necessary for long-distance trade could not be maintained when the Harappan urban centers were being abandoned. Or trade might suffer if, for example, the Mesopotamians avoided trading with a people known to be afflicted with a terrible plague, especially if the plague had a record of jumping from one city to another.

Independently from this prediction, a leading expert on diarrheal diseases in general and *V. cholerae* in particular, W. B. Greenough, III, concluded that an illness indistinguishable from cholera can be traced back to the second or third millennium B.C. from Sanskrit Vedic literature (W. B. Greenough, III, personal communication). If cholera was not present during this time period, some other severe diarrheal disease was, and severe diarrheal diseases of humans are typically waterborne (Table 5.1).

This circumstantial evidence raises the possibility that the disintegration of one of the first great civilizations on earth may have been the first example of how a culture's technological innovation sets in motion its own downfall, in this case by creating the cultural vector that favored the evolution of cholera or a disease like cholera. Other authors have suggested that infectious diseases may have contributed to the decline of the Harappan civilization (Dyson 1982, Kennedy 1982), but unlike the cultural vectors hypothesis, none of these suggestions explains how the named diseases (e.g, malaria) would be specifically linked to urban Harappan culture.

One might ask why cities of other early civilizations did not suffer the same fate. I expect that complete answers to this question probably would require many years of concerted effort by social scientists, archaeologists, historians, and biologists. The answers might or might not implicate evolutionary increases in virulence as factors contributing to the deterioration of other civilizations. It is noteworthy, however, that at least some other ancient civilizations did not have the same characteristics favoring waterborne transmission. Drains were rarely used in Egypt and were much less extensive in Mesopotamia (Mackay 1931). The Roman water system should have remained relatively uncontaminated by the high population density that it served because the water supplies were transported from relatively unpopulated elevated areas by aqueducts, and fecally contaminated wastewater was efficiently removed from areas of high density by their sewer systems.

The cultural vectors hypothesis also adds another dimension to the arguments about the history of cholera. For many decades experts have believed that cholera dates back thousands of years (Pollitzer 1959, De 1961). More recently, some scientists have proposed that cholera first arose less than two hundred years ago (Howard-Jones 1972, McNicol & Doetsch 1983). Advocates of a recent origin have emphasized that *V. cholerae* is a diverse species. Many *V. cholerae* survive and reproduce freely in marine environments with little evidence of continuous transmission between people (McNicol & Doetsch 1983). None of the existing evidence, however, is inconsistent with an ancient association between cholera-producing strains of *V. cholerae* and humans. The presence of free-living *V. cholerae* is no more compelling evidence against a significant evolutionary effect of humans on cholera-causing vibrios than is the presence of wolves evidence against a significant evolutionary effect of humans on dogs. The key issue is whether the difference between dogs and wolves is an evolutionary effect of associations with people.

One critical difference between free-living *V. cholerae* and cholera-causing strains involves toxin production. Strains isolated from water samples generally produce little if any cholera toxin unless they are in areas where there is substantial contamination from human infections (Minami et al. 1991)—and it is the cholera toxin that is central to any argument about increases in virulence as *V. cholerae* adapts to humans. The types that produce no toxin typically lack the toxin gene altogether (Miller & Mekalanos 1984, Minami et al. 1991). When the free-living types of *V. cholerae* enter the intestinal tract, they typically produce a mild illness if they cause any illness at all (Minami et al. 1991). Accordingly, fluctuations in the abundance of these free-living types are not associated with the extent of cholera in the local population, and the cholera-causing types tend to be isolated from water only when there are cholera cases close by (Khan et al. 1984b, Nair et al. 1988).

McNicol and Doetsch (1983) suggest a recent origin of cholera based on the absence of cholera in Europe prior to the early eighteenth century in spite of prior contact from medieval crusades, trade caravans, or boat routes. The cultural vectors hypothesis, however, explains how cholera could remain limited to south Asia even under these conditions: Highly virulent *V. cholerae* can be maintained only if the waterborne cultural vector is present in a fairly large population. On overland trade routes or among small crews on long voyages, this kind of transmission is unlikely; the populations of highly virulent *V. cholerae* in such groups would die out much as other virulent pathogens die out in small isolated populations. Other diseases could be transmitted in such settings because their characteristics differed; smallpox, for example, can survive in the external environments for many years (Wolff & Croon 1968). The classical biotype of *V. cholerae*, however, generally dies out in water within days to a few weeks, and rarely is shed in feces for longer than a week (Pollitzer 1959, Khan et al. 1984b).

McNicol and Doetsch (1983) suggest that *V. cholerae* acquired the capability to cause cholera suddenly about 200 years ago, whereas I argue above that the conditions favoring the enhanced production of toxin were probably present in south Asia four thousand years ago, and led to the evolution of an illness that is indistinguishable from cholera. Whether it was the same organism is perhaps not the most important issue. Insight into this question may come when the rate of *V. cholerae*'s biochemical clocks are used to estimate the growth rates of *V. cholerae*'s evolutionary tree, as has been done for the immunodeficiency viruses (Eigen & Nieselt-Streue 1990). The more compelling questions are, Why did this kind of virulent organism evolve, and what are the conditions under which its virulence could be favored or disfavored in the future?

The cultural vectors hypothesis argues that the various levels of toxin production represent adaptations to opportunities for waterborne or nonwaterborne transmission. This argument is quite different from recent interpretations generated by the widespread presence of free-living *V. cholerae* in aquatic environments. The similarity of some *V. cholerae* isolated from coastal waters with some isolated from human infections led some researchers to propose that *V. cholerae* may be best characterized as an incidental pathogen, its real niche being that of a free-living organism (Colwell et al. 1981, Hood et al. 1981, Miller et al. 1985). Occurring only incidentally in humans, it could therefore be considered poorly adapted to humans.

The lack of any known function of cholera toxin in the natural environment (Finkelstein 1973, Mekalanos et al. 1982) and the greater toxin production of strains isolated from people and from environments contaminated with human feces argue against this hypothesis. So does the biochemical variation across 260 strains of *V. cholerae* isolated from a wide range of sources (Salles & Momen 1991). The el tor and classical strains, which are responsible for human cholera, form one branch of the *V. cholerae* tree; the strains that are not commonly associated with human disease form the rest of the evolutionary tree (Salles & Momen 1991). The United States el tor strains, which provided most of the ammunition for the incidental pathogen hypothesis, collectively formed a single small branch off the main el tor branch (Salles & Momen 1991). The toxin-producing United States strains are all closely related and are distinct from most of the United States strains that do not produce toxin (Chen et al. 1991). In fact, it may be more appropriate to treat them as a group that is distinct from el tor *V. cholerae* (Salles & Momen 1991). If *V. cholerae* were a free-living organism producing toxin for some nonparasitic purpose, this branch of the evolutionary tree probably would not have been so clearly demarcated and the toxin-producing, cholera-causing *V. cholerae* would not be so distinctly separated from the other *V. cholerae*.

The following explanation seems more consistent with the available evidence. The toxin-producing strains found in the United States comprise a clone (*sensu* Chen et al. 1991) that by chance was stranded in the United States from an eastern endemic area. It has been barely able to sustain itself through its moderately successful survival in aquatic environments supplemented by occasional amplification in people. If this explanation is correct, the marginal existence of these pathogens in United States waters probably is not a very useful model for understanding maintenance of toxin-producing *V. cholerae* in endemic regions like India and Bangladesh. In these endemic areas the persistence of cholera is probably more dependent on continuing, though often restricted, transmission between people (Gangarosa & Mosley 1974). In the endemic regions where waterborne transmission is feasible, the *V. cholerae* that produce large amounts of toxin are maintained because of their greater potential for invading and multiplying in humans. In areas where waterborne transmission is less feasible, lower levels of toxin production are favored. In both of these pathogenic niches some pathogens that produce little if any toxin may be maintained because they have an advantage after an infection is established (see Chapter 2). But in either case the life cycles are largely separate from the life cycles of the genetically distinct, free-living *V. cholerae* that rarely have genes for toxin production (Nair et al. 1988, Pal et al. 1992). The former strains fill a pathogenic niche that often involves temporary survival during transmission, whereas the latter more heterogeneous strains live a primarily nonpathogenic aquatic existence, interrupted by accidental entrance into the human gastrointestinal tract.

WATERBORNE TRANSMISSION, RESEARCH, AND PUBLIC HEALTH POLICY

Resolution of contradictions: evidence and interpretations

The cultural vectors hypothesis helps resolve apparent contradictions in cross-specific studies and clarifies the degree of resolution needed in epidemiological studies. Current studies typically look for an association between risk factors and diarrheal disease, paying little if any attention to which diarrheal pathogens should show such an association. Not surprisingly, studies yield results that seem to contradict one another. Much of this ambiguity seems related to the kinds of pathogens under investigation. In a recent issue of the *Journal of Diarrheal Diseases Research*, for example, a study from southeastern China found an association between use of impure water and diarrhea, but a study from across the border in Myanmar (Burma) did not (Han et al. 1991, Kangchuan et al. 1991). The pathogens found in the Chinese study included *Shigella*, which, as Table 5.1 shows, is often waterborne, especially in China where *S. dysenteriae* 1 and *S. flexneri* are prevalent (Aoki 1968). The isolates from Myanmar included *E. coli* and nontyphoid Salmonella, but did not include any of the pathogens shown by Table 5.1 to be regularly waterborne (Kangchuan et al. 1991, Oo et al. 1991). By being cognizant of the relationship between waterborne transmission and virulence, researchers could be more efficient at searching for and identifying risk factors in particular geographic areas at various times. The ultimate result may be a bigger dent in the millions of diarrheal deaths that occur each year, as intervention programs are tailored to the local composition of pathogens.

During the latter half of the twentieth century, programs for controlling *V. cholerae* have been a source of controversy. One of the major disagreements concerns whether cholera is primarily a waterborne disease. On the basis of the long history of research, the widely accepted view during the 1960s and early 1970s was that cholera was almost exclusively waterborne (Mosley 1970, Gangarosa & Mosley 1974). This view was challenged by Feachem (1981, 1982), who pointed out that possibilities of non-waterborne transmission had been glossed over in many studies. But most of Feachem's analysis used data from the el tor biotype to reject generalizations that were based largely on the classical type. For example, Mosley and Khan (1979) stated that "the ease with which the disease has been eliminated worldwide simply through the provision of pure water supplies" is evidence that *V. cholerae* is a waterborne pathogen. Feachem questioned this contention, citing outbreaks of el tor *V. cholerae*. The cultural vectors hypothesis shows how both of these seemingly contradictory statements can be correct. Mosley and Khan's contention is consistent with the data if one restricts the statement to classical *V. cholerae*. Feachem's concern is well-taken but does not acknowledge the ease with which classical cholera has been eliminated through the provisioning of pure water supplies.

In addition to being a source of controversies, *V. cholerae* has been a source of confusion because it was sometimes the agent of epidemics that were inconsistent with traditional descriptions of cholera epidemics; for example, Gunn et al. (1981) stated, "The reason for the mild disease pattern observed in Bahrain and Saudi Arabia is unknown." According to the cultural vectors hypothesis, waterborne transmission should not occur in such geographic areas. Indeed, on the basis of their epidemiological investigation, they concluded that transmission did not occur through contamination of public drinking water.

The cultural vectors hypothesis therefore clarifies the epidemiology of cholera epidemiology by emphasizing that variation in virulence can be explained by variation in waterborne transmission. The traditional characterization of cholera as an extremely severe waterborne pathogen was largely accurate for the classical type, but not for the el tor type. As water supplies improved, the replacement of the classical type with the el tor type led to discrepancies between the traditional understanding of *V. cholerae* and the incoming data. The confusion and controversy over severity and transmission are thus attributed to the changing selective pressures resulting from purification of water supplies.

Alternative policies

The resolution of these issues adds another variable to evaluations of intervention strategies. Evaluation of alternative interventions currently focuses on frequencies of infection and disease without consideration of evolutionary effects. de Zoysa and Feachem (1985), for example, evaluated the cost effectiveness of immunization programs against diarrheal diseases caused by *V. cholerae* and rotavirus. They estimated that *V. cholerae* accounts for 0.4% of all diarrhea and 8% of all deaths in Bangladeshi children less than 5 years old, and that cholera immunization might reduce these rates by about one-fifth. They calculate that immunization at age 2 would cost about $500 (1993 U.S.) annually for each case of diarrhea averted and $10,000 for each death averted. These costs compared favorably with the costs of water purification, which tends to have a relatively small effect on the *frequency* of *V. cholerae* infections. But these estimates need to incorporate the numbers of diarrheal cases and deaths averted through the evolutionary changes in the virulence of *V. cholerae* that should result from water purification. If safe water were provided for the entire population in Bangladesh, strains with a virulence comparable to classical *V. cholerae* should die out. Since 1980, about one-quarter of the *V. cholerae* infections in Bangladesh have been caused by the classical type. The mortality per infection is about ten times greater for infections with the classical type than for infections with the el tor type. The introduction of clean water for all of Bangladesh should therefore cut the deaths due to cholera by more than half, a drop that is about twice as great as that expected from an intensive vaccination program. The annual cost per individual served by the purified water would be about $25 in rural areas and about $75 (including sewage disposal) in urban areas (Esrey et al. 1985, Feachem 1986).

The nonevolutionary analyses suggest that joint water supply and sanitation improvements reduce disease and death from all diarrheal pathogens by nearly one-third (Esrey et al. 1985). A much greater effect is attributed to sanitation improvements than to water supply (Feachem 1986, Esrey et al. 1991), but the estimates do not include any evolutionarily effects of water supply on virulence. How big might these effects be? When water supplies have been purified regionally, the most virulent killers—classical *V. cholerae*, *Salmonella typhi* and *Shigella dysenteriae* type 1—have virtually vanished. In Bangladesh, these three pathogens are responsible for about half of the mortality attributable to diarrheal diseases. Considering that the average virulence of the next most waterborne pathogens (el tor *V. cholerae* and *S. flexneri*) should also be reduced by water purification, we can expect that regional termination of waterborne transmission will reduce diarrheal deaths by at least 50%.

If true, the net cost would be about one-tenth the cost per life saved by vaccination (based on estimates of de Zoysa & Feachem 1985). The evolutionary attack would have some additional benefits that might be as important as the immediate reduction in cost per life saved from cholera. The benign infections will, to some extent, naturally immunize the children against any remaining virulent strains at a cost of $0.00 per "immunization." The shift from use of standing water reservoirs to underground or piped water should also reduce nondiarrheal diseases. Arthropodborne disease may be reduced by eliminating breeding grounds of mosquitoes. Wormy parasites may cause less damage because some are transmitted by water and others can be thwarted by frequent washing (Esrey et al. 1991).

The evolutionary approach also provides an important international benefit because vaccination of travelers is not cost effective. To save one life using routine cholera vaccination for North American travelers, the price would be about $20 million and 100 vaccine-associated adverse side-effects (MacPherson & Tonkin 1992). If *V. cholerae* and other diarrheal pathogens are forced to evolve to benignness, international travellers are protected from severe disease as are those whom they contact after leaving the areas where *V. cholerae* is present. In addition to all of these life-saving benefits are the aesthetic benefits of clean water.

Many variables could alter the rough estimates presented above. For example, the el tor strains in Bangladesh appear to be more virulent than el tor strains from other places (Khan & Shahidullah 1980), as one would expect from evolutionary principles; they too should evolve toward benignness as water supplies are purified, increasing the cost effectiveness of improved water supplies.

Oral rehydration therapy is considered the "flagship" of efforts to combat diarrheal diseases (see Feachem 1986). It is certainly one of the most cost-effective achievements of medical science. When given promptly and persistently, it can simply and inexpensively eliminate virtually all deaths from diarrheal organisms that kill through dehydration. Although oral rehydration therapy has been a major success story, it has some important limitations: Its effectiveness may be lessened in rural areas because it depends on ready access and perseverance by care-givers, and although it saves lives, it still leaves the patient vulnerable to tissue damage (Hirschhorn & Greenough 1991). It provides a great reduction in death from *Vibrio cholerae* (Varavithya et al. 1991), but because the most damaging effects of *Shigella* and *Salmonella* result from their invasion of the intestinal lining rather than dehydration, rehydration therapy has a relatively smaller effect on the mortality they cause. Purification of water complements rehydration therapy by simultaneously reducing the virulence of these three genera, which are most responsible for lethal diarrheal disease (see Table 5.1). Water purification may also increase the overall value of rehydration therapy in a more direct way. Oral rehydration solution can foster the growth of bacterial pathogens that are introduced when contaminated water is used during its preparation (Black et al. 1981).

Evolutionary assessments of alternative interventions are complicated because virtually any intervention may have some evolutionary effects on virulence. Vaccines that incorporate cholera toxin may cause the cholera organisms to evolve toward benignness (see Chapter 11). Traditional oral rehydration therapy might favor evolution toward increased virulence by allowing people infected with highly virulent strains to increase the contribution of these organisms into the environment. If, for example, a person dies of dehydration, the shedding of *V. cholerae* in stools will obviously be shortened (see Chapter 2). Among survivors, traditional oral rehydration therapy does not reduce the number of stools or duration of diarrhea, but the newer rice-based preparations do, apparently by reducing the efflux of fluids into the intestine (Rahman et al. 1991, Gore et al. 1992, Molla & Bari 1992). The newer rice-based preparations therefore may yield an unrecognized evolutionary benefit relative to the older preparations.

Long-term assessments also need to focus on the geographic and social contexts of disease. With limited funding, vaccination programs may be unable to reach rural inhabitants, who also may have less access to prompt treatment during the period between infection and death. Once in place, water supply programs protect without such a vulnerable period. Rural people may therefore be especially well protected by water supply. By altering assessments of the relative cost-effectiveness of the alternative investments, evolutionary considerations should eventually provide a more comprehensive understanding of which interventions should be used when and where.

CHAPTER 6

Attendant-Borne Transmission (Or How Are Doctors and Nurses like Mosquitoes, Machetes, and Moving Water?)

ATTENDANTS AS CULTURAL VECTORS

In hospitals and other institutions where some individuals physically attend to others in need of care, another kind of cultural vector occurs. While tending to patients, attendants may inadvertently carry pathogens from patient to patient without becoming infected themselves. They may do this by direct contact or indirectly through their use of hospital equipment. As with transmission by water and mosquitoes, attendant-borne transmission should favor the more rapidly replicating and hence more virulent pathogens.

Consider diarrheal diseases in hospital nurseries. From the pathogen's point of view, a neonate is very different from a nurse. Neonates are highly susceptible to infection because they lack the acquired immunity of adults, the protective bacteria inhabiting the gut and skin, and strongly acidic stomach contents, which can kill many pathogens before they can enter the intestine (Belnap & O'Donnell 1955, Sprunt & Redman 1968, Marcy 1976).

Although healthy attendants are relatively resistant to infection, hospital strains of diarrheal pathogens not only are present on the hands of attendants but persist and sometimes multiply there, even after extensive washing with disinfectants (Jameson et al. 1954, Boyer et al. 1975, Knittle et al. 1975, Bentley 1990). Strains cultured from babies are also cultured regularly from hands of attendants, which are frequently implicated as the immediate source of hospital acquired infections; the same strains generally are not isolated from the gastrointestinal tract of the attendants (Stevenson 1952, Wheeler & Wainerman 1954, Love et al. 1972, Boyer et al. 1975, Knittle et al. 1975, Marcy 1976). But even if attendants do occasionally become immobilized by illness, their duties are taken over by another attendant, and, hence, attendant-borne transmission continues.

Extensive pathogen reproduction in nursery ward neonates should provide the pathogen with high fitness benefits. Nurses typically touch babies 20 to 25 times per day (Love et al. 1963)—ample contact for attendant-borne transmission. Diarrhea may facilitate this transmission because attendants can avoid solid stools more easily than the diffuse fecal film that results from diarrhea. Contaminated hands inadvertently contact objects which can recontaminate hands after handwashing. Compounding these problems is the tendency to attend severely infected babies particularly frequently (Raju & Kobler 1991). Barring an increased effort at maintaining hygienic standards, this increased contact should yield increased dermal colonization of attendants (e.g., Love et al. 1963). Unlike their patients, attendants may avoid becoming intestinally infected by careful handwashing before engaging in activities like eating. In accordance with these considerations, epidemiological studies implicate contaminated hands of attendants as a major source of hospital-acquired diarrheal pathogens even though the attendants themselves tend not to suffer from infection (Mortimer et al. 1962, Love et al. 1963, Boyer et al. 1975, Thompson et al. 1982, Larson 1988, Bentley 1990).

The window of time available for attendant-borne transmission should also contribute to the virulence of hospital-acquired infections. When a mother takes her baby home from the hospital, the pool of susceptible hosts is greatly reduced. Like hospital attendants, the few adults and children that will contact the baby are relatively resistant to infection. But unlike hospital attendants, these household members have little potential for transporting pathogens from an immobilized infected individual to susceptibles. Hospital-acquired pathogens that have prolonged infectiousness by virtue of being benign should therefore gain few long-term transmission benefits. To the contrary, severe disease should tend to prolong the window of time available for hospital transmission because doctors tend not to release severely ill infants from hospital care (Hemming et al. 1976). Thus, as with mosquito-borne pathogens, severe symptoms may facilitate rather than inhibit attendant-borne transmission when hygienic standards are lax; sick babies will tend to release greater densities of pathogens, produce more diffuse and hence transmissible fecal material, be attended more closely in hospitals, and be kept longer in hospitals among larger numbers of susceptibles than well babies. Beyond yielding a great potential for transmission, the extensive reproduction and resultant severity of symptoms should impose relatively low fitness costs on the attendant-borne pathogen. A newborn baby would not be walking around to the beds of other newborns, even if it had a mild infection.

If attendant-borne transmission in institutions favors evolutionary increases in virulence, evidence of such evolution should be present in the medical literature. Specifically, strains of attendant-borne organisms in hospitals should tend to be more virulent than strains transmitted by direct contact outside of institutions; and, as the extent of continuous institutional transmission increases, so should virulence.

These predictions presume that pathogens can evolve on time scales of months to years in hospital environments. Evolutionary responses to antibiotics in neonatal nurseries lend credence to the possibility; a three-week preventative treatment of newborns with penicillin, for instance, rapidly increased the frequency of penicillin-resistant *Staphylococcus aureus* from a minority to 100% (Gezon et al. 1973).

ATTENDANT-BORNE BACTERIA IN HOSPITALS

Neonatal diarrhea due to *Escherichia coli*

Escherichia coli provide a data base suitable for evaluating these predictions. This bacterium usually has little if any negative effect on its human hosts, but some strains may immobilize or kill a substantial proportion of infected people.

In accordance with the preceding arguments about the fitness benefits associated with virulence, sick individuals typically excrete virtually pure cultures of the bacterium (Rogers 1951, Jameson et al. 1954, Thomson 1955, Belnap & O'Donnell 1955, Stulberg & Zeulzer 1956), especially severely ill patients (Shanks & Studzinski 1952, Hinton et al. 1953). Asymptomatically infected individuals generally release much lower densities of organisms and have not been identified as the source of nursery outbreaks (Shanks & Studzinski 1952, Marcy 1976). Most contacted objects in rooms housing infants with frank cases of *E. coli* diarrhea can become heavily contaminated within a day (Rogers 1951).

In accordance with the cultural vector hypothesis, virulent outbreaks typically occurred in hospitals and similar institutions. When large-scale community-wide epidemics occurred, transmission in hospitals often was strongly implicated. During an epidemic that progressed up the East Coast of the United States from October 1953 through February 1954, for example, "explosive outbreaks were limited to institutions, hospital wards, and newborn nurseries" (Belnap & O'Donnell 1955). Similarly, during the winter of 1961 an outbreak occurred in Chicago and adjacent communities in Indiana. About one of every 20 infants in these communities was affected, and nearly half of the affected infants had direct or indirect contact with one of the 29 involved hospitals just prior to their illnesses (Marcy 1976).   Direct transmission between hospitals has been incriminated (Rogers & Koegler 1951), but outbreaks are often introduced into hospitals from the outside community (Marcy 1976).

Are strains that have cycled in hospitals more virulent those that cycle in the outside community? Neonatal infections do tend to be less severe when they are derived from mothers who have been infected outside of the hospital. Nearly all of the maternally derived neonatal infections in a Cincinnati hospital, for example, were asymptomatic (Cooper et al. 1959). Three years earlier, in an outbreak in the same hospital, 32 of 33 hospital-acquired infections of infants were symptomatic and 3 were fatal (Cooper et al. 1955). Unfortunately, the presented data were insufficient to assess whether other factors, such as bottle-feeding, might have contributed to this difference.

Further evidence of high inherent virulence of hospital strains of E. coli comes from experimental studies, which showed that such strains can cause moderate to severe diarrheal disease in adults, although high dosages were required (Kirby et al. 1950, Neter et al. 1953, Ferguson 1956, Marcy 1976).

If attendant-borne transmission increases virulence, the severity of infections should increase as the extent of institutional transmission increases. I evaluated this prediction using nursery outbreaks of E. coli recorded since researchers began recognizing it as a hospital-acquired pathogen around 1940 (Ewald 1988, 1991b). The test confirmed the predicted association.   When nursery outbreaks of pathogenic E. coli were terminated within a week or so, few infected babies died. But when they continued for weeks or months, about one of every ten infected babies died (Ewald 1988). A summary of reported nursery outbreaks of diarrhea in upstate New York from 1946 to 1955 confirms a similar trend in a more restricted area. Mortality rates increased as the time between the onset of the first case in an outbreak and the reporting of the outbreak to the state health department increased (Harris et al. 1956, Ewald 1988).

At first glance one might speculate that the association between lethality and duration of outbreak was a nonevolutionary consequence of poor hygiene. Hospitals that put less effort into curbing outbreaks might put less effort into hygiene and, therefore, might have more severe infections because each patient tends to be infected with a larger number of pathogens.   The details of the outbreaks, however, are inconsistent with this interpretation. To terminate the outbreaks, hospital staff typically made intense, prolonged attempts to break the cycle of transmission by environmental decontamination. Certainly during these efforts the numbers of pathogens ingested must have been drastically reduced. Yet, severe infections persisted. Severe outbreaks were often eventually terminated only when the affected wards were closed and thereafter subjected to a comprehensive dousing with disinfectants (e.g., Jameson et al. 1954).

These considerations suggest that increased dosage is a weak explanation of the association between duration of hospital outbreaks and lethality. Nor can the association be explained by differences in the use of antibiotics (Ewald 1988).

The observed variation in virulence and the decline in the frequency of virulent outbreaks since the middle of this century has been a source of much confusion among epidemiologists (Hinden 1948, Taylor 1966, South 1971, Marcy 1976, Moon et al. 1980). Before *E. coli* was identified as the major etiologic agent, neonatal diarrhea was responsible for a staggering death rate. In New York City during the mid-1930s, for example, about one out of every 14 babies born in 15 surveyed hospitals died of diarrhea (Frant & Abramson 1938).

Such virulent outbreaks of *E. coli* are rare today. The cultural vectors hypothesis offers an explanation. By the mid-1950s there existed widespread recognition among public health workers that *E. coli* was a major cause of hospital outbreaks of neonatal diarrhea and that such outbreaks could be controlled by isolation procedures and antibiotics. Prolonged attendant-borne outbreaks therefore became rarer, although they were still severe when they did occur (e.g., Jacobs et al. 1970, Boyer et al. 1975). If prolonged attendant-borne transmission favors evolutionary increases in virulence, then a rarity of such transmission should translate into a rarity of virulent hospital strains of *E. coli*.

Strep, staph, and other bacteria

These arguments about attendant-borne transmission also apply to gastrointestinal pathogens other than *E. coli*. Prolonged outbreaks of nontyphoid *Salmonella*, for example, sometimes occur in hospitals. When acquired outside of hospitals, nontyphoid *Salmonella* are rarely lethal (Ewald 1991a), but hospital outbreaks are often severe; for instance, attendant-borne cycling of nontyphoid *Salmonella* was implicated in two outbreaks in Australian hospitals during 1946 and 1947. The outbreaks lasted about eight months. One death occurred for every seven infections in one of the outbreaks and for every three infections in the other (Mushin 1948, Rubbo 1948, Mackerras & Mackerras 1949). In contrast, hospital outbreaks with little or no attendant-borne transmission generally caused little or no mortality, even when antibiotics were ineffective (e.g., Kohler 1964).

Attendant-borne transmission also may influence pathogens infecting areas other than the gastrointestinal tract. Like *E. coli*, *Staphylococcus aureus* is primarily attendant-borne in nurseries (Wolinsky et al. 1960, Mortimer et al. 1962, Crossley et al. 1979, Thompson et al. 1982). *Staphylococcus aureus* colonizes about 20% of infants during their first year of life (Shinefield 1976), up to 40% of the people in the community at large and up to 70% of all people in hospitals (Gezon et al. 1973, Smith 1979, Norden & Ruben 1981). Although strains acquired within the community rarely cause severe infections in infants or mothers, hospital strains regularly cause severe infections: weeping pus-filled skin lesions (e.g., impetigo), breast infections in mothers, and sometimes the lethal scalded skin syndrome (Melish & Glasgow 1970, Shinefield 1976, Florman & Holzman 1980, Norden & Ruben 1981).

The destructive capacity of hospital strains is illustrated by an outbreak that was leapfrogging between hospitals in the Australian state of Victoria around 1980 (Pavillard et al. 1982). In the Royal Melbourne Hospital alone, antibiotic-resistant *Staph. aureus* infected over 500 patients. Approximately half of these infections had distinct symptoms, and about one-third of these patients died. About 1000 deaths may have occurred among all of the hospitals. The precise number is difficult to assess because many of the hospitals in the region were unwilling or unable to report their cases (Pavillard et al. 1982). Symptomatic infection was found not only among patients, but also among attendants, some of whom had severe disease. The outbreak was finally controlled by use of the only available antibiotic that was still effective: vancomycin.

As was the case with *E. coli*, relatively high virulence continued even after dramatic improvements in hygiene were enacted. In a severe outbreak in Malmö, Sweden, for example, extensive interventions were instituted to reduce the density of *Staphylococcus* in the hospital, yet the frequencies of symptomatic infection persisted for two years, even among personnel (Juhlin & Ericson 1965). When stringent guidelines for handwashing and glove use were followed, the frequency of infections begin to decline. Yet even at this point, those harboring the staph commonly showed symptoms of disease. The severity of hospital-acquired staph infections, therefore, does not appear to be simply a consequence of large infecting doses.

Infections that result from direct introduction of bacteria into the bloodstream also tend to be particularly severe in hospitals. Endocarditis is an inflammation of the heart lining, which occurs when injections or surgical procedures contaminate the bloodstream with bacteria such as *Staph. aureus*. Staphylococcal endocarditis in heroin addicts generally kills less than one-third of afflicted patients, whereas hospital-acquired endocarditis typically kills more than half (Norden & Ruben 1981). I am not arguing here that endocarditis is somehow beneficial to the staphylococcal organisms or that this difference in lethality proves that hospital strains are more virulent. Rather I am suggesting that the severity of endocardial infections is an indicator of how virulent a given strain of *Staphylococcus* is, and, by this indicator, hospital strains seem to be particularly virulent.

Additional studies of the genetic differences between hospital-acquired strains and community strains will be needed to clarify this matter. Some information along these lines however, is already available. One of the most severe manifestations of hospital-acquired staphylococcal infections is scalded skin syndrome, an often lethal disease that has been acquired in hospitals since the nineteenth century (Florman & Holzman 1980). The skin of afflicted babies flakes off as if the baby had been severely scalded; about one in five babies die.

Presumably the flakes of skin, like diarrhea, facilitate contamination of attendants and eventually infection of susceptible babies. The flaking is caused by a toxin, which is traceable to a gene in the bacterium (Rogolsky et al. 1974). The data from scalded skin syndrome therefore indicate that the virulence of at least some hospital-acquired infections is partly a consequence of virulent pathogen genotypes in the hospital environment.

During the 1970s, *Streptococcus agalactiae* (also called group B streptococci) became the leading cause of two often lethal infections of newborns: bacterial infections of the bloodstream (bacteremia) and inflammation of the spinal cord or brain membranes (meningitis) (Baker 1979). These bacteria asymptomatically infect from about 2% to 50% of the general adult population (Baker 1977, Concia et al. 1985). Hospital-acquired infections are especially prevalent in wards with large numbers of neonates where transmission occurs via nursery personnel (Aber et al. 1976, Green et al. 1978, Baker 1979, Concia et al. 1985). Those *Strep. agalactiae* categorized as type III are especially dangerous, and are disproportionately acquired from hospital sources in the United States (Baker 1979). In contrast, transmission from mother to infant occurs frequently but is rarely life-threatening (Baker 1979); only about one of every hundred infants colonized at birth will develop symptomatic infection (Manos 1982).

Because few otherwise healthy people harboring *Strep. agalactiae* develop disease, any tendencies for hospital-acquired organisms to be more virulent would be easy to overlook. In a study of neonatal infection in a Florida hospital, for example, none of about 45 babies colonized from their mothers showed any evidence of disease, whereas one case of severe disease occurred among about 30 babies who acquired their bacteria from the hospital. Although this difference is what one would expect from the overall trends, the small sample size obviously prohibits staff and researchers alike from drawing any conclusions about its significance.

In an Israeli hospital, transmission of *Strep. agalactiae* from colonized mothers to babies was similar to that found among U.S. hospitals, but the frequencies of infection consistent with attendant-borne transmission were substantially lower (Weintraub et al. 1983). In accordance with the evolutionary arguments raised above, the lethality per colonized infant was also lower. Only one case of severe infection occurred out of approximately 1000 colonized infants; in U.S. hospitals the corresponding figures were ten times greater (Manos 1982, Weintraub et al. 1983). Similar low levels of attendant-borne *Strep. agalactiae* and disease occur in Denmark (Carstensen et al. 1985). These differences are informative because they suggest the degree to which death might be lowered if attendant-borne transmission were blocked: one-half to one-tenth.

Patterns of lethality in adults are also consistent with a tendency for hospital-acquired *Strep. agalactiae* strains to be especially virulent. In a Hawaiian hospital, the probability of death among adults with *Strep. agalactiae* disease was 50% higher if the first isolation of this organism occurred later during the hospital stay as opposed to during the first two days in the hospital (Schwartz et al. 1991). The trend is consistent with the cultural vectors hypothesis because these late-isolated streptococci should tend to be hospital-acquired more frequently than the early isolated organisms.   Similar trends have been documented in other hospitals (Gallagher & Watanakunakorn 1985, Verghese et al. 1986).

One indicator of the severity of infection is whether the infecting organism has invaded the bloodstream.   Once this invasion has occurred, death commonly occurs in one-third to one-half of patients.   In spite of the far greater numbers of people outside of hospitals, patients whose bloodstream has been invaded, typically acquired their infections while in the hospital or similar institutional environment.   For a pneumonia-causing bacterium called *Klebsiella*, for example, from about 50% to 98% of bloodstream infections were acquired in the hospital, generally through the respiratory tract or urinary tract; and the mortality associated with hospital-acquired infections was twice that associated with community-acquired infections (Watanakunakorn & Jura 1991).   Other bacteria, such as *Serratia* and *Enterobacter*, similarly cause severe bloodstream infections in hospitals, but rarely cause severe disease outside of hospitals (Watanakunakorn & Jura 1991).

The differences in severity between hospital- and community-acquired infections are generally attributed to the compromised states of health and a greater exposure to invasive procedures among hospitalized patients.   These factors undoubtedly contribute to the differences, but researchers have not adequately investigated whether greater pathogen virulence contributes to the differences, presumably because they have not considered the evolutionary consequences of attendant-borne transmission.

The preceding analysis lends credence to the idea that attendant-borne transmission causes evolutionary increases in virulence, but it does not settle the matter.   Rather, it sets the stage for intervention studies in which experimental hospitals follow stringent measures to break the cycle of attendant-borne transmission.   Over a period of weeks to years, the frequencies of pathogenic strains and their effects can then be monitored.   Reduced attendant-borne transmission should reduce the frequency of virulence genes, the level of disease associated with infection, and, if infections are often lethal, mortality.   Long-term studies have been conducted to assess the effects of handwashing on the prevalence of particular hospital-acquired pathogens (e.g., Thompson et al. 1982). Expanding the scope of such studies to quantify the prevalence of virulence genes (e.g., using DNA hybridization techniques; Rademaker et al. 1992) could clarify the evolutionary effects of attendant-borne transmission. Frequencies of virulence genes should fall in such hospitals but not in control hospitals where the stringent measures have not been enacted.   It is important to realize that the virulence should fall in response to blocking of attendant-borne transmission, but the prevalence of a particular kind of organism may decline little if at all, because the reduced attendant-borne transmission of virulent organisms may be compensated for by increased transmission of benign organisms from other individuals.

If these ideas are correct, hospital-acquired infections should have been particularly dangerous prior to the recognition and control of attendant-borne transmission. They were. High lethality of hospital-acquired infections can be traced back to the origins of hospitals themselves. During the eighteenth and early nineteenth centuries, one death commonly occurred for every five admissions to the large urban hospitals; in the less crowded country hospitals the death rates were much lower (Jones 1776).

Although it is has not yet been determined whether the high death rates in hospitals is attributable to particularly virulent organisms, even the earliest studies of hospital-acquired disease incriminate attendant-borne transmission. In the mid-nineteenth century, the Hungarian physician Ignaz Semmelweis was trying to control an appalling death rate among new mothers in the obstetrical clinics at the University of Vienna. Noticing that lethality was about three fold higher among women attended by physicians than among those attended by midwives, he guessed that infections were transmitted by physicians and medical students who conducted physical examinations of women in labor after returning from the postmortem room where they examined women who had died shortly after giving birth. To break this cycle, he introduced routine handwashing with soap followed by rinsing with chlorine solution prior to patient contact. Introduction of this practice reduced the mortality rate from about 12% to 3% within a few weeks (Semmelweis 1861/1981).

We cannot now determine the importance of cadaver-to-patient attendant-borne transmission relative to patient-to-patient attendant-borne transmission in Semmelweis's patients. His evidence for postmortem transmission is noteworthy, however, because postmortem attendant-borne transmission should heighten the evolution of virulence beyond that occurring when attendant-borne transmission is restricted to living patients. If postmortem attendant-borne transmission occurs, even a pathogen strain that was so virulent as to kill its host could still be transmitted to susceptibles after host death.

Unfortunately, Semmelweis was biting the hand that fed him. He was telling people that the finest medical institutions were killing the people they were trying to help. The result was ostracism by powerful people at the University of Vienna and within the medical establishment of the day. The stress associated with this rejection may have contributed to his mental instability and his eventual downfall. In one of his tirades he carelessly cut himself during a postmortem examination and died of the infection that he spent his life trying to prevent in others.

ATTENDANT-BORNE TRANSMISSION AND ANTIBIOTICS

One needs only to open a medical text to see how modern medical science analyzes variation in disease severity in the context of variation in host resistance, antibiotic resistance, or random variation in pathogen virulence. In spite of centuries of death from hospital-acquired infections, I have never found a discussion of the possibility that the hospital environment may increase the pathogen's inherent virulence. The authors of a chapter on staphylococcal infections in a major medical text, for example, wrote that "the reasons why staphylococci are harmless commensals in most individuals and virulent pathogens in others remains a mystery" (Norden & Ruben 1981). They mentioned that hospital-acquired staphylococcal infections were generally more severe than community-acquired infection and then offered several explanations. They mentioned, for example, that patients in hospitals are already ill and frequently debilitated, but they did not consider the possibility that hospital environments might tend to have exceptionally virulent strains of pathogens.

This oversight may seem surprising, considering that evolution of antibiotic resistance has become well recognized in hospital environments. But unlike the evolution of pathogen virulence, the evolution of antibiotic resistance would be virtually impossible to ignore. Previously effective antibiotics were not working anymore. The antibiotics were the same and the patients were essentially the same; the pathogens, therefore, must have changed. In contrast, if a pathogen that rarely kills people, killed a substantial portion of the people in a hospital, this increased severity could be attributed to the patients' compromised condition. The patients had changed. Investigators therefore were not compelled to look any further for answers.

Severe disease may have been widely attributed to the patients' compromised states for several reasons. First, hospitalized patients *are* often especially vulnerable to infections because of wounds, surgical interventions, preexisting infections, and treatment with immunosuppressive drugs. Identifying and quantifying differences in vulnerability are crucial for understanding variations in severity of illness and for assuring high-quality medical care (Gross et al. 1991). But the importance of the compromised states of hospitalized patients does not justify the conclusion that compromised states are the only factor contributing to the severity of hospital-acquired infections. Consciously or subconsciously, people with a strong vested interest might discount the possibility that they played a role in creating the exceptionally high virulence of a bug that was killing their patients. Why open oneself to bad public relations, not to mention litigation? The difficulty that fellow hospital researchers have in obtaining information from microbiological records of local hospitals (e.g., see Pavillard et al. 1982) is a testament to the potency of this survival mechanism among hospital personnel. When I visited a nursery in a Boston hospital for a radio segment on disease evolution, I encountered similar resistance. The hospital's public relations representative was definitely in a defensive posture—like a hawk defending a nest of chicks. The representative insisted that the name of the hospital should not be used in the broadcast even though the hospital's neonatal care was a model of how to avoid attendant-borne transmission. The "problem" hospitals would not let us through the door.

Perhaps the underlying reason for blaming the compromised status of the patient is the general lack of understanding among medical researchers about evolutionary processes and the applicability of these processes to hospital settings. The rapid development of antibiotic resistance in hospitals—the phenomenon that could have alerted medical researchers to the feasibility of evolutionary changes in pathogen virulence—seems to have muddied rather than clarified the waters. Because antibiotic use is ubiquitous in hospitals, a relatively large proportion of hospital strains are resistant to antibiotics. This association between virulence and antibiotic resistance apparently led some investigators to suggest that antibiotic-resistant strains might be inherently more virulent (Craven et al. 1981). But at least one study of strains isolated in hospital settings indicates that antibiotic-resistant and antibiotic-sensitive strains do not have inherently different virulences (Holzman et al. 1980).

An evolutionary approach offers a resolution to this apparent discrepancy. Hospital strains may be more virulent than community strains because attendant-borne transmission favors increased virulence; hospital strains may be more resistant to antibiotics because of the pervasive use of antibiotics in hospitals. Antibiotic resistance and pathogen virulence therefore may be linked spatially, if one compares hospital strains with community strains. If one compares antibiotic-resistant hospital strains with antibiotic-sensitive hospital strains, however, one may find little if any difference.

Although there is no reason to believe that antibiotic resistance is obligately linked to increased pathogen virulence, antibiotic resistance might cause the evolution of increased virulence indirectly when the strains evolve resistance to all of the regularly used antibiotics. Antibiotic treatment should impose fitness costs on virulent, antibiotic-sensitive strains because a severe infection attracts the attention of hospital personnel. Antibiotic-resistant strains, however, will incur a relatively low fitness cost of virulence in the presence of widespread antibiotic use because their virulence does not bring about their own nemesis. Although their virulence attracts the attention of the antibiotic-wielding health worker, their antibiotic resistance makes the health worker's armaments impotent. The result should be an evolutionary increase in virulence, when resistance to all commonly used antibiotics evolves in the presence of attendant-borne transmission. The available data are not sufficient to test this idea. But it is noteworthy that the studies implicating a link between antibiotic resistance and virulence originated from pathogens that probably had experienced many cycles of attendant-borne transmission after evolving broad resistance to the antibiotics locally in use (Craven et al. 1981, Pavillard et al. 1982).

Throughout the antibiotic era, *Staph. aureus* has been killing patients and causing disease in attendants at high rates (Robertson et al. 1958, Juhlin & Ericson 1965, Hemming et al. 1976, Craven et al. 1981, Duggan et al. 1985). Whether or not the broad antibiotic resistance is evolutionarily linked to virulence, this threat has become more ominous as the range of antibiotic resistance has broadened without a concomitant increase in the classes of effective antibiotics. And the problem is not restricted to staph. Resistant hospital-acquired bacteria have now been found across taxonomic groups and in virtually all hospitals in the United States (Jones 1992).

Antibiotic resistance often arises repeatedly, even within a single species of pathogen responding to a single antibiotic. Resistance to penicillin is exemplified by *Strep. pneumoniae*, a common cause of hospital-acquired pneumonia (Bartlett et al. 1986). Its resistance to penicillin is generated by a change in enzyme structure, which reduces the capacity of penicillin to bind to and hence block the activity of the enzymes. Comparisons of variation in these enzymes indicate that resistance to penicillin has evolved many times independently (Hakenbeck et al. 1991, Muñoz et al. 1992).

If these arguments apply generally to hospital-acquired pathogens and the emphasis in combatting infections continues to focus on treatment of infection rather than prevention of attendant-borne transmission, we can expect recurring problems with virulent hospital-acquired pathogens. A pathogen population partially controlled with antibiotics may evolve resistance and then increased virulence. Alternatively, complete antibiotic control may pave the way for a new kind of pathogen to move into the virulent attendant-borne niche. If control is not achieved through antibiotic use, severe illness may occur until an appropriate antibiotic is found.

In accordance with these arguments, most of the dangerous attendant-borne pathogens are of little consequence outside of hospitals. They may colonize several people out of every hundred in the general population, but they rarely cause serious infections and often complete their life cycles without using humans as hosts. *Clostridium difficile*, for example, rarely causes severe disease in the general population even though it colonizes about one out of 50 adults (Bentley 1990). It is common in hospitals, particularly among infants who are not breast-fed (Cooperstock 1987) and in nursing homes, where it is attendant-borne and sometimes lethal (Bender et al. 1986; DuPont & Ribner 1986, Greenough & Bennett 1990, Bentley 1990). Like *Staph. aureus* and *E. coli, C. difficile* can be cultured from the hands of attendants, even after routine hand washing (Bentley 1990). It is particularly prone to invade after antibiotic treatment, and, as expected from the cultural vectors hypothesis, it spreads more pervasively from overtly symptomatic infections than from silent infections (Bentley 1990). Attendant-borne transmission within and between hospitals applies broadly to other dangerous bacteria, such as *Serratia, Pseudomonas, Proteus, Enterobacter,* and *Enterococcus* (Schaberg et al. 1976, 1981, Molavi & LeFrock 1984, Zervos et al. 1987, Kielhofner et al. 1992). Some of these organisms are best considered free-living bacteria that have only recently become pathogens cycling regularly from human to human. As Wallace (1989) has noted, highly vulnerable patients may act as stepping stones by which such species may evolve into full-fledged human pathogens.

Given that these newly recognized pathogens are emerging as problems in the midst of widespread antibiotic use, one might expect that they would be particularly resistant to antibiotics, and they are. Some, like *C. difficile,* are inherently resistant (Coudron et al. 1984, Greenough & Bennett 1990). Others, like *Serratia, Enterobacter,* and *Enterococcus,* can rapidly evolve resistance to new antibiotics (Schaberg et al. 1981, Manos 1982, Zervos et al. 1986ab, Jones 1992). These tendencies indicate that without stringent interventions, the hospital environment of the future will remain a dangerous place.

Hospitals may be an especially dangerous place for AIDS patients, whose compromised immune systems make them vulnerable to infection with bacteria that are often attendant-borne (Rolston et al. 1990, Weber et al. 1991, Turner & Ball 1992). The incidence of community-acquired pneumococcal pneumonia (caused by *Strep. pneumoniae*), for example, is about seven times greater in AIDS patients than in the general population (Polsky et al. 1986). AIDS patients face a similar increased risk of acquiring such life-threatening infections within hospitals (Weber et al. 1991). The highest mortality from pneumococcal pneumonia reported during the antibiotic era, has recently occurred among hospitalized AIDS patients (Pesola & Charles 1992). More than half of the patients died, even though the *Strep. pneumoniae* involved were sensitive to the antibiotics in use. Because immunologically compromised patients with pneumonia caused by *Strep. pneumoniae* are more prone to relapse (Kuhls et al. 1992), such patients may be a long-lived source of infections to others. Hospital-acquired, antibiotic-resistant *M. tuberculosis* is also growing problem in urban hospitals, especially for AIDS patients (Beck-Sagué et al 1992, Dooley et al. 1992ab, Edlin et al. 1992, Fischl et al. 1992ab, Pearson et al. 1992).

The heightened danger is not restricted to those HIV-infected patients who already have AIDS. Even the relatively slight immune suppression prior to AIDS symptoms seems to increase the risk of acquiring life-threatening infections caused by *Pseudomonas aeruginosa* and *M. tuberculosis* (Dooley et al. 1992a, Kielhofner et al. 1992, Lozano et al. 1992).

HIV-infected neonates are particularly susceptible because their already high vulnerability to infection is compounded by HIV. They often die within a few weeks of birth from *Staph. aureus* or other hospital-acquired pathogens (Rosenfeld et al. 1987). If attendant-borne transmission is making hospital-acquired pathogens particularly virulent, AIDS patients and HIV-infected newborns may often be better off if they are kept out of the hospital.

ALTERING THE EVOLUTIONARY COURSE OF
HOSPITAL-ACQUIRED PATHOGENS

A three-pronged approach

The considerations of this chapter suggest a three-pronged approach for avoiding or reducing the evolution of virulence in institutional settings: (1) Stringent hygienic standards should be maintained for all attendants who could transfer pathogens; (2) breast-feeding and other skin-to-skin contact should be encouraged between healthy mothers and their own babies, to allow transmission of benign protective bacteria; and (3) antibiotics should be used selectively for ill babies rather than for preventative treatment of entire wards. Each of these three actions involves disruption of a part of the attendant-borne transmission cycle.

Hygienic standards.   Improving standards of hygiene among attendants is a proven way of disrupting attendant-borne transmission (Easmon et al. 1981). In spite of the vast amount of evidence demonstrating attendant-borne transmission in hospital settings and the widespread acceptance of guidelines for curbing attendant-borne transmission, compliance with these guidelines is often poor (Larson 1988). A recent study of a nursery in a Chicago hospital, for example, showed that nurses followed good handwashing guidelines after only half of baby contacts and one-third of contacts with inanimate objects. Doctors were worse, following the guidelines after only one-third either kind of contact (Raju & Kobler 1991). These poor performances were dramatically improved with a more persistent advocacy of the guidelines (Raju & Kobler 1991). Increasing staff-to-patient ratios should also improve conformance to guidelines, and may even be more cost-effective over the long term.

Although frequent handwashing often fails to completely eliminate pathogens from the hands, it reduces their density, particularly if the handwashing is done with disinfectant soaps. The lower density of organisms on the hands should reduce the probability that a patient contacted by the attendant will become infected by an attendant-borne pathogen. Even if some organisms are transferred from that attendant, the lower number transferred should increase the chance that benign competitors on the patient will outcompete the transferred pathogens. An extremely high rate of handwashing is counterproductive, apparently because it compromises the natural defenses of the skin (Larson 1984).

Supplementing high rates of handwashing with disposable gloves can further reduce attendant-borne transmission. Use of disposable gloves for all personal contact reduced *C. difficile* infection rates, for example, by about 80% (Bentley 1990). Of course, disposable gloves have to be disposed of after each contact with a potential source of pathogens. To avoid glove-borne outbreaks (e.g.,

Patterson et al. 1991) attendants need to view gloves as objects to protect their patients rather than simply objects for their own protection.

Maternal contact.   The second complementary option is to enhance the competitive ability of benign organisms by actively favoring their transmission. A simple way to achieve this enhancement would be to *lower* the hygienic standards that inhibit transmission from people outside the attendant-borne transmission cycle. Transmission from mother to offspring, for example, could be facilitated. Mothers tend to harbor organisms acquired in the community at large. So long as conditions in the community favor benign variants (e.g., water supplies are uncontaminated), facilitating maternal transmission (e.g., by encouraging prolonged and close skin-to-skin contact and by not encouraging mothers to wash frequently or to wear hospital gowns) should help colonize the newborn with benign bacteria that inhibit infection by the more virulent hospital strains.

Advocating a reduction in the hygienic standards of mothers may sound rather heretical, but it is actually quite similar to other interventions that have proven successful. Severe staphylococcal outbreaks in nursery wards, for example, have been controlled by inoculating newborns with benign strains (Mackowiak 1983, Cooperstock 1987). Allowing transmission from mother to baby has two added advantages over this inoculation approach. Breast-fed babies receive, from their mothers, antibodies specific to the maternal organisms (Cooperstock 1987). These antibodies may help protect against any of the maternal organisms that by chance are moderately pathogenic. Because maternal transmission is inexpensive and easy to perpetuate indefinitely, attendant-borne transmission can be continuously disfavored, reducing the chances that attendant-borne enhancement of virulence will evolve in the first place.

In this sense, the evolutionary analysis of attendant-borne transmission provides additional reasons to support breast-feeding policies currently advocated by many epidemiologists. To date, this advocacy has been made on the basis of the short-term effects of breast-feeding on mortality and illness from neonatal diarrhea. Studies in less affluent countries have shown that a greater reliance on bottle feeding is associated with a greater infant death rate (Huffman & Combest 1990). A study from Brazil, for example, showed that the risk of death from diarrhea was nearly 25 times greater among infants who were not breast-fed during the first two months of life than among breast-fed infants (Victoria et al. 1987). Partial breast-feeding was associated with a proportional reduction in mortality. Although mortality rates are much lower in economically prosperous countries, similar benefits are apparent. A study of babies with rotavirus diarrhea in Buffalo, New York, showed that over half the exclusively bottle-fed babies had moderate or severe diarrhea. None of the breast-fed babies had severe diarrhea, and only 10% had moderate diarrhea.

Such findings have led to recommendations designed to enhance the protection afforded by breast-feeding: (1) frequent and intimate breast contact as soon as possible after birth; (2) breast-feeding without using any water, sugar solutions, milk, or formula as supplements; and (3) rooming-in of the baby with the mother to facilitate breast-feeding (Huffman & Combest 1990). Each of these activities should disfavor the virulent strains, (1) by giving the mother's relatively benign flora the competitive advantage gained from being first to colonize; (2) by reducing the contact with hospital personnel, thus reducing the doses of the more virulent hospital strains; and (3) by directly interfering with any virulent strains that enter the baby (the adherence of pathogenic E. coli to the gut lining, for example, is inhibited by colostrum and breast milk; Silva & Giampaglia 1992). Rooming-in policies are associated with a preponderance of transmission from mother to baby. In the Presbyterian Medical Center in New York City, where rooming-in has been extensively used, about 95% of the Staph. aureus isolated from newborns could be attributable to colonization from their mothers (Regan et al. 1987).

Termination of some infection-control guidelines is being considered on the basis of only short-term assessments. Studies have not revealed a lower frequency of infection with increased gown use, for example. On the basis of this information there has been a growing sense that gown use can be curbed, saving approximately 30 cents per gown used (Cloney & Donowitz 1986). Because this conclusion is based on short-term studies, it does not consider the possible evolutionary consequences of reduced gown use. Evolutionary considerations indicate that gown use should not be entirely abandoned without long-term studies designed to detect any evolutionary increases in pathogen virulence when gowns are not used. For newborn nursery wards, these long-term studies should encompass gown use by attendants but not by healthy mothers.

Selective antibiotic usage. Selective use of antibiotics may also help shift the competitive balance within institutions in favor of benign strains. If antibiotics are used selectively for dangerous infections, the milder strains are disproportionately left in the pool of organisms that remain in institutions. In contrast, nonselective, ward-wide treatment will reduce benign and virulent pathogens alike and, in the presence of attendant-borne transmission, might favor increased virulence by decimating the normal protective bacteria of patients in the ward, thereby increasing the pool of susceptibles; moreover, ward-wide use of antibiotics should more strongly favor the evolution of antibiotic resistance which, in the presence of attendant-borne transmission, can create virulent pathogens for which control is difficult or perhaps not even possible. Selective antibiotic use has proved effective over the short term, even against rare diseases in the general community (Kristiansen et al. 1992). Consideration of the long-term benefits associated with the increased prevalence of and protection by mild strains should enhance the effectiveness beyond the measured levels.

This last virulence-inhibiting intervention is the most expensive because it is best accomplished through establishment of surveillance and control programs. But these programs can be justified on the basis of their effect on the incidence of hospital-acquired infections. When enacted, the infection rates fall to about half of what would otherwise occur (Haley et al. 1985b). Long-term studies indicate that policies involving close tracking of resistant strains, as well as careful selection of antibiotics and restricted use, keep antibiotic resistance at low stable levels (Gerding et al. 1991). Any evolutionary damping of virulence through selective antibiotic usage should make these policies even more cost-effective.

Evaluation of interventions.

Although rigorous evaluation of these proposals requires studies that are better controlled than those currently in the literature, studies designed for other purposes have yielded promising results. Where stringent transmission prevention measures are enacted to preempt outbreaks, asymptomatic relationships predominate. In a New York City hospital, for example, where attendants adhered to rigorous handwashing and often used gloves and gowns in response to the presence of potential pathogens, attendant-borne transmission rates were very low, and only about one of 30 babies carrying *Staph. aureus* were symptomatic (Holzman et al. 1980). In contrast, in severe hospital outbreaks, symptomatic infections typically occurred in one-third to one-half of all patients carrying *Staph. aureus* (Craven et al. 1981, Dunkle et al. 1981, Pavillard et al. 1982).

Incorporating an evolutionary approach to hospital-acquired infections may become increasingly important in economically prosperous countries as antibiotic resistance in hospital settings reduces the usefulness of antibiotics. In poorer countries the importance of the evolutionary approach is heightened because ready access to the entire spectrum of antibiotics is often limited. In maternity hospitals in Rangoon, Myanmar, for example, neonatal diarrhea is the main reason for transfer to the sick baby unit and the largest cause of death in the unit (Aye et al. 1991). During the 1980s, changes in hospital policy improved hygienic conditions and increased the extent of rooming-in and breast-feeding. Overall, 12% of the babies acquiring diarrhea in the hospital died, but the rates of severe diarrheal disease declined steadily by nearly two-thirds for those babies born vaginally. Babies born by C-section, who are most likely to be colonized from the staff and fed less breast milk, did not show such a decline; they acquired life-threatening diarrheal disease nearly four times as frequently as vaginally delivered babies at the beginning of the period, and over seven times as frequently by the end of the period (Aye et al. 1991). Because the study was not carried out from an evolutionary point of view, the contribution of evolutionary changes in pathogen virulence was not addressed. But the dramatic decline in death rates attests to the ethical acceptability of instituting such changes to evaluate their evolutionary effects.

As these studies indicate, enactment of hygienic standards often reduces attendant-borne transmission. Although the goal of these activities is simply to reduce the frequency of new infections, blocking attendant-borne transmission should also favor evolution toward benignness and inhibit pathogens from evolving high virulence in the first place. Evolutionary considerations therefore indicate that investments in breaking cycles of attendant-borne transmission are more cost-effective than is currently thought.

In the United States, more than 1 in 20 patients admitted to hospitals and 1 in 7 intensive care patients acquire infections during their stay (Dixon 1978, Haley et al. 1985a, Raju & Kobler 1991). Even if one considers only pneumonia, the numbers are striking. Pneumonia has been the leading infectious cause of death during the antibiotic era; about one-third of the pneumonia is acquired within hospitals, and about one-third of these pneumonia patients die (Bartlett et al. 1986). By some estimates, hospital-acquired infections rank among the ten leading causes of death in the United States (Haley et al. 1985a). Even moderate reductions in the virulence of hospital-acquired pathogens might therefore translate into many thousands of lives saved each year.

ATTENDANT-BORNE TRANSMISSION OUTSIDE OF HOSPITALS

Homes for the elderly

The evolutionary effects of attendant-borne transmission may be applicable far beyond the specific case of attendants in hospitals. Increased virulence may be favored in any institutional setting in which attendants transmit pathogens mechanically from infecteds to susceptibles.

Severe outbreaks of many viruses and bacteria have occurred in long-term care facilities for the elderly, where attendant-borne transmission is common (Greenough & Bennett 1990). The incidence of hospital-acquired pneumonia mentioned above is matched by the incidence of pneumonia acquired in nursing homes (Bartlett et al. 1986). Serious bloodstream infections are also prevalent. In an Ohio hospital during the 1980s, 43% of the bloodstream infections by *Klebsiella* were acquired from the hospital and 16% were acquired in nursing homes (Watanakunakorn & Jura 1991). Nationally the 1.5 million infections acquired in nursing homes each year in the United States are only slightly less staggering than the 2 million infections acquired in hospitals (Haley et al. 1985a).

As with pathogens in hospitals, the pathogens' contribution to increased virulence in nursing homes may have been overlooked because the residents are especially vulnerable to infectious diseases. With regard to diarrheal diseases, for example, the physiological and behavioral mechanisms for maintaining fluid balance may be less effective in the elderly (Greenough & Bennett 1990). Undoubtedly, the increased vulnerability of these people is a major contributor to the virulence of their infections, but the available data do not justify ascribing all of this virulence to their compromised state. Careful measurements of pathogen characteristics are now needed to assess whether the strains circulating in nursing homes are more virulent and whether any increased virulence is attributable to attendant-borne transmission.

Attendant-borne transmission in kennels

The cultural vectors hypothesis is also applicable to attendant-borne transmission in nonhuman hosts. Canine parvovirus, for example, causes diarrheal disease in dogs, and is transmitted from cage to cage within kennels on the footwear and clothing of attendants (McCandlish et al. 1981). It is highly resistant to heat, disinfectants, and environmental exposure (Kramer et al. 1980), and can remain viable outside the body for over a year (McCandlish et al. 1981). The most lethal outbreaks typically occur in kennels, puppy farms, and veterinary hospitals (McCandlish et al. 1981, Meunier et al. 1981). The association of virulence and attendant-borne transmission, therefore, is consistent with the cultural vectors hypothesis.

The documentation of a prolonged outbreak in the Collaborative Radiological Health Laboratory at Colorado State University yields further evidence. The outbreak occurred from November 1978 through December 1980 in a population of about 1200 dogs (Studdert et al. 1983). At the beginning of the outbreak, most infected dogs did not develop clinical disease, but by the end of the outbreak infections regularly produced symptoms. Of the 151 symptomatic infections reported from the end of the outbreak, 27 were lethal (Studdert et al. 1983).

Agricultural attendant-borne transmission

Even though plants are not mobile, these arguments about attendant-borne transmission may be applicable. Obviously, increased pathogen reproduction does not impose a fitness cost on pathogens as a result of host immobilization, at least insofar as the rooted part of a plant's life cycle is concerned. Plants, however, do have a great potential for severely curtailing growth when infected by pathogens. The reduced amount of tissue available for pathogen reproduction and any reduction in the infected plant's competitive abilities as a consequence of this curtailment represent fitness costs of virulence for plant pathogens.

When pathogens are transmissible via seeds or pollen, pathogens incur additional fitness costs from high virulence. Plant gametes and seeds can typically be highly mobile by using, for example, wind or animals. If an infected plant dies or has severely curtailed reproduction, a primary avenue of pathogen transmission is impeded. More generally, as discussed in Chapter 3, this kind of vertical transmission from parent to offspring should favor evolution toward benignness.

Whether increased multiplication will be favored evolutionarily should depend on a tradeoff between short-term and long-term consequences. The long-term consequences involve decreases in pathogen transmission due to negative effects on the plant's growth, survival, and reproduction. These decreases are weighed against the increased transmission in the near future that results from the increased multiplication.

The hypothetical influence of attendant-borne transmission on this tradeoff is analogous to the influence of attendant-borne transmission in hospitals or transmission by mosquitoes. The presence of an insect vector should increase the fitness benefits associated with increased reproduction by providing a short-term opportunity for transmission and spread; moreover, increased reproduction and spread within a plant should increase the probability that a vector will obtain a dose sufficient to infect another plant. If different pathogen genotypes occur within a plant, increased reproduction should also increase the proportional representation of the genotype in the vector. Vectorborne plant pathogens should therefore tend to be more virulent than nonvectorborne pathogens, especially when nonvectorborne pathogens are transmitted by pollen or seed (in which case pathogen reproduction should be suppressed until pollen or seed formation). Although this prediction has not been adequately tested, it is consistent with the high virulence of many vector-borne plant pathogens such as the fungus that causes Dutch elm disease.

But are any plant pathogens attendant-borne? The cultural and physical characteristics permitting transmission by agricultural equipment or hands during cultivating, harvesting, or pruning conform to the definition of a cultural vector. The people conducting these operations attend to the plants much like a nurse attends to the babies in a nursery ward, even though the equipment and operations are quite different (thank goodness!). The operators therefore should have evolutionary effects on pathogen virulence that are analogous to those of hospital attendants.

One group of attendant-borne plant pathogens are viroids: infectious loops of RNA about 300 nucleotides long (Singh 1983). Some viroids have caused devastating outbreaks; others cause slightly pathogenic or asymptomatic infections. If this variation in severity results from the relative pervasiveness of attendant-borne transmission, one should find a positive association between these two characteristics.

This positive association occurs (Ewald 1988). At one extreme is the avocado sunblotch viroid, for which data implicate transmission only by tissue grafts and seeds (Wallace & Drake 1962). No tree-to-tree spread is apparent in field plantings by natural routes, through the operations of attendants, or by sap inoculations (Parker & Horne 1932, Wallace 1950, Wallace & Drake 1962). Infection by grafting does not involve an effective cultural vector because the transmission does not occur from diseased tree to healthy tree. Rather, as practiced in the nursery, grafting is analogous to subdividing an infected tree or simply moving an infected tree from one spot to another, for example, when the top of one sapling is grafted onto the trunk of another; moreover, diseased trees are generally avoided when selecting material for grafting. Pollen transmission has been experimentally demonstrated from asymptomatic and symptomatic trees (Desjardins et al. 1979, 1984). Vertical transmission through seeds can approach 100% for asymptomatically infected trees (Wallace & Drake 1962, Desjardins et al. 1979). The greater density of the viroid in flower buds than in leaves (da Graça & Mason 1983) reflects the relative importance of pollen/seed transmission.

Avocado sunblotch viroid causes disease when healthy buds are grafted to asymptomatic trees and in the infected seedlings of symptomatic trees (Wallace & Drake 1953, 1962). Symptoms are generally restricted to streaks and depressions in stems and fruit, roughened bark, and slight malformation of leaves (da Graça et al. 1981). Symptomatic trees often produce asymptomatic shoots or may become entirely asymptomatic (Desjardins et al. 1979, da Graça et al. 1981).

At the other extreme of virulence is the coconut cadang-cadang viroid, which is transmitted almost exclusively by attendants. Plantation workers move from tree to tree, using machetes to cut off coconuts and lacerate flowers to collect sap (Maramorosch 1987). The dependence of this viroid on attendant-borne transmission is illustrated by the pattern of infected trees on the Philippine Island, Luzon. For ethnic reasons workers do not move between plantations owned by two different ethnic groups. Cadang-cadang has spread through the plantations of one ethnic group but has not touched the plantations of the other even when plantations of the two groups are adjacent to each other (Maramorosch 1987).

Cadang-cadang means dying-dying. It has decimated the coconut industry in the Philippines since it was first observed during the 1920s and is considered to be "one of the most devastating plant diseases known" (Maramorosch 1987).

The other plant viroids are rather evenly distributed along the spectrum of attendant-borne transmission and virulence bounded by the avocado sunblotch viroid at one end and the cadang-cadang viroid at the other (Ewald 1988). As attendant-borne transmission increases, so does virulence.

If the limited genetic information in viroids can respond evolutionarily to the presence of attendant-borne transmission, then all other pathogens should have sufficient genetic material to respond. Although no comprehensive analysis of attendant-borne transmission and virulence of nonviroid agricultural pathogens has yet been conducted, the following examples suggest that attendant-borne transmission may be broadly relevant to the virulence of plant pathogens.

The bacterial agent of alfalfa wilt (*Corynebacterium michiganense* subsp. *insidiosum*) is transmitted by tractors during soil movement and by mowing machines (Chester 1942). Alfalfa wilt was unknown before 1925. It became progressively more devastating, eventually developing into the most important disease of alfalfa (Chester 1942). Similarly, the bacterial agent of bean blight (*Xanthomonas phaseoli*) is transmitted by the picking of beans and causes heavy or complete crop losses (Chester 1942). In contrast, when the related bacterium *Pseudomonas syringae* infects bean plants, it tends to cause spots on leaves, stems, and pods. Like the mild viroids, *Pseudomonas syringae* is transmitted from parent to offspring.

The sugar beet nematode (*Heterodera schachtii*) is transmitted by agricultural machinery. It kills rootlets, eliminating the beets or greatly reducing their size (Chester 1942). In contrast, the wheat and rye nematode (*Anguina tritici*), which is introduced to new fields by infested seed, causes relatively small losses (Chester 1942).

Tobacco mosaic virus is spread between tobacco and tomato plants through activities such as pruning, staking, tying, topping, harvesting, and hand pollinating (Chester 1942). Transmission occurs rarely, if ever, through insect vectors (aphids), seed, or soil (Chester 1942, Smith 1957). It is sometimes lethal, and the tissue damage and stunting it causes can reduce by more than half the per acre value of infected fields (Chester 1942).

These examples draw attention to the broad potential applicability of the attendant-borne transmission hypothesis. Rigorous tests will need to consider several alternative hypotheses, which are not applicable to the viroids. Pathogenic fungi, for example, are often durable and windborne; bacteria are often durable and waterborne; and viruses are often transmitted by insect vectors. Because each of these modes could permit transmission from infected plants to large numbers of susceptibles, each could act as a selective pressure to increase virulence.

CHAPTER 7

War and Virulence

DELIBERATE USE OF A LOOSE CANNON

It has become all too apparent that ruthless people will use scientific knowledge for ruthless purposes. Unfortunately, although most major scientific discoveries enrich human life, they also have the potential for degrading it. The insights developed in this book are no exception. I trust that collectively we shall prohibit the use of this knowledge for purposes of human destruction and suffering. Although this outlook would have been naive for much of this century when the various powers of the world were creating microbial weaponry using organisms like the anthrax bacterium (Doyle & Lee 1986), it is now more realistic. For one thing we now realize that microbes make poor weapons. They may be transmitted into human populations where their users do not want them to go. They act slowly and can mutate to infect those immunized against them, such as soldiers entering a contested area that has been contaminated by their own side.

Also, to be useful as weapons, microbes often need to be resistant to environmental destruction, especially if they are released by explosions. But this resistance can make contested areas uninhabitable for generations. Gruinard is a testament to that. In the summer of 1942, this small island off the northwest coast of Scotland was evacuated, except for about 30 sheep, which were tethered for an experiment. A small bomb containing anthrax spores was detonated nearby (Harris & Paxman 1982). Exposed sheep began dying from anthrax the next day. Now, a half century later, sheep and people might meet the same fate if they were allowed to visit the island unprotected. The spores distributed by the weapons testing of 1942 and 1943 lie dormant, and they may still be viable a century from now. What a prize this "Anthrax Island" would have been, had it been won through the use of such a microbial attack.

INADVERTENT EVOLUTION OF A LOOSE CANNON

Cultural vectors, host density, and influenza

The total amount of death and disease attributable to the development and use of microbial weapons has been minuscule compared with the pathogen-induced death and disease brought about by conditions of war. Until knowledge about germs was applied to curbing disease at the beginning of this century, infectious diseases regularly carried off far more soldiers than did weapons (McNeill 1976). Although the association between disease and warfare has long been recognized, it has been attributed solely to increased spread of pathogens and increased vulnerability of hosts. The possible effects of war on the evolution of pathogen characteristics have been overlooked.

One of the most dramatic historical examples of an evolutionary increase in virulence is the influenza pandemic of 1918. Ever since this pandemic, epidemiologists have been perplexed by its virulence and apprehensive about the return of a comparably virulent pandemic (Burnet & Clark 1942, Langmuir & Schoenbaum 1976). In the middle of this century MacFarlane Burnet wrote: "Influenza in its serious form as exemplified by the pandemic of 1918–1919 still remains the biggest unsolved problem of theoretical epidemiology and public health practice" (Burnet & Clark 1942). He identified "the essential objective of influenza research as the understanding of the conditions responsible for pandemic influenza of the 1918 type—and the establishment of conditions necessary to prevent its reappearance" (Williams 1959). Progress toward reaching this "essential objective" has been limited largely to improved understanding of the changes in the virus's external antigens (the parts of the virus attacked by our antibodies) and the influence of these changes and host immunity on the potential for epidemic spread. Little progress has been made toward understanding the conditions responsible for the extreme virulence "of the 1918 type" or the "conditions necessary to prevent its reappearance." The evolutionary approach to disease virulence can move us toward these objectives.

The environmental conditions associated with the trench warfare of World War I could hardly have been more favorable for the evolution of increased virulence of airborne pathogens like influenza. Soldiers in the trenches were grouped so closely that even immobile infecteds could transmit pathogens. When a soldier was too sick to fight, he was typically removed from his trenchmates.

But by that time trenchmates often would have been infected because rates of shedding are highest at the onset of illness, which typically occurs two to three days after exposure (Cate 1972, Berlin 1980).

The sick individuals were generally moved between a succession of crowded rooms by a succession of crowded vehicles. Severely ill soldiers were transported along with the wounded to field hospitals, where they were usually laid on blanket-covered straw inside tents. The severely sick and badly wounded were then sent within a few hours by trucks to one or more evacuation hospitals and then eventually by railcars to base hospitals. The large numbers of patients being moved give some idea of how these activities could increase the numbers of susceptibles contacted by an immobilized infected person. A 1300-bed medical unit of an evacuation hospital in Vaubecourt, France provided a 360-bed section for cases of influenza or mild respiratory disease. In one 24-hour period, this section received and passed along 824 people (Lynch et al. 1925). During the last six weeks of the war, this hospital admitted about 34,000 patients, of whom 24,000 had disease, about half of which were respiratory. Attempts to segregate infectious cases were not successful when influenza was epidemic (Lynch et al. 1925).

The potential for transmission from immobilized patients is perhaps best understood from the patients' point of view. Guy Emerson Bowerman Jr., an ambulance driver, fell ill with dysentery in August 1918. He described his transport in his diary.

> . . . they decided to evacuate us for three or four days. We left Vashe Noire at 6 just as the barrage for the attack on Hoyon commenced. Hub drove us to Villiers and only my condition prevented me from being frightened to death at the way he took corners. I was so weak that I was unable to sit on the little seat, but managed to stretch out a bit on the floor. Arrived at the evacuation hospital (a large tent) . . . I thot [sic] I suffered that night but a 20 kilometer jaunt in a camion to another evacuation hospital was so much worse that there was no comparison. I surely thot I would die before we reached the other hospital. We stayed here four hours and were then taken by ambulance to Crepy where they loaded us into a hospital train and we were off on a two day-two night trip to Toulouse, 75 miles from the Spanish border. The hospital train was a string of boxcars fitted with four tiers of three stretchers each . . . . At Toulouse we were taken by a woman ambulance driver to Hospital Auxiliaire No 1 and placed in a ward with 20 doughboys from the 1st and 2nd divisions who had been wounded at Soissons and Chateau Thierry. (Bowerman 1983)

The great potential for transmission of airborne respiratory viruses under these crowded conditions is apparent from the substantial transmission that occurred under the less crowded, more hygienic conditions of mid-twentieth century hospitals (Mufson et al. 1973).

Additional new susceptibles would be transported to the trenches to take the place of ill people who had been removed. As the trenchmates infected by an already removed soldier became ill, the process continued. In the camps away from the trenches, the high densities of soldiers and transport of sick and susceptible soldiers may have contributed to increased virulence by a similar mechanism.

The people and vehicles transporting the infecteds and susceptibles to and from the trenches and hospitals are components of a cultural vector because they permit transmission from an immobilized person to susceptibles. In this special case of attendant-borne transmission, the attendants (e.g., ambulance drivers, those moving patients into and out of hospitals and transport vehicles) transmit infections from immobilized infectious hosts to susceptibles by transporting to susceptibles the whole package—the pathogens and the immobilized host containing them—rather than just the pathogens.

The increased mortality in the trenches due to fighting or the other infectious diseases that typically accompanied such warfare should have, if anything, also favored a high level of virulence. Any deaths of recovered immune individuals would result in the transport of replacements into the trenches who would often be susceptible to the strains circulating in the trenches. In addition, one of the costs that a pathogen may incur from extremely rapid reproduction is a shortened duration of infection due either to a more rapid immune response or to host death. As the likelihood of host death from other causes increases, this cost of virulence should be lower. If your ship is about to be destroyed by enemy fire, then it might be better to abandon ship (using as much of the ship's resources as you can) now rather than later, even if abandoning the ship prohibits the ship's future usefulness. [Axelrod and Hamilton (1981) phrase an analogous argument more formally in terms of the "prisoner's dilemma."]

If the conditions and activities at the western front were responsible for the enhanced virulence of the 1918 pandemic, the timing and spatial pattern of virulent disease should accord with virulence enhancement at the western front. That is, the increased virulence should have occurred among troops at the western front when the mobility-independent transmission was occurring. When the activities allowing this transmission ended at the end of the war, the virulence should have gradually declined as the mobility-dependent transmission favored the milder strains.

Retrospective pinpointing of the origin of the highly virulent 1918 pandemic virus is extremely difficult (Burnet & Clark 1942), but the first appearance of influenza with the corresponding characteristics can be traced to troops in France near the western front (Burnet & Clark 1942, Crosby 1976). This origin is noteworthy because influenza pandemics typically spread from east Asia (Morse 1991). In typical influenza epidemics, less than one death occurs per 1000 infections. During the several months just before and just after the end of the war, mortality per infection was about 10-fold higher (Mulder & Masurel 1960, Neustadt & Fineberg 1983). During the three years after the war, the virulence gradually declined to normal levels (Burnet and Clark 1942). Our knowledge about the timing and spatial pattern of the pandemic therefore accords with virulence enhancement at the western front.

The age distribution of the pandemic was also different from that of other influenza epidemics. Normally, infections by the influenza virus are most lethal in the very young and very old. The 1918 pandemic was most lethal in young to middle-aged adults, the primary age group in which the enhanced virulence is hypothesized to have evolved. If physiology and tissue characteristics differ with age in ways relevant to pathogen reproduction, one would expect the strains evolving within a given age group to be of relatively high virulence in that age group. Fever and immune responses, for example, change with age and may also influence pathogen reproduction (Wade et al. 1988, Haq & Szewczuk 1991, Miller et al. 1991). The atypical age-specific attack rates therefore are consistent with the idea that the high virulence of the 1918 pandemic strain evolved in soldiers at the western front.

Molecular studies of influenza viruses have revealed how simple mutations can alter the virus's reproductive rate and virulence. The virus has protruding from its coat a molecule called *hemagglutinin*, which is part sugar and part protein, and allows the virus to attach and penetrate cells. A mutation in the hemagglutinin gene that causes hemagglutinin to be synthesized without a few of the sugar building blocks on its terminus allows the virus to multiply to higher numbers in cell cultures (Deom et al. 1986). Conversely, alteration of a single building block in the protein part of hemagglutinin can cause attachment to host cells to be reduced (Aytay & Schulze 1991).

Alternative explanations of the 1918 pandemic

Recent entrance into humans?   The reasons for the extraordinary virulence of the 1918 pandemic is still a source of concern and contention.   Current explanations continue to rely on recent entrance into humans as a reason for high virulence. These explanations are unsatisfying because they leave central issues unanswered. Gorman et al. (1991), for example, reconstruct from molecular data the evolutionary relationships among influenza viruses isolated from birds, mammals, and swine. Their analysis indicates that human and swine strains had a common ancestor during the second decade of the twentieth century. They suggested that the ancestor could have entered humans just prior to the 1918 pandemic. In parts of their argument, they emphasize how maintenance of the influenza virus is much more likely in humans than swine, but they then seem to prefer a swine ancestor for maintenance of the virus during the years prior to the 1918 pandemic. This preference apparently results from their predisposition to blame the high virulence of the pandemic on recent entry of a strain into humans. Aside from this inconsistent use of swine as influenza sources, they leave a central issue unresolved. Human influenza epidemics occurred for about a half-century before 1918, but after the ancestral influenza virus diverged into bird and human lineages during the nineteenth century. If all of the human influenza strains originated from a lineage established in humans around 1918, where did the strains causing the human epidemics before 1918 come from? It seems unlikely that all became extinct, especially considering the much lower rate of extinction of post-1918 lineages and the poorer infection control measures prior to 1918. The similarity of these early epidemics to the post-1918 epidemics make it doubtful that the early epidemics were all caused by the other two major groups of influenza virus.

The hypothesis of war-enhanced virulence provides a more parsimonious explanation. The lineages of human and avian influenza viruses split from a shared ancestor prior to the twentieth century. The human lineages then generated several swine lineages, one of which branched off during the second decade of this century. The key issue is that there is no evolutionary basis for supposing that transmission from swine to humans should be associated with particularly high virulence in humans. To the contrary, transmission into new hosts should often be associated with low virulence in the new hosts because the ability of our immune systems to block novel pathogens should tend to be greater than the ability of novel pathogens to invade new hosts species (see Chapter 3).

Another pathogen?   Stevens (1981) offered a different proximate explanation for the high virulence of the 1918 pandemic; he ascribed the high death rate to simultaneous infection with the bacterium *Hemophilus influenzae*. He mentioned that a bacterial contribution was ruled out in later epidemics, but his analysis does not explain why such a co-occurring virulent strain of *H. influenzae* has been absent since that time.

Also troublesome is the low isolation rate of *H. influenzae*. Stevens believes that influenzal pneumonia is the key manifestation of co-infection and the cause of the increased mortality. Yet, only about half of the patients with influenzal pneumonia were positive for *H. influenzae* (Rapoport 1919, Stevens 1981).

A final concern is timing. Why did this virulent form of *H. influenzae* arise at the end of World War I and then gradually recede during the year following the war? If Stevens's proximate explanation is at least partially correct, the evolutionary explanation for war-enhanced virulence of influenza virus may also apply to *H. influenzae* and might resolve this question about timing.

Attendant-borne transmission and rapid passage.   Shortly after World War I, the official record from the U.S. Office of the Surgeon General offered an evolutionary explanation based on inductive rather than deductive reasoning: Virulence was enhanced by "rapid passage"—that is, transmission among the large numbers of recruits in rapid succession. Later scholars echo this argument (Burnet & Clark 1942, Crosby 1976). This explanation, however, does not provide an evolutionary mechanism; rather, it is based on the observations that rapid passage of pathogens among laboratory animals often increases a pathogen's virulence. The cultural vectors hypothesis provides an evolutionary mechanism deduced from basic principles of natural selection.

Rapid passage of pathogens in laboratory animals, like the passage of pathogens among soldiers in World War I, may favor increases in virulence because it eliminates the requirement that hosts be mobile to transmit their infections. In the lab, the researcher and the inoculating tool comprise the cultural vector favoring the more highly reproductive and hence more virulent pathogens. By permitting transmission from immobilized hosts, this cultural vector may have increased the virulence of strains that had been rapidly passaged in the lab.

Rapid transfer might, however, cause an enhancement of virulence directly. Transfer soon after the onset of infection selects for those pathogen variants that reproduce rapidly and early during the infection; damage late in the infection may be a direct consequence of this rapid early multiplication.

These two alternatives could be distinguished in a general sense by experimentation. The cultural vectors hypothesis could be evaluated by transferring pathogens (e.g., malarial organisms infecting rodents) from randomly selected animals in experimental groups of hosts and at the same rate from only mobile animals in control groups. According to the cultural vectors hypothesis, the former should become more virulent than the latter. The passage rate hypothesis could be assessed directly by transferring pathogens at different rates from mobile animals.

The relevance of the answer. The mortality figures for the 1918 pandemic dramatically illustrate the need to distinguish these selective mechanisms and, more generally, to understand the evolutionary forces favoring virulence. We are horrified by the ten million killed during combat throughout the four years of World War I. But twice as many were killed by the influenza pandemic that spread across the world during the two years following the war (Kilbourne 1979). The cultural vectors hypothesis proposes that most of these influenza deaths were caused evolutionarily by the war rather than being just coincidental with the war.

If we fail to recognize the evolutionary changes in pathogen virulence that our activities may inadvertently cause, then we will pay the price in sickness and death not just until our activities change the environment back to a state that favors the benign forms, but rather until the evolutionary change toward benignness is completed.

On the positive side, the cost/benefit argument based on host mobility indicates that the 1918 virulence will not be repeated in the absence of conditions such as those in the western front. We are now passing through a time period during which the 1918 antigenic type would be able to create another pandemic owing to loss of immunity to the 1918 antigenic combinations (Neustadt & Fineberg 1983). The "swine flu" of 1976 may have been the first such revisitation; the antigens of this strain were very similar to those of the 1918 pandemic (Langmuir & Schoenbaum 1976). The low mortality of this 1976 outbreak (Neustadt & Fineberg 1983) accords with the idea that the virulence of the 1918 pandemic was an evolved response to wartime conditions rather than simply an inflexible characteristic of this antigenic type.

But what about the chickens that I mentioned at the beginning of this book? If this conceptual foundation for understanding the 1918 pandemic can be generalized, it ought to provide a basis for understanding the 1983 Pennsylvanian chicken epidemic. The molecular evidence indicates that the virulent chicken virus evolved from milder viruses that had been circulating for many years in North America (Kawaoka & Webster 1988). The epidemic virus was not simply a mutant that by chance had generated a virulence that was too high for its own good. Although it killed up to 100% of the chickens it infected, its control required drastic measures: the destruction of over 17 million birds (Kawaoka & Webster 1988). But the more critical point is something that chicken farms have in common with the western front: large numbers of hosts packed so closely that even immobilized hosts can transmit the virus to susceptibles.

Virulence in wars before the germ theory

The effects of warfare on virulence should have been especially pronounced prior to the establishment of the germ theory because virulence-enhancing cycles of transmission were rarely blocked. Although the absence of knowledge about germs during this period makes evaluation of this idea difficult, the trends observed in the pre–germ-theory wars accord with the hypothesized effects of warfare on the evolution of virulence.

In the American Civil War, for example, the troops were densely packed into camps by the hundreds of thousands for months without pure water and adequate sanitation. The war caused more deaths of American soldiers than any other war, most of them from diarrheal diseases (Steiner 1968). Perhaps more telling, however, was the progressive increase in the lethality of diarrheal diseases over time. During the first year, 4 out of every 1000 Union soldiers died of diarrheal disease. By the last year of the war, the diarrheal death rate had increased to 21 out of every 1000 (Steiner 1968). Death rates from chronic cases increased steadily from 3 out of every 100 cases in 1862 to over 20 deaths out of every 100 cases in 1865 and 1866 (Woodward 1879). A similar rise in mortality occurred among acute diarrheal infections (Woodward 1870, 1879). This increase was apparently not due to increased numbers of ingested organisms resulting from a decline in hygiene. If anything, the hygienic conditions were improving slightly toward the end of this period. Guidelines for improving camp hygiene were circulated, but implementation was poor, and no effective control of waterborne transmission was ever put in place. Long-term accumulation of pathogens in the environment is not feasible because the organisms that could have caused these diseases typically die in the external environment within a few days and almost never survive longer than several weeks (Dudgeon et al. 1919, Block & Ferguson 1940, Cruickshank & Swyer 1940, Felsen 1945, Gispen & Garr 1950, Hutchinson 1956, Andre et al. 1967, Geldreich 1972, Rosenberg et al. 1976, Blaser et al. 1980). One could also argue that the increased mortality resulted from increased vulnerability to infectious disease as the war dragged on, but this argument is inconsistent with data from other nondiarrheal diseases. The mortality per unambiguous case of malaria did not increase significantly over the duration of the war (Woodward 1870, Smart 1888). Because the agents of malaria are transmitted by mosquitoes, their inherent virulence should not increase as a result of the conditions of war. These considerations suggest that the increased deaths from diarrheal diseases are better explained by an increase in the inherent virulence of the diarrheal pathogens than by compromised defenses of the soldiers or large numbers of ingested pathogens.

A U.S. medical official, James Tilton, recorded a similar increase in deaths largely from diarrheal diseases and pneumonias, during the second and third years of the American Revolutionary War. Tilton recognized an association between centralization of soldiers in hospitals and death from "camp disease" across armies during this period. The American armies experienced more centralization and death than the French armies, which experienced more than the English, which in turn experienced more than the German armies (Tilton 1813). He estimated that 10 to 20 soldiers died of camp diseases for every one killed in combat and that at least half of the army was "swallowed up" by disease in the general hospitals (Tilton 1813).

To remedy the situation, Tilton enacted decentralized care. Patients were arranged in small circular wigwams like the spokes of a wheel, with heads to the periphery and feet to the central fire. Heads of patients were thus spread apart from one another, with the fire bringing fresh air to the patients and exhausting the stale air through the roof (Tilton 1813). The small size and one-way air currents must have reduced the potential for airborne spread of pathogens. Army regulations called for burning of straw, washing of bedding, and exposure of bedding to the sun (Rush 1777); these procedures probably reduced the potential for transmission of both directly transmitted diarrheal pathogens and virulent airborne pathogens that might have been wafted into the air from dust in bedding material (Cruickshank 1941). By this time, the medical authorities were also prescribing more careful burial of fecal material, especially during outbreaks of dysentery (Jones 1776). As the practice of crowding patients in large hospitals was supplanted by these procedures, mortality from hospital-acquired disease gradually declined (Tilton 1813, Wilbur 1980). Guidelines for water consumption were also circulated during this period, but their effects on waterborne outbreaks are unclear. The guidelines probably reduced consumption of the most contaminated water supplies, but promoted stream water over well water because the medical officials believed that coldness of well water caused disease (Wilbur 1980).

The hospital conditions may have favored increased virulence, or they may have permitted the spread of pathogens whose virulence had been enhanced in the camps, or both. The higher lethality associated with hospital-acquired infections (Jones 1776) suggests that hospital transmission was a major contributor to the lethality. The decline in mortality after improvements in hospital and camp procedures similarly suggests, as does the high lethality among doctors and nurses, that the preponderance of death was not simply a result of a common soldier's compromised state of hygiene and stress (Jones 1776, Tilton 1813).

Details of a dysentery outbreak provides further evidence that the condition of soldiers was not the underlying cause of the increased mortality. Washington's army marched from Boston to New York on April 1, 1776, leaving behind their sick in hospitals. "The whole army was in perfect health" upon their arrival in mid-April (Beardsley 1788). Upon their arrival, the troops were housed by residents and in barracks, but were transferred to tents around May 10, except for one regiment, which continued living in overcrowded rooms. Dysentery attacked this regiment during a week in mid-May. The long period before the first cases of dysentery, and the absence of the disease in the rest of the army and in some other companies in the regiment suggest that the dysentery was not caused by a typical camp strain. Only two deaths occurred among over 100 cases (Beardsley 1788). Under the congested conditions one would expect the dosage to be high and living conditions poor, yet the lethality was comparable to that of a typical community outbreak of dysentery (Ewald 1991a). Dysentery was absent for the following two months, but by the end of summer it again began ravaging the army (Beardsley 1788).

The circumstantial evidence from these wars is consistent with the idea that wartime conditions may enhance the virulence of pathogens, and that this enhancement may be responsible for much of the death that has resulted from wars during the premicrobial era. By blocking cycles of transmission from immobilized, infected people during more recent wars, we may have inadvertently avoided the virulent wartime epidemics that took so many millions of lives during our history. But the same might not be true of other diseases. In fact, we may now be paying the price of our ignorance with the human immunodeficiency virus (HIV), which through its destruction of the immune system leads to AIDS, the acquired immune deficiency syndrome.

CHAPTER 8

AIDS: Where Did It Come from and Where Is It Going?

WHERE IT CAME FROM

Evolutionary trees

Over ten million people are now infected with the human immunodeficiency virus; over one million have AIDS or have died from AIDS. These numbers are still small relative to the tolls imposed by other disease organisms: Over 20 million were carried away by the influenza virus in little more than a year during the pandemic that began at the end of World War I. Although the lives claimed by AIDS are few compared with the lives claimed by influenza, the plague, malaria, or the diarrheal diseases, there is no end to the AIDS pandemic in sight, nor is there any recognized therapy that can cure AIDS or even postpone death for more than a year or so. If the evolutionary approach can help resolve vexing epidemiological problems, its application to HIV would be especially timely. Why is HIV so lethal, and what can be done to change its future evolutionary course?

Current molecular evidence suggests that HIV has been infecting humans for decades to centuries. Most of the evidence derives from differences in the sequences of building blocks along the length of the viral RNA. According to one statistical technique for interpreting these differences, the two major groups, HIV-1 and HIV-2, diverged from a common ancestral virus about 900 years ago

(Eigen & Nieselt-Struwe 1990). Another technique based on different assumptions (Myers et al. 1992) leads to a more recent date, a century or two ago. HIV-1 strains diverged from each other before 1960 (Li et al. 1988, Eigen & Nieselt-Struwe 1990) and diverged from a virus isolated from chimpanzees (Peeters et al. 1989) roughly a half-century to a century or more ago, depending on statistical assumptions. [The more recent date of divergence is suggested by Myers et al. (1992), and the more distant date is generated from the evolutionary tree of Eigen & Nieselt-Struwe (1990) and the nucleic acid sequence data of Huet et al. (1990).] It is unclear whether this chimpanzee virus entered chimps from humans or humans from chimps, but an HIV isolated from Cameroon (called ANT 70; De Leys et al. 1990) branched off the human–chimp lineage before the chimp/human divergence (Myers et al. 1992 and Fig. 8.1). If the transmission occurred from chimps to humans, two jumps between species therefore would be needed to explain these two groups of HIV-1. If the transmission occurred from humans to chimps, only one jump would be required. The evolutionary trees suggest that most HIV-2 strains and their closest relatives among the simian immunodeficiency viruses (SIVs) had a common ancestor at about the same time as the common ancestor to the HIV-1 and chimpanzee viruses (Eigen & Nieselt-Struwe 1990, Myers et al. 1992).

These findings yield evolutionary scenarios that fall between two extremes: The extreme assuming the longest association with humans is that HIV-1, HIV-2, and their unshared ancestral HIVs have been evolving in humans for about a millennium with occasional entry into various monkeys and chimps. The extreme assuming the shortest association with humans is that the immunodeficiency viruses have been evolving primarily in nonhuman primates, and that by midcentury, two separate viruses had entered humans, yielding HIV-1 and most of the HIV-2 lineages.

Until additional data are obtained, the best we can do is to identify the evolutionary history that is most parsimonious with the available information. The nucleic acid sequence data indicate that the simian immunodeficiency virus (SIV) isolated from Gabonese mandrills (*Mandrillus sphinx*) is the most divergent virus within the HIV–SIV group. This divergence suggests that the common ancestors of the group were present in mandrills (or another host species from which the mandrill lineage was derived) before they occurred in humans. Using this as the starting point, one can use the existing evolutionary trees (Eigen & Nieselt-Struwe 1990, Khan et al. 1991, F. Gao et al. 1992, Myers et al. 1992, Novembre et al. 1992, Tomonaga et al. 1993), a composite of which is diagrammed in Figure 8.1, to determine the scenario with the fewest number of jumps between species. According to this scenario, the virus jumped from mandrills into humans. Soon thereafter (working from left to right in Figure 8.1), the ancestors of HIV-1 and HIV-2 diverged. The viruses in the HIV-1 half of the tree yielded the ANT 70 lineage and a virus that jumped from humans to chimpanzees as suggested above. In the HIV-2 half, a virus jumped from humans into green monkeys (*Cercopithecus aethiops*). A green monkey SIV then moved into white-crowned mangabeys (*Cercocebus torquatus*; Tomonaga et al. 1993). The viruses in humans then split into two branches.   One of these branches eventually led to several descendants isolated from humans, called GH-2, D205 (or ALT), and 2238 (Dietrich et al. 1989, Miura et al. 1990, F. Gao et al. 1992, Kawamura et al. 1992, Kreutz et al. 1992). An additional isolate (called 7312A) probably represents a recombination of a virus from this branch and the other branch (F. Gao et al. 1992). This other branch generated the vast majority of the HIV-2 viruses.   [Howell et al. (1991) present direct evidence for such recombinations.]   From the first of these two branches, another HIV lineage separated, leaving a descendent called FO784 (F. Gao et al. 1992). At about the same time, an HIV entered a monkey to generate the viruses that have been isolated from sooty mangabeys (*Cercocebus atys*) and macaques.

FIG. 8.1   An evolutionary tree derived from viral nucleotide sequences. HIV refers to viruses isolated from humans and SIV to viruses isolated from non-human primates. The closer the branches are in time, the less reliable the order of branching; for example, as described in the text, the HIV lineages may have branched off before or after the african green monkey lineages.   The branch containing the vast majority of HIV-1 isolates is labeled HIV-1. The same is true for HIV-2.

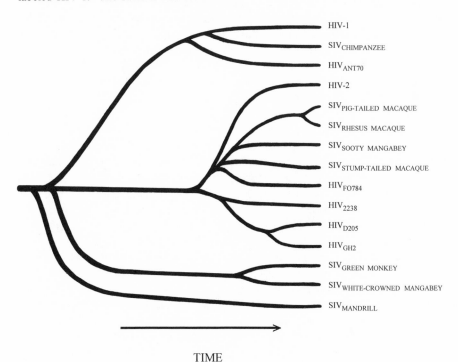

TIME

Researchers have suggested that sooty mangabeys were the source of HIV-2 (Doolittle 1989). But this suggestion raises a problem: Where are the sooty mangabey lineages that branched off after the green monkey branch and before the F0784 branch. HIV lineages are there, but not sooty mangabey lineages (Figure 8.1).

Other evolutionary trees suggest that the SIVs from mandrills and African green monkeys are more closely related to each other than to any of the other viruses (Tsujimoto et al. 1989, Miura et al. 1990). According to these trees, the fewest jumps between species would occur if the mandrill–green monkey branches were derived from humans, or if all human viruses were derived from the mandrill-green monkey group soon after the split between the mandrill and green monkey lineages.

If the common ancestor of the human and simian immunodeficiency viruses are far more ancient than the oldest estimates generated from molecular data, the african green monkey viruses could have evolved from a common ancestral virus as the ancestral green monkeys evolved into the present-day varieties of green monkeys during the last 10,000 years (Allan et al. 1991). This interpretation requires that a major error has been made in the setting of the molecular clock by which the molecular divergences are translated into time periods. If mutations have been accumulating among the immunodeficiency viruses at a greater rate during recent decades or centuries than during the earlier millennia, or if the mutations that are used to set the clock are not representative, the clock could have been set at much too fast a rate (Coffin 1990, Hahn & Shaw 1990, Allan et al. 1991). If the clock has been set incorrectly, the fewest-jumps scenario suggests the possibility of an even longer period over which immunodeficiency viruses have been evolving in humans—perhaps for millennia rather than decades or centuries.

Changes in the rates of evolution could also alter the sequences of these branches, thus altering conclusions about the direction of the jumps. If viruses undergo rapid evolution when first entering a new species, they may have left behind molecular footprints revealing the direction of the jump. These footprints may be observed by dividing the changes in nucleic acid sequence into two categories: those that cause a change in the virus's structure and those that do not. When a virus evolves quickly in a new species, the ratio of the former to the latter should increase. David Mindell, Jeffrey Shultz, and I found that these ratios indicate movement from humans to chimpanzees and from humans to sooty mangabeys. Surprisingly, the results suggested a movement from humans to mandrills, calling into question whether the mandrill lineage is more ancient than the human and green monkey lineages. Perhaps the mandrill virus gives the illusion of antiquity because it evolved at a more rapid rate. The results could not provide any information about the direction of viral movement between humans and green monkeys. This ambiguity may result from a reduction in the discriminating power of the ratios as the time since divergence increases.

Modes of transmission between species

If the fewest-jumps scenario is valid, HIVs have been infecting humans for a relatively long time, and humans have been sources of viruses for other primates rather than simply recipients. But is it useful to focus on the number of jumps between species? The answer depends on how the virus is jumping. If the jumps from monkeys to humans are much easier than the jumps from humans to monkeys, then the fewest-jumps scenario is not particularly useful. If the probabilities of jumping from humans to monkeys and from monkeys to humans are similar, then the fewest-jumps scenario offers a most reasonable hypothesis.

Unfortunately, how the viruses jumps between species is still a mystery. Some have proposed that biomedical activities may have transferred a SIV to humans. Because polio vaccines were produced using monkey cells, they could have been infected with any SIVs that were infecting these cells (Kyle 1992). Similarly, SIVs might have been transferred to humans when monkey and chimp blood was being transferred to humans early in this century by experimental inoculations of the malaria protozoa that naturally infect these animals (Gilks 1991).

Several considerations argue against these biomedical accident hypotheses. If the virus is jumping between monkey species and between humans and chimps in nature, there is no *need* to invoke biomedical accidents to explain transmission of the virus from monkey to human. More importantly, neither hypothesis corresponds well to current evolutionary trees of HIV and SIV. With regard to the vaccine hypothesis, most trees indicate that the viruses in the suspect monkeys branched off the tree *after* the HIV-1 lineages. With regard to the malaria transfer hypothesis, the chimp SIVs appear to branch off the HIV-1 limb of the tree after the most ancient lineage of HIV-1: that generating ANT 70 (Figure 8.1). Moreover, the time scale over which the vaccinations and blood transfers took place is not broad enough to cover the span of time implicated by the evolutionary trees (see also Schulz 1992). The first apparent HIV-positive AIDS patient left the alleged site of vaccine transmission (in the Congo) before the vaccination occurred there (Corbitt et al. 1990, Anonymous 1992).

The limitations of the vaccine and malaria-transfer hypotheses are also apparent when one considers another group of retroviruses: the T cell lymphotropic viruses. Geographic patterns of infection indicate that members of this group have been transferred between humans and other primates at least three times over a period that probably spans millennia (Hunsmann et al. 1983, Schatzl et al. 1992, Saksena et al. 1992, 1993). If these retroviruses have been jumping between humans and other primates without biomedical accidents, then there is no need to invoke biomedical accidents to explain HIV's interspecies transfers.

I assume that sexual transmission of retroviruses between humans and other primates can be ruled out. That leaves two hypotheses as viable, general explanations. The hunting and eating of simians could provide one route for transfer to humans (Southwood 1987, Fox 1992), but this hypothesis seems less feasible as an explanation for transfer among other primates. Some of these primates might hunt others, but behavioral and ecological differences among other species pairs make any interspecies transmission by hunting extremely difficult to envision (e.g., transmission from green monkeys to white-crowned mangabeys, Figure 8.1) (T. M. Butynski, J. Kingdon, personal communications). If something other than hunting is responsible for these interspecies transfers, then the need to invoke the hunting hypothesis to explain transfer to humans evaporates.

Perhaps the most viable hypothesis presumes vectorborne transmission. Mosquitoes and other biting arthropods rarely if ever transmit HIV from person to person (Humphery-Smith et al. 1993). But even extremely rare transmission via arthropods could account for the known jumps between species, and could explain the presence of immunodeficiency viruses in a wide spectrum of primates and other mammals. The naturally infected primates have been distributed within arthropod-biting distance in central and west Africa, an area with a great potential for transmission by arthropods. If vectorborne transmission is occurring, the minimum-jumps scenario may be useful because transmission to humans from simians and transmission to simians from humans may occur at comparable frequencies.

Divergent HIV continue to be isolated from people. One of these isolates was recently obtained from a French AIDS patient with no known risk factors (Agut et al. 1992)—and France does not offer much potential for simian-to-human transmission. When such isolates branch off the evolutionary tree prior to simian branches (e.g., ANT 70 or D205 in Figure 8.1) they lend credibility to the idea that HIV has been diverging in humans for a long period of time, and weaken the idea that the divergent isolates are different because they are actually simian viruses that have recently entered humans.

If rare vectorborne transmission from humans to simians is responsible for some of the SIV branches, and the molecular clocks have not been misset, we can expect to see similar jumps from humans to other primates within the next decade or so, because the pool of HIV that can be transmitted from humans is now greater than it was in the past. South African researchers did recently find a virus indistinguishable from HIV-1 in a captive vervet green monkey, but they did not discuss possible routes of transmission (Lecatsas & Alexander 1992).

The origin of HIV-1

On the basis of the nucleic acid sequences of HIV-1, Gerald Myers proposed that the western region of central Africa might be the evolutionary epicenter of the HIV-1 viruses (Sternberg 1992). This proposition is particularly intriguing because the most divergent SIV were isolated from mandrills inhabiting this region. As mentioned above, evolutionary trees indicate that this SIV diverged from the HIV evolutionary tree before HIV-1 and HIV-2 lineages split from a common ancestor (Figure 8.1). HIV isolated from this area during the mid-1980s differed substantially from the pandemic strains (Fleury et al. 1986). The most divergent isolate in the HIV-1 branch (ANT 70) was also isolated from this region, as was one of the chimp viruses (Peeters et al. 1989). A second closely related virus was isolated from a chimp that apparently was infected just to the east in Zaire (Peeters et al. 1992). The evidence is therefore consistent with an early transfer between mandrills and humans in west central Africa.

Myers's proposition brought him criticism from epidemiologists, virologists, and others, who doubted that west central Africa could be the homeland of HIV-1, because a small percentage of people there are infected with HIV-1 (Sternberg 1992, Mavoungou 1992). According to traditional epidemiological thinking, the prevalence of HIV-1 should be at least moderately high in its homeland. But, as we shall see, Myers's proposition accords with epidemiological principles, particularly after evolutionary processes are accounted for.

PARTNER CHANGE AND THE EVOLUTION OF VIRULENCE

Partner change and viral replication

What can considerations of fitness costs and benefits tell us about the evolution of HIV's virulence? Consider a sexually transmitted pathogen in a population of relatively monogamous humans. If it infected a couple, it would have to remain infectious until one member engaged in sexual activity outside the pair. If such outside activity occurred, say, only once every 5 years, the typical durations of infectiousness of directly transmitted pathogens (i.e., several days to a few weeks) would leave the pathogen in a dead-end. Only those pathogen variants that have some way of prolonging infectiousness would be maintained venereally.

To extend infectiousness, pathogens must avoid being destroyed by the host's immune system, while maintaining access to new hosts. One option is to remain latent inside long-lived cells. By integrating into the host chromosome and suppressing production of viral products, a virus can wait out the time period between partner changes. Herpes simplex virus, for example, hides out in neurons and periodically reacts to host stress by activating its reproduction, traveling down the neuron to the skin, and erupting through the skin by way of a blister (McLennan & Darby 1980, Whitley 1990, Banks & Rouse 1992). Retroviruses such as HIV hide out in our white blood cells, which may be long-lived (Spiegel et al. 1992). They can then be transmitted within white blood cells or as recently shed virus during intimate sexual activity. Evolutionarily, the benefits to the virus of extending infectiousness by such means would have to be weighed against the higher rate at which progeny would be produced without latency.

HIV has the raw material for either strategy. Most of infected cells in a person appear to be latently infected (Pomerantz et al. 1992, Embretson et al. 1993a), but throughout each infection, at least some of the viruses are actively reproducing (Schnittman et al. 1991, Michael et al. 1992, Piatak et al. 1993, Pantaleo et al. 1993). Many of the latent viruses have made a DNA copy of their RNA instructions, which has been inserted into the cell's DNA (Seshamma et al. 1992, Zack et al. 1992). The messages for making regulatory proteins appear to be transcribed from this DNA, but messages for the building blocks of new viruses tend not to be (Seshamma et al. 1992); hence few viral components are made. Other HIV appear to produce viral progeny slowly, if at all, by having restricted the process even earlier, before the insertion of viral DNA into the cell's DNA (Ma et al. 1990, Stevenson et al. 1990). A study of SIV indicates that the ease with which strains are differentially activated is at least partly genetically determined (Anderson & Clements 1992).

Imagine a mutation that increases replication rate of the virus either by reducing the tendency of the virus to remain latent or by increasing the replication rate of an actively replicating virus. The mutant virus generally will be similar in structure to its unmutated brethren, but the mutant will generate more progeny within the host during a given amount of time. Its progeny may be decimated by the immune system, but its brethren, which reproduce more slowly, will be especially decimated so long as their structure has not been changed (by mutation and recombination) sufficiently to evade the defenses triggered by the more rapidly reproducing mutant. The important point is this: Mutations that increase viral reproduction rate are continuously favored within an individual host.

Indeed, evolutionary trends toward increased replication within HIV-infected patients have been repeatedly documented, with the highest rates accompanying immune cell depletion and the late symptomatic stages of infection (Åsjö et al. 1986, Cheng-Mayer et al. 1988, Albert et al. 1989, Fenyö et al. 1989, Levy 1989, Tersmette et al. 1989, Schneweiss et al. 1990, Gruters et al. 1991, Schellekens 1992, Connor et al. 1993). Differences between HIV strains in their replication rates are attributable to high reproduction rates within cells and to viral interactions with the cell membrane during entrance into the cell or during fusion of infected cells with uninfected cells (Ma et al. 1990, Fernandez-Larsson et al. 1992, Chowdhury et al. 1992, Hirsch et al. 1992). Viral propagation in cell culture is 100- to 1000-fold greater when transmission occurs through cell fusion than through infection by free virus (Dimitrov et al. 1993).

Rapidly reproducing strains tend to be especially damaging to the cells that house them (Ma et al. 1990, Schneweiss et al. 1990, Hirsch et al. 1992), and both replication rate and cell damage can be readily altered by just a few mutations

(Sakai et al. 1991, De Jong et al. 1992, Fouchier et al. 1992). The potential for variation in reproduction rates within cells is illustrated by the copies of HIV instructions per infected cell. A cell infected with particularly damaging HIV may contain hundreds of copies of the HIV's DNA and millions of copies of the HIV's RNA (Somasundaran & Robinson 1988), and the rate of viral RNA production from viral DNA can increase about 1000-fold over the course of an infection (Michael et al. 1992). Actively replicating HIV normally diverts about 1% or 2% of a cell's protein production, but particularly active HIV may monopolize nearly half of the protein produced in the cell (Somasundaran & Robinson 1988).

The displacement of slow replicators by fast replicators during the course of an infection raises a critical question. What keeps the slowly replicating HIV from being displaced by the rapid replicators in the HIV population as a whole? Answering this question requires an analysis of how AIDS influences transmission.

During AIDS, HIV and its components tend to be more abundant in the blood than they are prior to the onset of AIDS and ARC (AIDS-Related Complex) symptoms (Ho et al. 1989, Fauci et al. 1991, Bagasra et al. 1992). People with AIDS probably have a higher chance of infecting a partner in a given instance of sexual contact than they would prior to symptomatic infection. Accordingly, source individuals who are symptomatic or soon to be symptomatic infect their contacts more frequently than do source individuals who have a longer AIDS-free future (Perkins et al. 1987, Puel et al. 1992, Rossi 1992, Saracco et al. 1993). During ARC and AIDS, however, HIV and its components in the blood increase only slightly, if at all, apparently because the increased numbers of viruses inside cells are offset by the decimation of these cells (Fauci et al. 1991, Hendrix et al. 1991, O'Shea et al. 1991, Schnittman et al. 1991). At some point during infection, the person becomes too ill to engage in sexual contact. At this point, barring any other routes of transmission, the group of HIV within the person is excluded from the evolutionary contest. A process of group selection (*sensu* Wilson 1980) therefore places an upper limit on the virulence to which HIV can evolve. In short, the high replication rates and virulence of AIDS and ARC are selected *for* by competition among genetically different HIV *within* a host, and selected *against* by group selection *among* hosts.

This analysis leads to a key prediction: As sexual partner rates increase, the net benefits to HIV from immediate reproduction should increase. The result should be increased reproductive rate, and hence, increased virulence. By "sexual partner rates," I mean the number of sexual partners weighted by the potential for transmission per partner. This potential reflects the number of unprotected sexual contacts per partner and the kinds of sexual contact (Padian et al. 1987, de Vincenzi et al. 1992).

Infections transmitted from symptomatic versus asymptomatic people

This proposed association between sexual partner rate and HIV virulence assumes that the HIV present at the end of the infection will tend to be the most virulent HIV found during the course of the infection. If this assumption is true, increased virulence should be apparent among people who acquired their infections from people with overt disease.

The time between seroconversion and onset of AIDS is certainly variable enough to find such an association between the disease status of the source individual and the rate of progression to AIDS among the recipients. Although the median time between seroconversion and the onset of AIDS is about ten years, it can be as short as a few months (Isaksson et al. 1988, Pedersen et al. 1989, Rutherford et al. 1990, Kuo et al. 1991). Is this variation solely a consequence of differences among patients, or is it at least partly due to differences in virulence among infecting viruses?

The evidence indicates that the source of virus does influence the outcome. People who were infected from transfusions progressed to AIDS more rapidly when the asymptomatic donors were closer to the onset of symptoms (Perkins et al. 1987, Ward et al. 1989). Similarly, people whose history involved sexual contact with AIDS patients progressed to AIDS more quickly than did people who were infected by asymptomatic individuals (van Griensven et al. 1990). The differences between these sexually infected groups could not be explained by any apparent psychological or behavioral differences between individuals. The more rapid progressors did not have more sexual partners, greater drug use, different psychological states, or more complications from other infectious diseases (van Griensven et al. 1990). These findings therefore support the hypothesis that viruses transmitted late during infection cause accelerated progression to AIDS in recipients because the viruses are particularly virulent.

An alternative explanation for this accelerated progression proposes that the viral dosage increases as the infecting individuals reach more advanced stages of infection. The density of virus in the blood increases by about 10- to 100-fold during the year or so prior to the onset of symptoms and then levels off during the symptomatic period (Ho et al. 1989, Fauci et al. 1991). The rapid progression of infections that were acquired from people with advanced infections therefore could have been a consequence of high dosages.

For sexually transmitted infections, this dosage hypothesis depends on an increasing density of HIV in semen or vaginal fluids. Measurements of HIV in semen have given mixed results, but the measured amounts of HIV do seem to be at least marginally higher when infections progress to AIDS (Coombs et al. 1990, Krieger et al. 1990, Mermin et al. 1991, Anderson et al. 1992). But the rates of unprotected sexual contact during AIDS are probably much lower than during the asymptomatic periods; ill individuals tend to be less interested in sex, and susceptibles probably are less willing to have unprotected sex with them. The total number of HIV entering a susceptible from all sexual contact with a partner suffering from AIDS, therefore, is probably little if any greater than the total from asymptomatically infected individuals. This contention is consistent with the evidence. The chances of having infected a partner rise rapidly when the immune system falters prior to AIDS, but not after progression to AIDS (de Vincenzi et al. 1992). The dosage hypothesis is also weakened by data from hemophiliacs. The rate at which HIV-infected hemophiliacs progressed to AIDS was not significantly associated with the amount of plasma concentrate they had used (Goedert et al. 1989).

The studies correlating the rate of disease progression in source and recipient individuals did not measure the intrinsic replication rate of the transmitted HIV, but a recent study of maternal transmission did (De Rossi et al. 1991b). Children infected with the rapidly reproducing strains that characterize symptomatic disease had higher densities of virus in their blood and progressed more quickly to severe disease than children infected with the more slowly reproducing strains.

The rate of progression to disease is predictable from disease indicators during the first few months of HIV infection. Individuals that have prolonged or intense illness at the beginning of their infections progress to AIDS more rapidly, as do patients who experience the early hints of the immunological suppression that characterizes AIDS (Pedersen et al. 1989, Lifson et al. 1992b, Krämer et al. 1992, Keet et al. 1993). Rapid and slow progressors show similar increases in virus density over the years of an infection, but the rapid progressors have higher levels of virus and greater depletion of target cells during the early months of infection (Ascher et al. 1991, Weiss et al. 1992). Although differences between people appear to explain part of this trend (Sheppard et al. 1991, Fabio et al. 1992, Hentges et al. 1992), they cannot explain it all. Differences in host resistance cannot explain why progression to AIDS is shorter when the source individual has more advanced disease and when the infecting strain is a fast replicator; nor can differences in resistance explain why the early symptomatic disease occurs more frequently when the source individual is at a more advanced stage of infection, or why some particularly benign infections can be traced to a benignly infected source individual (Perkins et al. 1987, Ward et al. 1989, van Griensven et al. 1990, De Rossi et al. 1991b, Learmont et al. 1992). Comparison of viral growth characteristics in source and recipient individuals also suggests that variations in both host and viral characteristics determine the future course of infection (Roos et al. 1992).

Because HIV has the ability to generate variation rapidly, the HIV population that infects a person may be genetically heterogeneous, with rapidly reproducing viruses tending to be shed from infected cells sooner after transmission than more slowly reproducing viruses (Geelen & Goudsmit 1991). This sequence of events has been presented as somehow weakening the predicted correlation between sexual partner rates and virulence (Groopman 1991). Recent evidence, however, suggests that the group of HIV in a newly infected host is relatively homogeneous either because a bottleneck effect occurs during transmission or because disproportionate replication by a small proportion of infecting viruses occurs (Wolfs et al. 1992, Wolinsky et al. 1992). Moreover, any heterogeneity of replication rate within each infecting dose should, if anything, enhance the selection for increased replication as sexual partner rates increase, because more sexual contact will occur shortly after transmission; hence, more of the rapid reproducers in a heterogeneous infecting dose will be transmitted. Both the variation in replication rates within infective doses and the balance between transmission requirements and evolution within hosts therefore lead to the same prediction: Higher sexual partner rates should increase the viral reproductive rates and, hence, the virulence of HIV.

The geographical evidence

HIV-1, HIV-2, and sexual partner rates. The data gathered since the early 1980s are consistent with this prediction. One batch comes from the most fundamental division of HIV: into HIV-1 and HIV-2. Current evidence indicates that HIV-2, like HIV-1, can initiate infections that eventually progress to AIDS (Odehouri et al. 1989, Nauclér et al. 1991). But current evidence also indicates that HIV-2 is less virulent than HIV-1 (Romieu et al. 1990, Pepin et al. 1991, Kanki 1992). Although HIV-2 in Senegal, for example, is associated with some immune suppression and AIDS, 400 person-years of follow-up on HIV-2-infected women revealed only one case of AIDS and one case of ARC (Kanki 1992, Le Guenno et al. 1992). This risk of progression to AIDS is about one-tenth the risk among those with HIV-1 infections (Kanki et al. 1990, Nagelkerke et al. 1990, Kanki 1992). This slow progression of HIV-2 infections to AIDS accords with observations of HIV-2-infected Europeans (Ancelle et al. 1987, Bryceson et al. 1988, Dufoort et al. 1988).

The asymptomatic HIV-2 infections cannot be dismissed as recent infections that have not spanned the amount of time needed for HIV-1 to progress to AIDS. Rates of HIV-2 infection increase steadily with age, a trend indicative of protracted infections with a virus that has been stably present for decades (Essex & Kanki 1988, Poulsen et al. 1989, Kanki et al. 1990, Romieu et al. 1990, Kanki 1992). Individual case histories and stored sera also suggest that HIV-2 has been widespread along the west coast of Africa for decades or longer (Ancelle et al. 1987, Saimot et al. 1987, Bryceson et al. 1988, Kawamura et al. 1989). Yet the frequency of AIDS relative to the frequency of HIV infection in Africa is much lower where HIV-2 predominates than where HIV-1 predominates (Romieu et al. 1990). Among patients with AIDS or AIDS-like symptoms, the occurrence of HIV-1 relative to HIV-2 was greater than that found in the general population;

and patients with AIDS or AIDS-like symptoms tend to deteriorate more rapidly when they are infected with HIV-1 than with HIV-2 (Essex & Kanki 1988, Gody et al. 1988, Romieu et al. 1990, Kanki 1992, Whittle et al. 1992). Similarly, HIV-1 appears to increase vulnerability to tuberculosis more than does HIV-2 (Romieu et al. 1990) and is disproportionately present in cadavers (De Cock et al. 1991).

Differences in enzyme activity may contribute to this difference in virulence. One of HIV's most critical enzymes, reverse transcriptase, transcribes the virus's RNA information into DNA. The reverse transcriptase of HIV-1 works faster than that of HIV-2 (Hizi et al. 1991). Experimental substitutions of reverse transcriptase genes suggest that faster reverse transcriptases lead to faster manufacture of progeny virus, and greater virulence (Hirsch et al. 1992).

Another contributor to this difference between HIV-1 and HIV-2 may be the number of sites in the viral genetic material that activate replication (Cullen & Garrett 1992). Active cells produce a compound, called NF-κB, that stimulates replication of latent HIV by binding to these target sites. HIV-2 has only one viable target site; HIV-1 has two. HIV-2's latency is also more deep-seated: HIV-2 requires activators besides NF-κB that HIV-1 does not require (Leiden et al. 1992). Yet another factor is an accessory gene (called "*vif*") which can enhance virulence in HIV-1, but not in HIV-2 or in the SIV from mandrills (K. Sakai et al. 1991, H. Sakai et al. 1992)

Whatever the biochemical reasons for differences in replication and virulence, data from mother–offspring pairs indicate that HIV-1 is more transmissible than HIV-2 during a given amount of contact. In the Ivory Coast, mothers harboring HIV-1 infected about half of their babies, but mothers with HIV-2 infected less than 10% (Gayle et al. 1992). Mathematical models similarly suggest that transmission per sexual act is four times more likely for HIV-1 than for HIV-2 (Kanki 1992). Apparently, the higher densities of HIV-1 inside people cause the higher probabilities of transmission per contact.

The divergences and variations in RNA sequences (Eigen & Nieselt-Struwe 1990) indicate that HIV-1 was present in humans at least two decades before the pandemic. This conclusion is bolstered by an HIV-positive blood sample drawn in 1959 in Zaire and the presence of HIV in seamen, one who died in the United Kingdom in 1959 from a disease resembling AIDS, and another who apparently was infected during the early 1960s and died of AIDS in the early 1970s (Nahmias et al. 1986, Frøland et al. 1988, Corbitt et al. 1990). AIDS-like diseases were recorded in Europe and North America during the first half of this century and might have resulted from circulating HIV that tended to be relatively asymptomatic until host defenses became compromised (Lange & Klein 1991). Conversations with clinicians in Africa indicate that AIDS cases were very rare prior to the pandemic. Had they occurred in a large proportion of infections, they would have been difficult to overlook unless the number of infections was extremely small (Biggar 1986). The absence of viral isolations prior to 1959 does not mean that the virus was not present in people, because few large samples remain from blood taken prior to the 1960s, particularly in Africa (Biggar 1988). The scarcity of clinical AIDS in central and east Africa before the pandemic is therefore consistent with the idea that pandemic HIV-1 emerging during the 1980s had increased in virulence from an ancestral HIV. The realization that HIV has been circulating in humans for time periods of several decades to many centuries has led researchers to such conclusions, but left them without any clear explanation for when and why such changes in virulence have occurred (Eigen & Nieselt-Struwe 1990).

According to the cost/benefit argument presented above, higher sexual partner rates provide an explanation because they favor evolution of higher virulence. Relative to HIV-1, HIV-2 therefore should have tended to occur in areas with lower sexual partner rates; and the increase in the virulence of HIV-1 should have occurred after an increase in rates of such sexual contact. The available evidence supports this argument.

Historically, HIV-2 tended to occur in west African countries and HIV-1 in central African countries (Essex & Kanki 1988). HIV-1 was inadvertently brought into west African countries during the mid 1980s, largely from residents of those countries who had traveled to central African countries (Böttiger 1988). If the higher virulence of HIV-1 resulted from increased sexual partner rates, the greatest frequency of partner changes should have occurred in the central and east African countries and should have increased there during the years or decades before AIDS began to appear as a common manifestation of HIV-1 infection.

During the 1960s and 1970s extensive migrations occurred from rural areas in central and east Africa because of socioeconomic problems. This mobility in response to economic forces was partly a legacy of the colonial period, during which a migrant labor force developed in response to centralization of jobs. When agricultural options deteriorated, men left the agricultural areas to obtain industrial jobs. The large populations of men without families created a market for sexual commerce, drawing young women from rural into urban areas (Dawson 1988, Schoepf 1988, Clumeck 1989, Hunt 1989). People in west Africa generally did not experience such massive migrations or such increases in sexual contact during the few decades before the AIDS pandemic (Hunt 1989).

The frequency of contacts through prostitution in central and east African countries has been extremely high. In Nairobi, Kenya during 1985, for example, prostitutes averaged nearly 1000 sexual encounters per year in economically poor areas and just over 100 in wealthy areas; about two-thirds of the former and one-third of the latter were seropositive (Kreiss 1986, Piot et al. 1990). Sexual partner rates of prostitutes were slightly lower in Kinshasa, Zaire, where over one-third of the prostitutes were infected by 1987, and where about one-quarter of men at work sites visited prostitutes (Piot et al. 1990, Nzila et al. 1991). Male clients of prostitutes averaged about 30 regular partners per year; males not visiting prostitutes averaged 3 (Cohen & Wofsy 1989).

Contact with prostitutes has been one of the greatest risk factors of HIV-1 infection in Africa. In the mid-1980s, about 80% of HIV-infected men in Rwanda, for example, had sexual contact with prostitutes over a two-year period. Similarly, men that visited prostitutes were more frequently infected with HIV and represented an increased risk of infection for their other sexual partners (Carael et al. 1988, Lindan et al. 1991). For a variety of social and historical reasons high sexual partner rates occurred rather broadly across both rural and urban populations of central and east Africa (Larson 1989, Konings et al. 1989). These high sexual partner rates generated a high potential for HIV transmission, particularly because condoms were used infrequently and other sexually transmitted diseases were prevalent there during the 1970s and early 1980s (Osoba 1981, Moses et al. 1991). Besides being an indicator of high rates of unprotected sexual contact, the other sexually transmitted diseases appear to increase the risk of HIV transmission by causing lesions that permit viral entry into the bloodstream (Carael et al. 1988, Neequaye et al. 1991, Nzila et al. 1991, Martin et al. 1992).

The regional differences in sexual contact inadvertently created an evolutionary experiment. In central and eastern Africa, where sexual contact increased substantially, infections in the HIV-1 lineage changed from being unnoticed to being clearly associated with severe immunodeficiency disease. In most west African countries, where sexual contact did not increase so strongly, HIV-2 did not become as rapidly lethal as HIV-1. This association therefore bolsters the idea that the harmfulness of HIV-1 at the outset of the pandemic resulted from increases in sexual partner rates.

This interpretation assumes that evolutionary changes in virulence occur over a time scale of a few years to a few decades. This assumption is consistent with our current knowledge about HIV's potential for rapid evolution. The mechanism by which HIV replicates inside cells promotes mutations and recombinations (Temin 1989ab, Hu & Temin 1990, Howell et al. 1991); such alterations of HIV's genetic instructions can modify replication rate in a graded way (Luciw et al. 1987, Fujita et al. 1992b). HIV can therefore generate a great deal of variation on which natural selection can act, fostering a high rate of evolution toward increased or decreased virulence.

Variation in virulence within HIV-2. The potential for graded changes in virulence in response to genetically determined changes in replication rates appears to be pervasive throughout the HIV–SIV group. The SIV from mandrills experiences a twofold change in replication rate—with a corresponding change in its destructiveness inside cells—in response to a single mutation in its *transactivating protein* (called "tat") (H. Sakai et al. 1992). HIV-2 also seems to have variations in virulence that accord with replication rate and the generation of symptoms (Albert et al. 1989). Increases in virulence and propagation potential appear to occur readily as a result of simple alterations in one of the virus' envelope proteins (called gp41; Mulligan et al. 1992). Accordingly, the SIV from African green monkeys tends to be asymptomatic in green monkeys and generates a relatively low virus density, comparable to that found among asymptomatic HIV-1 infections in humans (Hartung et al. 1992).

The favoring of rapidly replicating, highly virulent HIV by increased sexual partner rates should apply more strongly within than between HIV groups; viruses that are more similar should tend to trigger stronger immune responses against each other. This cross-reactivity among viruses in the HIV-2 group is generally strong. Immunological protection generated against HIV-2, for example, protects against monkey SIVs (Putkonen et al. 1990). The evolutionary arguments presented above should therefore apply within the HIV-2 group, given sufficient time and sufficient geographical differences in sexual partner rates.

No rigorous attempt has yet been made to determine whether geographical variations in virulence are associated with differences in sexual partner rates, but emerging trends accord with this prediction. Although the data are scanty, a difference seems to be taking shape in the two most extensively studied areas of endemic HIV-2 infection: Senegal and the Ivory Coast.

In Senegal, HIV-2 infections are associated with an especially low progression to AIDS (see above). This mildness is mirrored at the cellular level by the limited data available. A healthy prostitute in Senegal was the source of a strain called HIV-2$_{ST}$, which replicated slowly and caused little damage in cell culture (Kong et al. 1988). This strain was readily converted into a more pathological virus with increased propagative potential by simple genetic changes (Kumar et al. 1990, Mulligan et al. 1992). Researchers have experienced difficulty isolating HIV-2 in Senegalese subjects, apparently because of its reduced rate of entrance into and propagation from cells (Kong et al. 1988).

Senegal did not experience the kind of social change experienced in urban areas of the Ivory Coast, where conditions have been favorable for the spread of HIV-1 (Odehouri et al. 1989, Benoit et al. 1990, Gershy-Damet et al. 1991). In Senegal, several cultural factors may have favored relatively low rates of sexual partner change: an extended family structure encompassing rural and urban residences, an agricultural infrastructure that has survived intact over the past few decades, and Islamic traditions that discourage premarital and extramarital sexual contact (O. F. Linares, personal communication). The Senegal government has also provided incentives to encourage rural youth to remain in the countryside (Gellar 1982). Accordingly, the few direct quantifications of sexual contact in Senegal suggest a low sexual partner rate (Pison et al. 1993).

In Abidjan, HIV-2 seems relatively virulent but heterogeneous. Some but not all strains show cytopathic effects on infected cells (Evans et al. 1988). HIV-2 appears to cause AIDS less frequently than HIV-1 but more frequently than the Senegalese HIV-2 (Odehouri et al. 1989, De Cock et al. 1990ab, Gayle et al. 1992, Kanki 1992). This comparison of Abidjan and Senegal therefore accords with the predicted association between sexual partner rate and HIV-2 virulence.

More precise and detailed analyses are needed both for the Senegal–Abidjan comparison and for other comparisons among regionally distinct HIV-2. The HIV-2 isolated from different geographic regions, and even from neighboring countries in west Africa are often distinct (Albert et al. 1987, Hasegawa et al. 1989). The HIV-2 infections in Guinea Bissau appear to be relatively virulent (Nauclér et al. 1989, 1991), more like those of Abidjan than those of Senegal. On the basis of this difference one would predict that sexual partner rates in Guinea Bissau have been higher than those in Senegal.

Although the HIV-2 in Abidjan, Senegal, and other areas may have been diverging from one another for just a few decades, the evolution from a slow reproducer to a fast reproducer can occur in a much smaller time frame. Just a few passages of one mild HIV-2 strain in cell culture transformed it into a virus that caused cell death more frequently, spread more rapidly among cells, and multiplied to higher numbers (Hoxie et al. 1991).

Variations in virulence within HIV-1.   The argument for evolutionary changes in virulence among HIV-2 strains also applies to HIV-1 strains. When an HIV-1 lineage has had a recent history of particularly rapid transmission through high rates of sexual contact, it should be particularly virulent. During the early years of the epidemic in the United States, the highest rates of transmission apparently occurred among male homosexuals in urban centers, who typically had about ten different sexual partners during a six-month period (Koblin et al. 1992). By 1985, about half of the male homosexuals in San Francisco had become infected (Montgomery & Joseph 1989). If this rapid transmission enhanced virulence, then the viruses infecting male homosexuals during the mid-1980s should have caused especially virulent disease. Most of the HIV that infected hemophiliacs by way of clotting factor was derived from HIV-infected individuals in the late 1970s and early 1980s (Goedert et al. 1989, Lee et al. 1989, Zhang et al. 1991, Fricke et al. 1992). Because most of the untreated homosexuals were infected later in the epidemic, the HIV lineages from the homosexuals should have experienced, on average, a greater degree of rapid cycling through homosexuals than those viruses that contaminated the clotting factor. In accordance with this line of reasoning, the period of time between initial infection and AIDS was shorter among untreated homosexual men than among untreated hemophiliacs (Biggar 1990).

Several other factors may be contributing to the difference in AIDS progression experienced by these two groups. Differences in age, route of transmission, and co-occurring infections could all play a role. Analyses have found correlations between age and more rapid progression (Lee et al. 1991, Eyster et al 1993), but effects of differences in inherent virulence of the infecting HIV have not been adequately evaluated.

Much the difference in progression is attributable to Kaposi's sarcoma, which is a cancer that occurred as an indicator of AIDS more commonly among the homosexual group (Biggar 1990). This difference may represent increased virulence in the sense of a reduced symptom-free period rather than increased mortality, because Kaposi's sarcoma is often associated with earlier onset of AIDS but not earlier death (Hessol et al. 1990). Patients whose AIDS begins with Kaposi's sarcoma may experience reduced severity during the first year of AIDS because Kaposi's sarcoma can occur when the immune system is less suppressed (Hessol et al. 1990, Barillari et al. 1992). Early treatment may also slow the deterioration of Kaposi's patients. The difference in survival between Kaposi's patients and other AIDS patients vanishes, however, after two years of AZT treatment, by which time the HIV tends to become largely resistant to AZT (Moore et al. 1991a, Richman et al. 1991a, Gotzsche et al. 1992; see Chapter 9, this volume). On the other hand, the prolonged survival of Kaposi's sarcoma patients may have been overestimated. One recent study found that Kaposi's sarcoma patients had just as short survival as patients whose AIDS begins with other diseases (d'Arminio Monforte et al. 1992).

This association of Kaposi's sarcoma with homosexuality has perplexed researchers. One most widespread belief is that Kaposi's sarcoma results from the presence of another pathogen (Beral et al. 1991, Wahman et al. 1991). To support this idea, researchers point to the high prevalence of Kaposi's sarcoma (1) in primary epidemic centers, (2) during the first half of the 1980s, (3) among heterosexual and homosexual partners of men with Kaposi's sarcoma, and (4) among homosexual men who had more oral–anal contact (Abrams 1991, Beral 1991, Schechter et al. 1991a, Wahman et al. 1991, Beral et al. 1992).

One or more other pathogens may well be involved, but all of the preceding risk factors are consistent with the possibility that the increased frequency of Kaposi's sarcoma results at least in part from infection with viruses that evolved high rates of replication in response to high sexual partner rates. Since the early days of the epidemic, Kaposi's sarcoma has been particularly prevalent among people who had many different partners (Montgomery & Joseph 1989, Beral 1991). The decline in Kaposi's sarcoma since the mid-1980s can be explained by the lower sexual partner rates disfavoring the most rapidly reproducing strains. Similarly, according to the evolutionary arguments of this chapter, the faster reproducing HIV should have been more common in the primary epidemic centers and among people who acquired their infection from men with Kaposi's sarcoma. Because men who engaged frequently in oral–anal contact tended to be more sexually active (Beral et al. 1992), they should also tend to have acquired rapidly replicating HIV. Accordingly, a recent study showed that men with many partners progressed to AIDS more rapidly even when the occurrence of Kaposi's sarcoma was comparable to that among slower progressors (Phair et al. 1992).

When viewed in isolation, a fecally transmitted co-infecting organism seems to provide a reasonable explanation for the preponderance of Kaposi's sarcoma among male homosexuals (Beral 1991, Beral et al. 1992). But this explanation is weakened by recent results from Sydney, Australia: Kaposi's sarcoma declined strongly among homosexual and bisexual men even though oral–anal contact did not (Elford et al. 1992). The argument based on orally-acquired fecal pathogens also fails to explain the high rates of Kaposi's sarcoma among heterosexuals infected with HIV-1 in Africa. Because these high rates occur in areas of central Africa that have had high rates of sexual contact (see above and Beral 1991), the rapid replication argument offers a feasible explanation. The decline in Kaposi's sarcoma among American heterosexuals is also consistent with an evolutionary reduction in virulence, because these Kaposi's cases tended to be infected by bisexuals who had Kaposi's (Beral 1991).

The occurrence of Kaposi's sarcoma among people who are not infected with HIV has been offered as evidence that some pathogen other than HIV is responsible for the high rates of HIV among homosexual men. But the presence of Kaposi's sarcoma in the absence of HIV infection means only that the abnormal growth of cells that manifests itself as Kaposi's sarcoma can result from processes that can occur in the absence of HIV. It does not negate the idea that more rapidly replicating HIV can cause a higher incidence of Kaposi's sarcoma among male homosexuals by contributing to such processes or by triggering similar processes.

Efforts to find some cofactor responsible for the high rate of Kaposi's sarcoma among homosexual men have not identified a culprit despite more than a decade of investigation (Drew 1986, Biggar 1990, Gallo 1991, Peterman et al. 1991, Wahman et al. 1991). This lack of success lends credibility by default to the possibility that the higher rates of Kaposi's sarcoma among male homosexuals early during the pandemic reflect at least in part a more virulent character of the infecting HIV-1.

Biochemical knowledge about Kaposi's sarcoma also lends credibility to this hypothesis. Current evidence indicates that growth of Kaposi's sarcoma is stimulated by HIV's tat protein, which helps transform latent or sluggishly replicating HIV into actively replicating HIV (Ensoli et al. 1990, 1993, Barillari et al. 1992, Buonaguro et al. 1992). High rates of sexual partner change should favor HIV that replicate early during infection; and early replication means greater overall production of tat—cells that are infected with rapidly replicating HIV may produce more tat (Ma et al. 1990) and rapid replication may lead to a greater number of infected cells. The role of tat in HIV replication and Kaposi's sarcoma, together with the evolutionary effects of sexual partner rates, therefore offer an explanation for the disproportionate occurrence of Kaposi's sarcoma among men who were very active sexually in urban centers during the early 1980s.

This tat mechanism also offers an explanation for an apparent paradox. Kaposi's sarcoma gradually became a less common early indicator of AIDS, but the occurrence of Kaposi's sarcoma after the onset of AIDS declined little, if at all, in some groups (Rutherford et al. 1989, Peters et al. 1991). This continuing presence of Kaposi's sarcoma is difficult to explain if the changes in Kaposi's sarcoma as an early indicator of AIDS resulted solely from the presence or absence of an infectious cofactor. The continuing presence of Kaposi's sarcoma, however, makes sense if the probability of developing Kaposi's sarcoma depends on increased exposure to tat. As AIDS wears on, the exposure to tat accumulates.

Even if another infectious cause of Kaposi's sarcoma is found, its existence does not imply that it is solely responsible for Kaposi's sarcoma as an early indicator of AIDS among homosexuals. Indeed the mechanism by which tat stimulates Kaposi's sarcoma appears to depends on activation of the immune system by other pathogens (Barillari et al. 1992). Evidence also suggests that another retrovirus, called HTLV-I (human T-cell lymphotropic virus type I; see Chapter 11), can trigger Kaposi's sarcoma (Veyssier-Belot 1990, Morozov et al. 1992). HTLV-I produces an activating protein (called "tax") that is similar in structure and function to tat. The identification of HTLV-induced Kaposi's sarcoma may therefore strengthen rather than weaken the argument that the higher rate of Kaposi's sarcoma among homosexuals results directly from HIV and the tat it produces. The specific cofactor alternative would be strengthened only if the cofactor is associated with the increased incidence of Kaposi's sarcoma among male homosexuals.

The tat mechanism also helps explain why people whose AIDS begin with Kaposi's sarcoma develop AIDS sooner after infection but do not die sooner (Hessol et al. 1990). Most current hypotheses propose that prolonged viral activity triggers the destruction of the immune system. The immune system seems well-equipped to deal with a burst of replication by HIV during the first few months of infection, but not with the prolonged assault that HIV imposes. The problem for the immune system is compounded by the increasing rate at which the viruses tend to reproduce and damage cells as the infection drags on (Tersmette & Miedema 1990, Roos et al. 1992, Schellekens 1992). If the prolonged infection and steadily increasing viral replication rate are primary causes of immune decimation, the active replication early during infection may bring about Kaposi's sarcoma more rapidly [because more tat is produced; see, for example, Ma et al. (1990)], without bringing about a more rapid decimation of the immune system.

This tat mechanism provides a basis for the decline in Kaposi's sarcoma that occurred during the latter half of the 1980s. After sexual partner rates among gay men declined around 1984, virus variants with lax requirements for breaking latency would tend to be destroyed by the immune system before being passed on, leaving a higher proportion of viruses that tend to enter latency upon infection. The result would be a lower proportion of Kaposi's sarcoma as the AIDS-defining event during the ensuing years. This selection against nonlatent viruses would occur sooner after the reduction in sexual contact than any selection due to the disease itself, particularly if the reduction in sexual contact reduced the general level of immune activation, which primes cells to generate Kaposi's sarcoma in response to tat (Barillari et al. 1992).

In proposing this scenario I acknowledge that there may be several factors contributing to Kaposi's sarcoma. Infectious organisms other than HIV may be one such factor. My argument stresses, however, that the declining rates of Kaposi's sarcoma can be explained without invoking declining rates of infection by a specific undiscovered organism. Because these two hypotheses are not mutually exclusive, both demand further testing.

One might argue that the selective process has been too weak to cause such a marked change in Kaposi's sarcoma within a few years of the drop in sexual partner rates. Perhaps so, but it is important to realize that this selective process would be amplified by active avoidance of people with the visible markings of Kaposi's sarcoma. This avoidance probably began when the purplish spots of Kaposi's sarcoma were first associated with AIDS, two or three years before the major decline in rates of sexual partner change. This early selection against Kaposi-producing pathogens would occur, whether the pathogens were rapidly replicating HIV alone, or HIV in conjunction with some other pathogen.

Geographic comparisons are also consistent with the idea that HIV-1 is more virulent where rates of sexual contact are high. In Kinshasa, Zaire, for example, high sexual partner rates have been associated with high mortality rates and high rates of progression to AIDS following transfusion of infected blood (Cohen & Wofsy 1989, Colebunders et al. 1991). Similarly, during the rapid rise of the AIDS pandemic, Nairobi prostitutes experienced some of the highest unprotected sexual partner rates in the world (Kreiss et al. 1986), and they tended to progress very rapidly to severe disease (Colebunders et al. 1991). Accordingly, HIV isolated from these areas can be particularly damaging when grown in cell culture (e.g., Hirsch et al. 1992). Of course, these comparisons do not take into account several other possible influences on the severity of HIV infections, but they do demonstrate the need to assess whether HIV-1 is inherently more virulent in geographic areas in which sexual partner rates are relatively high.

Geographic invasions by HIV-1. The patterns of HIV virulence described above certainly do not prove that the evolutionary arguments are correct, but they do represent variation in disease severity consistent with the evolutionary arguments, and not predicted by any other general theory. Besides drawing attention to the need for more precise measurements of virulence and sexual partner rates, these patterns provide a basis for investigating the outcome of geographic invasions by HIV-1.

The geographic patterns of HIV-1 and HIV-2 fit with the idea that HIV-2 is adapted for slow transmission in areas with lower sexual contact and HIV-1 for more rapid transmission in areas with higher sexual contact. Areas where HIV-2 predominates tend to have lower prevalences of HIV infection than adjacent areas where HIV-1 predominates. This trend occurs on a broad geographic scale from western to central African countries (Hughes & Corrah 1990) as well as on a finer scale within countries (Gershy-Damet et al. 1991).

These differences in geographic distribution of HIV-1 are attributable largely to differences in its ability to invade areas where HIV-2 has predominated. HIV-1 has invaded the west African cities whose growth most strongly resembles the growth of central and east African population centers. Abidjan, for example, is a west African city that has experienced massive urban immigration and social disruption. After quadrupling since the mid-1970s, its population now stands at about two million. HIV-1 is about twice as prevalent as HIV-2 within the greater Abidjan area, but in rural areas of the Ivory Coast the two HIVs are similar in abundance (Odehouri et al. 1989, Gershy-Damet et al. 1991). A few hundred miles northwest of the Ivory Coast is Guinea-Bissau, whose largest city is less than one-tenth the size of Abidjan. In Guinea-Bissau, HIV-2 is common and HIV-1 rare (Nauclér et al. 1991, Ferro et al. 1992).

An alternative explanation for this geographic trend is that HIV-1 has recently entered western Africa by chance in urban areas and is in the process of spreading to rural areas. Information gathered during the next decade should reveal whether this greater prevalence of HIV-1 in urban west Africa reflects competitive superiority of more virulent HIV in certain urban areas and more benign HIV in rural areas, or whether these differences are just a timing artifact. The limited comparisons that have been done to date suggest that the prevalence of HIV-1 and HIV-2 are remaining relatively stable in areas of west Africa where HIV-2 predominates, such as Gambia, Guinea Bissau, and rural areas of Ivory Coast (Ouattara et al. 1989, Del Mistro et al. 1992, Ferro et al. 1992). The prevalence of HIV-1 has been similarly low and stable in some rural areas of central Africa (Montagnier 1986, Nzilambi et al. 1988). In Senegal and in Abidjan, HIV-1 has spread among prostitutes over the past decade, but only in Abidjan has it spread extensively in the general population; the prevalence of HIV-2 among prostitutes has been relatively stable in both Senegal and Abidjan during this period (Le Guenno et al. 1991, Kanki 1992, Koffi et al. 1993).

As HIV-1 invades areas with different rates of sexual contact, its virulence should become lower in the low-contact areas. I predict, for example, that a decade or two from now, any HIV-1 lineages endemic to Senegal will be less virulent than those endemic to nearby areas where rates of transmissible sexual contact remain higher.

What will happen to HIV-1 after it enters areas in which HIV-2 has predominate may depend partly on the degree to which the two interfere with each other. Such interference probably does occur to some extent when both viruses occur within an individual. Because the viruses cross-react immunologically (Barin et al. 1987, Tedder et al. 1988), infection by one virus could hinder the development of the other; however, this cross-reactivity is much less than that occurring between viruses in the HIV-2 group and its SIV relatives (Robert-Guroff et al. 1992). Whatever immunological interference exists would probably be highest after the primary infection but before severe immune suppression sets in, because during this window of time virus levels are suppressed by the still-intact immune system.

HIV-1 and HIV-2 also directly interfere with each other when they attack the same cell; infected cells block or eliminate the receptors to which other viruses outside the cell need to attach in order to enter the cell (Hart & Cloyd 1990). Although the numbers of infected cells are low early in infection, they rise rapidly as infections approach the symptomatic stage, thus increasing the potential for this interference. HIV-2 seems to interfere more with HIV-1 than vice versa (Hart & Cloyd 1990). When rates of sexual contact are low, HIV-2 therefore may have a greater ability to stand its ground against HIV-1 than one would expect on the basis of replication rates. When rates of sexual contact with susceptibles are high, however, the fast replicating HIV-1 should spread to susceptibles at a faster rate than HIV-2.

The strength of this competition might seem minuscule if one considers only the overall prevalences of the two HIVs. But much of the transmission occurs within high-risk groups in which HIV prevalences may be high. In Abidjan, where HIV-1 predominates, about one in ten prostitutes over the age of 30 are infected with both HIV-1 and HIV-2 (Diallo et al. 1992). In Senegal, the scarcity of HIV-1 (Kanki et al. 1992) generates a lower ratio: about one joint infection for every 100 prostitutes. Such simultaneous infections with HIV-1 and HIV-2, and at least one case of sequential infection indicate, however, that the interference between the pathogens is not strong enough for one HIV to prohibit spread of the other, even within infected individuals (Boudart et al. 1992, George et al. 1992).

Geography, adaptation, and the origin of HIV

The origin of HIV-1. If we trace invasions of HIV-1 back through time, we should ultimately arrive at the homeland of HIV-1. As I mentioned at the end of the first section of this chapter, the HIV researcher Gerald Myers was recently criticized for proposing that west central Africa is this homeland. The criticism was based on the low prevalence of HIV-1 infection there (Sternberg 1992). This low prevalence, however, is consistent with the preceding evolutionary analysis. HIV-2 in west African countries has a lower level of replication, a lower virulence, a more smoldering transmission, and a lower prevalence than HIV-1 in eastern and central Africa (Kanki et al. 1990, Romieu et al. 1990, Ewald 1991b). The same should be true of HIV-1 strains that have evolved endemically in populations that did not experience a surge in sexual contact. The surge in central and east Africa was driven by a paucity of jobs (Schoepf 1988, Hunt 1989), a paucity which did not occur in west central Africa. In Gabon, for example, there have been labor shortages (U.S. Department of State 1986). In Cameroon, the economy has remained relatively stable during the past three decades; it has provided relatively favorable economic opportunities for women, resulting in less prostitution than in those central and east African countries that have been particularly hard-hit by AIDS (Azevedo et al. 1989). Because the west central African countries did not experience the increase in sexual contact experienced by their neighbors to the east, evolutionary considerations suggest that the epidemiological characteristics of HIV-1 lineages long endemic to west central Africa will resemble those of west African HIV-2 strains more than the pandemic HIV-1 strains. That is, we can expect such strains of HIV-1 to have a lower, more stable prevalence than the HIV-1 strains in mid-central and east Africa.

If this stable prevalence has occurred, infections with these central west African lineages of HIV-1 should progress steadily with age, as infections with HIV-2 do in west African countries, rather than showing the steep epidemic hump among people between 20 and 40 years of age that typifies HIV-1 infections in east central Africa. The data in the literature are not yet sufficiently precise to test this prediction, but they are suggestive. HIV-1 in Gabon, for example, peaks in the 30–39 age group, with the 40–54 age group and 20–29 age group having lower but similar rates (Schrijvers et al. 1991). These rates, however, do not separate any long endemic lineages from non-endemic lineages that have reinvaded west central Africa.

This evolutionary argument also can be tested by assessing the virulence of the long-endemic west African HIV-1 lineages in humans by quantifying, for example, the time between the onset of infection and the onset of AIDS. The evolutionary theory predicts that the virulence and replication rates of these lineages should be lower than those of the lineages in mid-central and east Africa.

Is immunodeficiency a sign of recency?   The arguments developed in the preceding sections help explain why researchers were so ready to conclude that the HIVs recently jumped from nonhuman primates to humans, in spite of the consistency between the available evidence and a long association of HIV with humans. The first part of this explanation is psychological. The question researchers asked shaped the answer they found. People wondered where this pandemic came from. The isolation of related viruses from green monkeys, mandrills, mangabeys, macaques, and chimpanzees provided an answer: the HIVs jumped into humans from these simians. Had the green monkeys or mangabeys been conducting the research, they might have concluded prematurely that humans were the source of their SIVs.

The second part of this explanation invokes the idea that old associations are benign. HIV causes AIDS in humans. SIVs do not seem to cause AIDS in mangabeys, green monkeys, or chimpanzees, but can cause an AIDS-like disease in rhesus monkeys and macaques. If old associations are benign, green monkeys, mangabeys, and chimps must be the older hosts.

The logic presented in this chapter offers an alternative. Because immunodeficiency viruses are venereally transmitted, they must survive in the host for a period comparable to the time between partner changes. Generally this requirement means that they must infect long-lived cells without triggering immunological destruction of the cells. Specialization on cells of the immune system allows them to do so, but also requires suppressed reproduction if partner changes are infrequent. If, however, rates of partner change increase, natural selection should favor increased rates of viral reproduction, such as those exhibited by HIV-1. Yet even among HIV-1 variants, these rates must be relatively restricted because the virus has specialized on critical cells of the immune system. If HIV were to replicate explosively, the infected person would probably die during the early symptomatic stage rather than after many years of infection. Indeed, a variant of SIV that was transmitted experimentally in a way that favored such variants, soon replicated explosively, causing death of infected macaques within two weeks of inoculation (Lewis et al 1992). Such a rapid progression rarely, if ever, occurs among HIV infections of humans.

The evolutionary approach presented here suggests that specialization on immune cells generally favors the evolution of suppressed growth rates, and that increases in sexual partner rates relax this suppression; even a slight relaxation may be enough to destroy the immune system after ten years of infection. The growth of HIV-1 in cell culture offers evidence of how strong this suppression may be. The slowly growing viruses that tend to be isolated during the asymptomatic periods of infection are difficult to grow continuously in most cell cultures. The more rapidly replicating viruses that are typical of the later stages of infection can be propagated more easily in a variety of cell types (Åsjö et al. 1986, Fenyö et al. 1989, Korneyeva et al. 1993).

If an SIV or HIV is transferred into a new species, it will tend to be eliminated by the immune system because immune systems must be able to deal with a wide variety of would-be pathogens. This argument is analogous to that presented in Chapter 3 to explain why vectorborne pathogens will tend to be relatively benign in new host species. But unlike vectorborne pathogens, immunodeficiency viruses should generally evolve toward very restricted reproduction because they are infecting critical cells of the immune system. In those relatively few situations in which the virus has the ability to productively infect a new host species, it is unlikely also to have, by chance, a finely tuned mechanism for restricting its reproduction in the new biochemical environment. These considerations suggest that HIV and SIV will tend to be relatively severe when they first take hold in new host species. But this tendency does not necessarily mean that severe immunodeficiency indicates a new virus/host association. Severe immunodeficiency could develop in an old association, as a result of increases in sexual partner rates causing evolution of increased virulence.

THE FUTURE OF AIDS

Altering sexual transmission

By understanding the evolution of HIV one can assess not only why a high level of virulence evolved in the past, but also how virulence may evolve in the future, and, most importantly, how human activities can influence this future evolution. If rates of unprotected sexual contact decline, so should the virulence of HIV. Because it is the illness and death that ultimately disfavor the most virulent strains, a slowing of the progression to AIDS in response to reductions in sexual contact cannot be detected until a sufficiently high proportion of infected individuals become ill. What is sufficiently high depends on the sensitivity of detection.

The rates of transmissible sexual contact among urban male homosexuals began to decline sharply around 1984, in response to improved knowledge about sexual transmission of HIV (Stall et al. 1988). About 10% of the male homosexuals infected around this time developed AIDS within four years (Curran et al. 1988, Phair et al. 1992). If AIDS developed early in these 10% largely because they were infected with the most virulent strains, and if transmission from them was drastically reduced as a result of the drop in sexual contact, the time between the onset of infection and the onset of AIDS might have been lengthened detectably by the end of the 1980s. The ability to detect such a trend is confounded by the effects of AZT treatment, but Rosenberg et al. (1991) have published a statistically sophisticated analysis that accounts for these effects. They found that the lengthening of the time between the onset of infection and AIDS that occurred among male homosexuals prior to 1988 could be explained entirely by AZT treatment. After mid-1988, however, there was an additional lengthening that could not be explained by AZT treatment. In an attempt to explain this lengthening, Rosenberg and his colleagues (1991) suggested that physicians might have been treating AIDS patients effectively without recognizing that the patients had AIDS. But generally the reverse is considered true: As an epidemic proceeds, physicians become more familiar with diagnostic criteria and identify disease entities sooner. In contrast with such *a posteriori* hypotheses, the evolutionary hypothesis of HIV virulence predicted, *a priori*, that such a lengthening would eventually occur in response to reduced rates of partner change (Ewald 1991b).

The evolutionary hypothesis also predicts that the HIV isolated just before the decline in sexual partner rates should be more virulent than those HIV isolated earlier, before this rapid cycling among homosexual men. The infections among homosexuals tabulated by International Registry of Seroconverters (supplied by R. J. Biggar) support this prediction. Men who were infected prior to 1980 progressed to AIDS at a slower rate than those men who were infected between 1982 and 1984.

The evolutionary hypothesis also may help resolve a finding that Rosenberg and his colleagues (1991) found anomalous. Homosexual intravenous drug users had unexpectedly slow progression to AIDS near the end of the decade, even though they almost never used AZT. This pattern is consistent with the evolutionary hypothesis so long as a large proportion of these people acquired their infections homosexually.

Data gathered during the next few years should firmly resolve whether the predicted evolutionary decline in virulence is occurring. The nonevolutionary, post-hoc explanations predict that the slower than expected progression should vanish as reporting and diagnostic techniques are standardized and any artifacts are accounted for.

A sustained lengthening in the asymptomatic period is expected from evolutionary considerations because risky contact by homosexuals declined consistently during the mid-1980s. Among homosexual men in Chicago, for example, the frequency of unprotected anal intercourse dropped from about 40% in 1986 to about 20% in 1988 (Adib et al. 1991). In San Francisco, a comparable drop occurred among nonmonogamous homosexuals, from about 50% in 1984 to 12% in 1988 (Sittitrai et al. 1990); the number of partners declined similarly during this period (Winkelstein et al. 1988). The use of condoms has increased dramatically among homosexual men in San Francisco; the proportion always or nearly always using condoms is now about five times greater than among single San Franciscan heterosexuals of similar age and race. For people with two or more sexual partners, condom use is ten times greater among homosexuals (Catania et al. 1992). The reductions are somewhat weaker than these figures indicate, however, because about half of those who begin safer sexual practices at one point may relapse into unsafe sexual practices at a later time (Adib et al. 1991). Although heterosexuals have initiated safer sexual practices over the last decade, the reductions that have occurred are still small relative to the potential for further reductions (Catania et al. 1992).

The reductions in unprotected sexual contact are associated with declines in new infections among urban homosexual and bisexual men (Kingsley et al. 1991). The seroconversion rates leveled off during the late 1980s to about one-tenth of the rate that had occurred among these groups before knowledge about HIV transmission became widespread (Kingsley et al. 1991). In San Francisco, the fall has been even more precipitous (Winkelstein et al. 1988, Bacchetti & Moss 1989).

Rates of unprotected sexual contact have been declining generally in North America, Europe, and Africa since the mid-1980's (Ijsselmuiden et al. 1988, van Griensven et al. 1989, Samuel et al. 1991). In other parts of the world, rates of unprotected sexual contact have shown smaller reductions in response to improved knowledge about AIDS. Brazil, for example, reported one of the highest prevalences of AIDS in the world during the 1980s. Among poor prostitutes in Rio de Janeiro, 80% did not change their sexual practices in response to AIDS prevention campaigns there (De Meis et al. 1991). They typically had more than five sexual contacts per day, most of them without condoms. In 1989, about 10% were infected with HIV (De Meis et al. 1991). Heterosexually infected AIDS patients in Brazil survive for half as long as comparable groups of AIDS patients in the United States and Europe (Chequer et al. 1992), but the relative contributions of HIV virulence and lack of effective treatment are yet to be determined.

These geographic differences suggest that an unplanned, global, evolutionary experiment is now occurring. The geographic areas in which transmission rates are being reduced are the experimental groups. The areas in which transmission rates are not being reduced are the controls. The HIV in the control areas are predicted to remain virulent relative to the experimental areas. In India and Thailand, for example, independent lineages of HIV-1 have recently spread rapidly, suggesting rapid sexual transmission (Clements 1992, Lenihan 1992, McCutchan et al. 1992, Pfützner et al. 1992, Dietrich et al. 1993). Sexual partner rates among Thai prostitutes and their clients appear comparable to the high rates observed in central and east Africa (Rehle et al. 1992). If high rates of transmission continue, HIV-1 should remain highly virulent or increase in virulence in these countries. HIV-2 also has been found recently in India and appears to be spreading rapidly (Pfützner et al. 1992, Babu et al. 1993). If the tradeoffs analysed in this chapter are correct, HIV-2 may now be evolving increased virulence in India.

I am certainly not advocating that we should try to keep the transmission rates high in these areas to foster this global experiment. Considering the ethical issues involved, I would use the evolutionary approach to advocate just the opposite: that we should invest heavily in programs to reduce HIV virulence by reducing rates of transmission. Such interventions would, however, alter the predictions. For example, if recent campaigns to reduce HIV transmission in Thailand (Lenihan 1992) prove successful, we can expect the virulence to eventually fall.

One of the most cost-effective ways of reducing rates of HIV transmission is to focus intensive educational programs and condom distribution efforts among those individuals with the highest rates of sexual contact. Such a program was enacted in 1985 among prostitutes in Nairobi, Kenya. Calculations indicate that the program spends about $10 for each HIV infection prevented; thus, about 10 to 100 infections could be prevented for the cost of treating a single person there with AIDS (Moses et al. 1991). Targeting couples with one HIV-infected partner has been successful in Rwanda: When condom use increased from 4% to 57% over a two-year period, the infection rate fell by half (Allen et al. 1992). Expanding the program to reach individuals with lower rates of sexual contact will undoubtedly increase the cost per life saved from AIDS. But considering the massive difference between the high costs of caring for AIDS patients and the low cost of preventing HIV infection, such an expansion could certainly be justified solely on the reduced frequencies of infection. The added benefit from the evolutionary reductions in pathogen virulence that should accompany this kind of intervention (not to mention the lives saved and the demonstrated reductions in other sexually transmitted diseases; Moses et al. 1991) makes such expansions even more cost effective. Condom use and accessibility have been low in most African countries, and other sexually transmitted diseases (which can increase vulnerability to HIV) have been common (Harrison et al. 1991, Lindan et al. 1991, Moses et al. 1991, Neequaye et al. 1991, Allen et al. 1992, Miller et al. 1992). Programs to increase the use of condoms, particularly those with antiviral additives, therefore offer great potential for reducing HIV transmission and hence virulence.

Altering needleborne transmission

Transmission of pathogens through hypodermic needles, like transmission by mosquitoes (and like needleborne malaria; see Chapter 3), should favor virulent genotypes. Unlike a potential sexual partner, needles do not shy away from contact with AIDS cases, nor do needles get ill or protect themselves against infection. Moreover, an intravenous drug addict, severely ill with AIDS, probably is more motivated to obtain a fix than sex. Needleborne transmission of HIV may therefore involve a cultural vector. The most obvious analogy to mosquito-borne and attendant-borne transmission occurs when injection equipment is transported to and from users by drug dealers or friends. But the transport of an ill, infected person to a "shooting gallery" also fulfills the definition of a cultural vector because it permits transmission from an immobilized infected person to susceptibles. The definition of a cultural vector is similarly fulfilled by the transport of ill people to traditional healers, if the healers then transmit HIV infection by skin-piercing procedures. Such transport of ill patients to traditional healers in conjunction with reuse of unsterile surgical equipment commonly occurs, for example, in west African countries, but any association with HIV infection remains unclear (Harrison et al. 1991, Neequaye et al. 1991).

Because HIV may remain viable on injection equipment for several days (Resnick et al. 1986, Tjøtta et al. 1991) and because drug addicts typically have many injections per week, needleborne transmission offers a great potential for HIV transmission. This potential was tragically demonstrated during the last eight months of 1988 in Elista, a Russian city near the Caspian Sea. When sterilization procedures were neglected in a hospital there, over fifty children were infected by needleborne HIV from a single infected patient; seven women apparently contracted infection from breastfeeding their infected children (Belitsky 1989, Pokrovsky 1989, 1990).

The potential evolutionary importance of needleborne transmission depends on its frequency relative to other modes of transmission as well as its absolute frequency.   At the very beginning of the AIDS pandemic, needleborne transmission was apparently rare, but this situation began to change in many regions soon after the pandemic took hold. Intravenous drug transmission has been responsible for much of the transmission in the United States since the early years of the pandemic (DesJarlais & Friedman 1988). By the end of the 1980s, New York City had nearly a quarter million intravenous drug abusers infected with HIV, with about 20,000 people added annually to the total. HIV has surged similarly among drug users in the United Kingdom, Italy, and Thailand (DesJarlais & Friedman 1988, 1989, Blattner 1991, Salmaso et al. 1991). During the past few years, intravenous drug users have comprised about one-quarter to one-half of all AIDS cases in the United States and Europe, and they are increasingly infected in developing countries such as Brazil and Thailand (DesJarlais & Friedman 1988, 1989; Piot et al. 1990, Guiguet et al. 1991). In Italy, for example, the lower rates of sexual transmission make intravenous drug transmission relatively more prevalent (Cargnel et al. 1991). In recent years the situation in the United States has been moving in this direction (Centers for Disease Control 1989).

In Europe, Australia, and the United States, the time interval between infection and AIDS among intravenous drug users has tended to be shorter but not significantly shorter than that among male homosexuals (Biggar 1990 as corrected by personal communication, Mariotto et al. 1992, Rezza et al. 1992a). Interpretations of this difference are ambiguous because of the small numbers of drug users in these studies. A recent study from New York City (Selwyn et al. 1992) found a progression of untreated asymptomatic infections to AIDS among drug users that was nearly twice as great as that found among homosexual men (Volberding et al. 1990). This difference draws attention to the need for further study of drug users using statistical methods that distinguish inherent virulence of HIV from other variables that might increase the vulnerability of intravenous drug users to rapid progression of HIV infection.

Intravenous drug users were not as quick as male homosexuals to change their risky behavior during the early 1980s, and the subsequent progress at reducing risk among intravenous drug users has also been less consistent (Fisher & Fisher 1992, van den Hoek et al. 1992). Accordingly, the interval from the onset of infection to AIDS has not lengthened more than predicted on the basis of AZT use (Rosenberg et al. 1991). That is, in contrast to the situation among male homosexuals during the late 1980s, there is no evidence that virulence of HIV infections among intravenous drug users has diminished.

In this regard, it is interesting that heterosexuals also did not experience this AZT-independent lengthening of the interval between the onset of infection and AIDS (Rosenberg et al. 1991). This lack of reduction is consistent with the evolutionary interpretation of HIV virulence because reductions in risky behavior among heterosexuals were not as early nor as dramatic as those found among homosexuals, and heterosexuals are frequently infected from intravenous drug users (van den Hoek et al. 1992).

Reductions in needleborne transmission should lead to evolutionary reductions in virulence. Epidemiological data indicate that risky behavior and needleborne transmission can be reduced through education, needle exchange, and rehabilitation, without increasing the number of addicts (Des Jarlais & Friedman 1988, Barthwell et al. 1989, Magura et al. 1989, van den Hoek, et al. 1989, Skidmore et al. 1990, O'Keefe et al. 1991, West 1991, McCusker et al. 1992). But even participants in programs may often take part in high-risk activities. In a methadone treatment program in New York City during the late 1980s, patients averaged five shots in a shooting gallery and eight shared uses of injection equipment in a typical month (West 1991). Particularly relevant is the finding that addicts often share needles because of the scarcity and cost of needles on the street and fear of arrest for possession of needles. These factors force many to risk the kinds of needle borne transmission that should especially favor the evolution of increased virulence: the use of house works provided by drug dealers and the rental of equipment in shooting galleries (O'Keefe et al. 1991). Accordingly, in areas where needles can be purchased or exchanged legally, high-risk needle-sharing tends to be lower (Calsyn et al. 1991).

The reductions achieved by intervention programs may be partially negated when funds are inadequate: drawing addicts together in programs may increase transmission when follow-through on testing, counseling and rehabilitation is delayed (West 1991). Fully funded intervention measures should, conversely, reduce virulence by reducing transmission rates. Because intravenous drug users tend to have higher than average rates of unprotected sexual contact (Guiguet et al. 1991, Saxon et al. 1991), interventions combining reduced needleborne transmission and reduced sexual transmission are needed.

Increasing the limited funding for such programs may have a far greater positive effect on health than is presently estimated, because current estimates do not take into account evolutionary decreases in virulence. Measuring virulence indicators during long-term interventions such as needle exchange and education programs could provide direct tests of the predicted decline in virulence. Specifically, measurements of reverse transcriptase activity, viral load, blood indicators of disease progression, and time until onset of symptoms could be used in concert to estimate virulence throughout the intervention.

Compared with the costs of treatment, interventions designed to reduce needleborne and sexual transmission are relatively inexpensive, even if one considers only the reduction in the spread of HIV attributable to nonevolutionary processes (Moses et al. 1991, O'Keefe et al. 1991). The evolutionary approach outlined above simply draws attention to a generally unrecognized dimension of the problem. So long as our basic principles of evolution are correct, these interventions should provide an added benefit that will make them even more worthy of funding: The HIV in these regions should become more benign.

Psychological studies suggest that changing high-risk behavior necessitates a three-pronged approach: (1) education about transmission and prevention, (2) motivation to reduce risky behavior, and (3) skills that allow the educated, motivated individual to reduce transmission (e.g., communication and negotiation with sexual partners; Fisher & Fisher 1992). The limited effort at developing these three prongs on a broad geographic scale translates into a great potential for further reductions in transmission rate, and hence for reductions in virulence.

How benign could HIV-1 become?

The answer to this question depends on how strongly the overall rates of sexual and needleborne transmission are reduced. In the absence of precise knowledge about the evolutionary determinants of virulence, I can offer only an educated guess. We may be able to reduce the virulence to that of the other evolutionarily related retroviruses—the milder strains of HIV-2 and perhaps the HTLVs. A recent study from Australia suggests that mild HIV-1 strains are currently being transmitted (Learmont et al. 1992). The variation in virulence therefore seems to be present; our task is to enact prevention policies that favor the mild competitors over the virulent ones. Just as importantly, by enacting such policies we may keep other retroviruses from evolving into pathogens as virulent as pandemic HIV-1 (see Chapter 11).

PATHOGENESIS OF AIDS AND EVOLUTION OF HIV

Diversity thresholds and replication rate

Levin (1992) offered a *diversity threshold hypothesis* as an alternative to the *replication rate hypothesis* that forms the basis of this chapter. His hypothesis is based on a mathematical model by Nowak et al. (1990), which emphasizes destruction of the diversity of white blood cells as the underlying cause of AIDS. Levin interprets the evolutionary increases in viral replication rates as side effects of infection that have little if any relevance to the generation of symptoms.

In accordance with the model by Nowak and his colleagues, HIV populations inside of people do generate variants that can escape at least temporarily a person's immune system (Albert et al. 1990, Tremblay & Wainberg 1990). When the immune system eventually develops an attack directed specifically against these escape mutants, the attack appears to be damped (Arendrup et al. 1992). This damped response may reflect a gradual overwhelming of immune cell diversity (Nowak et al. 1990, 1991), accelerated perhaps by an effect referred to as Original Antigenic Sin, whereby the immune system reacts particularly strongly to the antigenic variants encountered early during an HIV infection (Nara et al. 1991). As HIV variants continue to emerge within an individual, the immune cells that muster attacks on specific variants have progressively diminished capacities to defend against each new variant. Eventually the allocations are spread so thinly that the new escape mutants can no longer be controlled. Virus density then rises rapidly, and the individual progresses to AIDS (Nowak et al. 1990, Goudsmit et al. 1991, Nara et al. 1991).

This diversity threshold hypothesis is also supported by changes in an external part of HIV that is attacked by the immune system. This part shows greater evolutionary change among children who progress slowly to AIDS than among children who progress rapidly (Wolfs et al. 1990). Apparently, the immune systems of these slow progressors are better at tracking and destroying mutant HIV, keeping HIV on the run evolutionarily, thereby generating a longer trail of change over a given amount of time.

The diversity threshold concept may well prove central to the progression of HIV infection to AIDS, but all of the interactions described above and all of the evidence presented by Levin (1992) are consistent with the replication rate hypothesis. The diversity threshold and replication rate hypotheses are complementary rather than mutually exclusive. The diversity threshold hypothesis offers a proximate, immunological mechanism for the progression to AIDS within infected individuals, rather than an ultimate, evolutionary explanation for the origin of high virulence. It does not address whether the characteristics of HIV that promote its destructiveness are evolutionary accidents or adaptations to environmental conditions such as rapid rates of sexual partner change. The diversity threshold hypothesis does suggest that the decimation of the immune system may be a cause rather than a consequence of the increased viral replication that occurs late in disease (Nowak et al. 1991). The current evidence indicates, however, that the transition to more damaging, rapidly replicating HIV precedes rather than follows immune decimation (Åsjö et al. 1990, Connor et al. 1993, Koot et al. 1993). Even if the diversity threshold hypothesis proves to be a primary reason for progression to AIDS, higher inherent replication rates should facilitate this progression (Nowak et al. 1991). A similar role for replication rate can be made for the other hypothesized mechanisms of HIV-induced immune deficiency, which generally involve overkill of white blood cells by the virus or by the immune system itself. [Hypothetical mechanisms are described by Capon & Ward (1991), Fauci et al. (1991), Grant (1991), Hoffmann et al. (1991), Imberti et al. (1991), Kion & Hoffman (1991), Arthur et al. (1992), and Marcuzzi et al. (1992); Tersmette & Miedma (1990) describe how rapidly replicating viral types could potentiate some of these mechanisms.]

Early measurements of HIV density suggested that a very small proportion of cells were infected by HIV: only one to ten out of every 100,000 cells. Pointing to this small percentage, many investigators have discounted the importance of replication rate, but sensitive measurements of HIV in infected people show that one in twenty or even one in ten target cells in the blood of AIDS patients may house HIV (Hsia & Spector 1991, Bagasra et al. 1992, Embretson et al. 1993a, Wood et al. 1993). The densities of virus in the plasma are far greater than was previously thought; and in lymph nodes and other lymphoid tissues, where most of the target cells reside, one out of three cells may be infected (Piatak et al. 1993, Embretson et al. 1993b). Although most of these HIV will be quiescent at any point in time and many may be incapable of continued cycles of replication because of the mutations they have acquired, many of these relatively inactive viruses may eventually adversely affect the cells in which they reside (Bukrinsky et al. 1991). The high densities of virus, particularly in ill people, therefore further emphasize the importance of focusing on rates of viral reproduction.

The link between advanced disease in the source individual and rapid progression to AIDS in the recipient is yet another reason for attributing a role to rates of viral reproduction. This link is expected if the rate of HIV reproduction inside a host determines the time until onset of symptoms, because those individuals with AIDS should have more rapidly reproducing viruses than those without. One could explain this finding in the short run by the diversity threshold hypothesis if individuals with AIDS have evolved a greater diversity of HIV. The infections generated from these individuals would therefore start with a greater diversity of HIV and progress to AIDS more quickly (Nowak et al. 1990). However, measurements do not reveal any clear increase in viral diversity as patients progress to AIDS (Goodenow et al. 1989). Very early during infection the diversity seems to be low, perhaps because of a bottleneck during transmission (McNearney et al. 1992, Wolfs et al. 1992, Wolinsky et al. 1992). This diversity increases during the intermediate period, but once the immune system is decimated, the diversity of the virus population is often low (Nowak et al. 1991, Wolfs et al. 1991, McNearney et al. 1992). The most rapidly reproducing variants apparently comprise an increasing proportion of the overall population during the late stages of infection because they are no longer held in check by the immune system. The apparent bottleneck and the lack of increased diversity during late stages of infection therefore weaken this application of the diversity threshold hypothesis: severe disease does not seem to result from the transmission of a more diverse group of viruses from AIDS patients.

These considerations taken together justify focusing on evolutionary changes in HIV reproductive rate, even though we do not yet know precisely how HIV cripples the immune system. As is often the case when evolutionary hypotheses are applied to new disciplines, resolution comes from drawing the distinction between proximate mechanisms on the one hand (how HIV infection leads to decimation of the immune system) and evolutionary explanations on the other (why the virus evolved characteristics that lead to this decimation).

Rates of replication and mutation: the interplay

Relationships between replication rate and mutation rate are critical to integration of the evolutionary basis for HIV virulence with mechanistic hypotheses about AIDS pathogenesis. The most obvious relationship results from the effects of replication rate on generation time, that is, the time needed to complete a full cycle of viral replication. More rapid replication can foster a more rapid evolutionary divergence of HIV lineages because the potential for divergence increases as generation time decreases (Coffin 1990). The variation across different lineages was generated originally by mutations; hence, the evolutionary divergence reflects one relationship between mutation and replication rate.

A second relationship between mutation and replication rate is less obvious. High mutation rates are often costly for organisms because they tend to untune finely tuned machinery. But for genes that code for external structures of viruses, high mutation rates can provide a great benefit by making the mutant viruses "look" different to the immune system. A virus whose external structure is different may escape detection and destruction by an immune system that has "learned" to recognize the parental viruses.

A high mutation rate would be especially beneficial to viruses like HIV, which often enter a latent state upon infecting a cell (presumably as an adaptation for sexual transmission under moderate rates of partner change as mentioned above). By the time most of these latent viruses start reproducing, the person's immune system will have been stimulated to defend against the viruses that had previously begun active replication. A rapid mutation rate could therefore increase the chance of diverging from the earlier viruses sufficiently to escape destruction by the immune system (Coffin 1990).

Direct measurements of mutations and the reverse transcription events that generate mutations show that HIV's reverse transcriptase tends to generate mutations at greater rates than the reverse transcriptases of other retroviruses (Preston et al. 1988, Roberts, et al. 1988, Takeuchi et al. 1988, Bakhanashvili & Hizi 1992ab, Hübner et al. 1992, Ji & Loeb 1992, Monk et al. 1992, Varela-Echavarria et al. 1992). The reverse transcriptase of HIV-1 generates mutants at a greater rate than that of HIV-2 (Bakhanashvili & Hizi 1992ab). HIV-1's reverse transcriptase might generate mutations faster simply because it works faster whenever it is synthesizing DNA strands (Hizi et al. 1991, Bakhanashvili & Hizi 1992ab, 1993), or it might be more mutation prone because it may be better able to connect mismatched building blocks during the construction of the new strand of DNA (e.g., see Goodman et al. 1993).

The relevance to human infections of these high mutation rates has been questioned because such high rates would make virtually all of the progeny viruses from an infected cell different from the parental virus, and many of progeny nonfunctional (Temin 1989b). Indeed, HIV pays this cost: A substantial proportion of the HIV in infected cells appear to be so altered by mutation that they are incapable of completing their reproductive cycle (Bagasra et al. 1992). But the costs of losing some of the successful parental combinations must not be considered in isolation. Natural selection will weigh this cost against the benefits of divergence from the parental virus: a temporary escape from immune detection. As argued above, this benefit should be particularly great when high sexual partner rates favor increased replication rate among viruses that often cause prolonged quiescent infections.

HIV therefore seems to make use of two mechanisms to increase net reproduction inside of a host: a high replication rate within cells and rapid generation of genetic variation, which increases net reproduction over many cell infection cycles by generating structurally novel viruses that can at least temporarily evade attack from the immune system.

For increased mutation rate to evolve in response to increased sexual contact, one must have genetically heritable variation in mutation rate. It could be argued that the necessary genetically based variation in mutation rate is implausible because mutations are generally detrimental. But recent studies confirm that mutation rates of envelope proteins vary by several fold among influenza A viruses (Suárez et al. 1992), which typically undergo a slightly lower overall rate of mutation than HIV (Goodenow et al. 1989).

The role of nef

One mechanism by which HIV may evolve higher rates of replication during a single infection involves a protein called "nef" (for *negative regulatory factor*), which is produced by the virus using instruction from a viral *nef* gene. During the early stages of infection, at least some versions of nef suppress HIV's reproduction (Terwilliger et al. 1986, Luciw et al. 1987, Ahmad & Venkatesan 1988, Ameisen et al. 1989, Niederman et al. 1989, Venkatesan 1992). Although additional studies show that nef proteins do not always suppress HIV and sometimes even accelerate its replication (Hammes et al. 1989, Kim et al. 1989, Bachelerie et al. 1990, Akari et al. 1992, Kirchhoff & Hunsmann 1992, Zazopoulos & Haseltine 1993), suppression by one version of nef has been confirmed by some genetic tinkering. When the normal *nef* gene was neutralized and a mutant *nef* gene inserted, rates of HIV reproduction were five times as great as when a normal *nef* was inserted (Maitra et al. 1991).

The long period of time that typically occurs between initial infection and AIDS may be attributed at least partly to suppression by nef (Fauci et al. 1991), which blocks activation by NF-κB (see above; Niederman et al. 1992). At the later stages of an infection, when replication rates are high and symptoms appear, the *nef* gene is no longer effective at suppressing the virus' reproduction (Cheng-Mayer et al. 1989). Accordingly, antibodies to nef are often less abundant in the blood during the late symptomatic stages of infection than during the asymptomatic period (O'Shea et al. 1991, Rezza et al. 1992b). Production of nef declines, or mutated nef proteins occurring in the later stages do not react as well with the antibodies that attach to normal nef. In a few individuals, the unsuppressed viruses are apparently destroyed by the immune system, yielding the occasional disappearance of serological signs of HIV. Accordingly, nef is sometimes detectable in such individuals when they temporarily become seronegative, much as they are in some people prior to detection of viral products in the blood (Montagnier 1988, Ameisen et al. 1989).

Apparently then, during the course of infection, mutant viruses that experience reduced suppression by nef tend to reproduce faster and make up a progressively greater proportion of the viruses within the person. Early during infection, nef is produced by a large fraction of the HIV in a person, but this fraction steadily diminishes as mutations erode this suppression.

Considering the variability among HIV infections, one can expect the evolutionary outcomes found in one person to differ from those in another. In some people the viruses may evolve toward a loss of suppression by nef, whereas in others the nef suppression may, by the luck of the draw, remain intact. Indeed the existing studies are consistent with such a diversity of outcomes (Cheng-Mayer et al. 1989, Delassus et al. 1991). It is just this kind of variability that provides raw material for evolution toward increased or decreased virulence in response to changes in sexual partner rate.

Suppression of replication by nef makes evolution of increased replication rates particularly easy. Increased replication may result from mutations that damage rather than refine nef's function, and such damaging mutations appear to be common among the nef versions that would otherwise suppress replication (Niederman et al. 1989). But a particularly strong form of group selection (*sensu* Wilson 1980) may counter this evolution. Illness and death arrest the transmission of groups that contain rapidly reproducing mutants, thereby preferentially allowing transmission from people whose HIV replication is still lowered by intact nef or other genetic instructions.

The rapid evolution of nef and its group-selected maintenance may help explain not only the progression of HIV infection toward AIDS but also the controversy among different teams investigating nef. The early reports of *nef*'s controlling effects on reproduction were contradicted by later studies which failed to show a suppressive effect (Hammes et al. 1989, Kim et al. 1989). But these contradictory results came from strains that had been cycled for long periods of time in laboratory cultures. Depending on how this laboratory cycling is conducted, it may select for or against suppressive *nef*. If the cycles involve frequent transfers of both free virus and infected cells to populations of susceptible cells, the laboratory environment should select against *nef* that suppress replication, much like the population of HIV inside of a person should evolve to be controlled less and less by *nef* over the duration of an infection. Such prolonged cycling in the laboratory should also select against extensive production of nef; once nef no longer provides a benefit, its production represents a drain of resources that can be used for viral production. Accordingly, one of the most extensively lab-propagated isolates of HIV produced small amounts of nef that did not inhibit viral production (Hewlett et al. 1991). The change to a nonsuppressing mutant nef may occur rapidly, within a few cycles of passage through cell cultures (Laurent et al. 1990)

If, however, the cycling in the lab involves transfer of infected cells that grow for long intervals between transfers, then the less destructive nef-suppressed viruses may have a competitive advantage. This advantage is possible because a cell's nef production is associated with a shedding of the cell's receptor molecules, which other HIV would need to gain entry into the cell (Niederman et al. 1989, Gama Sosa et al. 1991). A virus inside a cell that is suppressed by nef is therefore protected against invasion by competing viruses. If long periods of time occur before infected cells are transferred to a population of susceptible cells, the actively replicating viruses would destroy the available uninfected cells and eventually be without new cells to infect. Cells infected with nef-suppressed viruses would be able to reproduce, thus reproducing the latent HIV at each division. When the transfer of infected cells to new medium or to a new population of susceptible cells eventually occurs, the nef-suppressed HIV would therefore tend to be disproportionately represented. Just this kind of trend seems to have occurred when infected cells were serially transferred in cell culture (Zweig et al. 1990).

The different cycling methods and the differing selective pressures on nef production inside of people apparently has caused the evolution of different functions of the *nef* gene. Some versions of nef suppress whereas others accelerate replication (De Ronde et al. 1992, Terwilliger et al. 1991, Zazopoulos & Haseltine 1992, 1993). This diversity of nef function helps to explain the different patterns of nef production during infections (Amiesen et al. 1989, Reiss et al. 1989) and controversies about nef. The most vehement critics (e.g., Kirchhoff & Hunsmann 1992) implicitly assume that the function of nef remains constant across HIVs. Like HIV's external proteins, its nef proteins have parts that are highly variable (Roberts et al. 1988, Zazopoulos & Haseltine 1993), and hence can rapidly generate the variation upon which natural selection acts. More importantly, measurements of the changes in the *nef* genes that occur within infected hosts sometimes indicate selection according to the function of the nef proteins they encode (Kestler et al. 1991, Blumberg et al. 1992).

Both the nef issue and the more general topic of HIV virulence illustrate well why virologists and molecular biologists, like epidemiologists and physicians, need to be cognizant of ongoing evolutionary processes. It is perhaps no surprise that molecular biologists and virologists studying HIV were especially quick to recognize the relevance of evolutionary processes over short periods of time (e.g., Åsjö et al. 1986, Cheng-Mayer et al. 1988, 1989; Kim et al. 1989; Meyerhans et al. 1989).   Like physicians encountering antibiotic resistance, they were faced with results that seemed contradictory, but made sense in the light of evolution. Now it is the epidemiologists' turn to investigate whether the HIV that they are studying may change in virulence in response to the policies that can be enacted. To understand and control this network of cause and effect may be the next century's most formidable challenge at the interface of the social, natural, and health sciences.

CHAPTER 9

The Fight Against AIDS: Biomedical Strategies and HIV's Evolutionary Responses

ANTIVIRAL CHEMICALS

Suppression of HIV by AZT

In the last chapter I proposed that behavioral changes may alter the evolution of HIV's virulence. The practical significance of this proposition depends on the success of nonevolutionary strategies for treating the disease and control its spread. If these more conventional options were to prove completely successful in controlling and eradicating AIDS, the evolutionary control of HIV would be of theoretical rather than practical importance. What is the outlook for these options?

Because viruses complete their life cycles by becoming integrated with the cellular machinery, they are notoriously difficult to control by drugs that block viral activity. If a drug blocks some critical function of the virus, it also may be blocking some critical function of our cells. The general approach of HIV researchers therefore has been to identify steps in viral invasion and reproduction that are uniquely viral. If these critical steps can be blocked, then we may be able to block HIV's reproduction while keeping intact the processes that our cells need to perform.

One target for controlling HIV is reverse transcriptase, the enzyme that HIV uses to transcribe the information coded in its RNA into DNA. Because the DNA version of this information must be used for building new HIV, blocking reverse transcriptase would prohibit HIV's reproduction. Not surprisingly, scientists have been intensively studying chemicals that shut down reverse transcriptase. The first of these compounds with demonstrated effectiveness against AIDS was AZT (azidodideoxythymidine, also known as zidovudine). AZT is built almost but not quite like a component of DNA. Its similarity allows it to bind to reverse transcriptase like the normal components of DNA, but its slight differences make it like a Chrysler part in a Ford engine. The mismatch makes the transcriptase stall. AZT can slow the progression of AIDS and prolong the survival of AIDS patients by a year or so (Fischl et al. 1987, 1990, Swanson & Cooper 1990, Moore et al. 1991b).

This success of AZT among AIDS patients raised an intriguing question. Given that AZT can suppress viral replication during the asymptomatic period prior to AIDS (DeWolf et al. 1988), might it postpone the onset of AIDS when used before AIDS symptoms appear? The answer is yes, at least in some cases. The protocol of the study that provided this answer (Volberding et al. 1990) has been used as the basis for current guidelines for AZT use in the United States. The researchers categorized patients according to the blood's abundance of T4 cells, which are helper lymphocytes—white blood cells that stimulate other white blood cells to produce appropriate defenses. T4 cells are attacked by HIV, and the decline in the density of T4 cells is an indication that the HIV infection is progressing toward AIDS. Because a delay in the onset of symptoms occurred only the AZT-treated group that had less than 500 T4 cells per cubic millimeter of blood, this threshold density was accepted as the primary criterion for treatment (Friedland 1990, Hecht et al. 1990, National Institute of Allergy and Infectious Diseases 1990, Food and Drug Administration 1991, Kess et al. 1991; although extremely variable, T4 densities are generally near $1000/mm^3$ in healthy people and below $100/mm^3$ in people dying from AIDS).

Resistance to AZT and disease progression

While generally supportive of these or similar recommendations, researchers have appropriately cautioned that resistance to AZT and side effects of AZT could negate its beneficial effects over the entire course of an infection (National Institute of Allergy and Infectious Diseases 1990, Ruedy et al. 1990, Swart et al. 1990, Volberding et al. 1990, Graham et al. 1991). European researchers and policymakers have been particularly cautious; the British Department of Health, for example, advocates treatment when T4 counts are between 200 and 500/mm^3 and rapidly falling (Anonymous 1989b, Swart et al. 1990, Gazzard 1992).

In spite of the cautionary statements, assessments of the proper timing of AZT treatment have given only a sketchy view of the evolutionary pros and cons associated with early treatment. A more complete consideration of these pros and cons leads to the conclusion that the available data do not justify the guidelines for treatment that are currently accepted in the United States. To the contrary, analysis of the available data with reference to the evolutionary processes involved leads to the conclusion that asymptomatically infected individuals who are several years away from the onset of symptoms probably should not be treated with AZT, even if their T4 counts are less than 500/mm^3.

As I mentioned in the previous chapter, HIV has a vast potential for generating genetic variation. This genetic variation, when purged by the great differences in survival between the genetically distinct viruses, results in rapid rates of evolutionary change. Such rapid evolution occurs in two characteristics of HIV that are critically relevant to AZT treatment. The first is replication rate, which increases during the course of a single infection (Cheng-Mayer et al. 1988, Levy 1989, Tersmette et al. 1989, Schellekens 1992). The second characteristic is resistance to AZT, which also increases during the course of a single infection. This resistance was first confirmed when AIDS patients were treated with AZT (Larder & Kemp 1989, Larder et al. 1989). Shortly thereafter, it was demonstrated in asymptomatically infected people who were treated with AZT to retard the onset of AIDS (Boucher et al. 1990). One of the resistance-conferring mutations was present in nearly half of the patients after six months of treatment. After two years of AZT treatment, nearly 90% of the patients housed HIV with this mutation, which along with other mutations conferred partial resistance (Boucher 1992).

Years of observation are needed to document both increased resistance of the HIV inside people, and whether these people will progress toward AIDS faster than those whose HIV are less resistant to AZT. The process can be expedited by observing neonatally infected children because progression of infection to AIDS occurs more rapidly among them than among adults. A study of 23 children with symptomatic HIV-1 infection revealed that increased resistance to AZT in cell culture was strongly associated with more rapid deterioration of health (Tudor-Williams et al. 1992). Although the available evidence does not prove that AZT resistance causes a deterioration of patients by reducing the effectiveness of AZT (Boucher & Lange 1992, Richman 1992), the associations between increased resistance and deterioriation certainly support the idea (Tudor-Williams et al. 1992, Gøtzsche et al 1992, Montaner et al. 1993).

In another recent study, 18 infected adults were tested for four mutations that confer AZT resistance (Boucher et al. 1992b). The presence of mutations was associated with more advanced disease, but the association was not statistically significant. This lack of statistical significance may have resulted from the small sample size. Or it may have resulted from a more ominous problem: mutations besides the four that were studied may increase AZT resistance. This possibility is theoretically credible because resistance to AZT could be conferred by many different changes in shape of reverse transcriptase, which in turn could be caused by many different mutations. Measurements confirm that resistance to AZT is more variable than would be expected if resistance resulted from just the four sites of resistance-conferring mutations that were originally identified; seven mutations at five sites are now known to confer resistance, and evidence indicates that more are still to be discovered (Gingeras et al. 1991, Richman et al. 1991a, Darby & Larder 1992, Q.Gao et al. 1992a, Kellam et al. 1992, Richman 1992). A recent isolate, for example, was over 10,000 times more resistant to AZT than typical AZT-sensitive strains (Muckenthaler et al. 1992). This isolate could be distinguished from typical strains by 11 mutations in the reverse transcriptase gene. Eight of these mutations occurred in the active regions of reverse transcriptase, but of the four mutations originally associated with HIV resistance only one was found. Because the resistance was far higher than the resistance ascribable to that single mutation, one or more of the additional mutations were probably conferring the observed resistance (Muckenthaler et al. 1992).

Resistance, replication rate, and timing of treatment

Collectively these findings have important implications for AZT treatment of asymptomatic infections, as well as for the broader use of antiviral compounds against HIV. To appreciate these implications, first consider the evidence for an AZT-induced delay in the progression of asymptomatic infections to AIDS (Volberding et al. 1990). This delay owes its statistical significance to a biased sample of asymptomatic HIV infections. Specifically, the difference between AZT treatment and placebo can be attributed only to those individuals who would have become symptomatic during the study period had they not received AZT. The average duration of treatment was about one year. The results of the study therefore show only that for every 20 asymptomatic people, one person who would have become symptomatic within a year will have this progression postponed. Because AZT resistance tends to be only partially developed after one year of treatment (Boucher et al. 1990), AZT treatment is justifiable for these individuals: Severe symptoms are postponed and AZT will still be at least partially effective at the time when it otherwise would have been needed for treatment of ARC and AIDS.

But what about the other 19 out of every 20 asymptomatic individuals with T4 counts below 500? Prior to the use of AZT, AIDS developed within 18 months in 4%, 8%, and 16% of patients whose T4 counts were 500, 400, and 300 per cubic millimeter, respectively (Fahey et al. 1986). These figures, being gathered from asymptomatic homosexual men in Los Angeles in the mid-1980s, probably overestimate the progression rates of recent years which have slowed even after the effects of AZT have been accounted for (Rosenberg et al. 1991). A person has about a 50/50 chance of developing AIDS within ten years after becoming infected, but the timing of this progression varies greatly from person to person (Isaksson et al. 1988, Rutherford et al. 1990, Kuo et al. 1991, Lee et al. 1991). These figures indicate that the asymptomatic periods of the vast majority of the study's placebo-treated patients probably would have ranged broadly across durations of many years.

The broadness of this range is important because the available data do not justify AZT treatment of those individuals who would be more than a year or so from progressing to AIDS if left untreated. The most relevant data come from a large study of pre-AIDS patients, who were grouped according to manifestations indicative of differential probabilities of progression to AIDS (Graham et al. 1991). AZT postponed the progression to AIDS over a two-year period in patient groups whose untreated members experienced substantial progression to AIDS during the first year of treatment, but not in patient groups whose untreated members showed negligible progression to AIDS during the first year.

In a small group of asymptomatic patients treated with AZT, progression to symptoms over a two-year period occurred at 8% per year (Mulder et al. 1990). This rate is about the same as the rate among the placebos and double that of the asymptomatic patients treated with AZT for an average of one year (Volberding et al. 1990, as described above). The tendency for AZT to postpone death also diminishes as duration of treatment increases, until the two-year mark, when the lower death rates attributable to AZT treatment fall short of statistical significance (Graham et al. 1992). Although additional study is needed to assess alternative explanations, these results accord with the idea that HIV's increasing resistance to AZT during the first two years of treatment can offset the positive effects of AZT documented over the first year of treatment.

A recent study (Hamilton et al. 1992) of patients in the early stages of symptomatic infection strengthens this argument. Patients treated with AZT during these early stages of pre-AIDS symptoms progressed more slowly to AIDS than did patients whose AZT treatment was begun about a year later. But these benefits vanished as the total duration of treatment lengthened to about two years, and early-treatment patients did not live longer than late-treatment patients. A similar diminishment of a treatment benefits appears when patients treated with and without AZT are compared: AZT treated patients survive longer on average, but this advantage disintegrates after about two years of treatment (e.g., D'Arminio Monforte et al. 1992).

AIDS experts consider the accelerated deterioration of early-treatment patients to be paradoxical (Corey & Fleming 1992, Fackelmann 1992), but the results make sense in light of the two evolutionary processes described above (i.e., evolution of AZT resistance and increased rate of replication during the course of an infection) together with HIV's potential for geometric growth inside of a patient. Specifically, early treatment of symptomatic infections should initially delay the progression to AIDS because the geometric growth of HIV is held in check by AZT treatment. Symptomatic patients whose treatment is begun later should initially pay the price of more rapid progression in the absence of treatment. But when AZT treatment is initiated, these late-treatment patients should reap the benefits of more effective control of HIV by AZT because their HIV will be less resistant. At this point in time, the AZT-resistant HIV in the early-treated patients can undergo geometric growth if the patient's immune system permits it. But because evolution toward increased replication rate should have continued during early AZT treatment, the HIV in early-treatment patients should have a greater intrinsic replication rate at the onset of late treatment than at the onset of early treatment. The viruses in the late-treatment patients should also have this potential for more rapid growth when the late treatment is begun, but the virus population, still being sensitive to AZT at this time, can be held in check temporarily by AZT treatment. The initial postponement of AZT among early-treatment patients is thus offset by improved effectiveness of AZT among late-treated patients at a time when HIV has evolved a greater potential for replication. According to this interpretation, the net result is that early-treatment patients start to show a marked clinical improvement relative to late-treatment patients, but this initial advantage dissipates soon after the late treatment begins.

This interpretation presumes that progression to AIDS may depend on both AZT resistance and the evolutionary changes in virulence that occur during the course of an infection. These influences are still being assessed, but the evidence suggests that the increased virulence during the course of infection influences the progression of AZT-treated asymptomatic individuals, and that the partial resistance generated during this treatment may be a prerequisite for this progression (Boucher 1992, Boucher et al. 1992a).

Recognition of these evolutionary tradeoffs is largely of interpretative value insofar as treatment of symptomatic disease is concerned; it fosters improved assessments of the costs and benefits of early versus late treatment of symptomatic patients, but does not warrant a shift away from early treatment of symptomatic infections (see also Graham et al. 1992, McLean & Nowak 1992). In contrast, understanding the evolutionary processes underlying these results provides predictive insights with practical consequences for treatment of asymptomatic patients. If early treatment of symptomatic patients fails to prolong survival because of evolutionary increases in AZT resistance and replication rate, then extending the onset of treatment into the asymptomatic period is dangerous because AZT treatment during the asymptomatic period favors further evolution of AZT resistance, albeit at a slower rate (Richman et al. 1990, Richman 1991a). The absence of a long-term survival advantage associated with early treatment of symptomatic infections (Hamilton et al. 1992; see above) suggests that the evolution of resistance during the symptomatic period is sufficient to offset some of the positive effects of AZT on survival. If so, the additional resistance generated prior to the symptomatic period will probably exacerbate the problem because mutations conferring resistance contribute additively to the overall degree of resistance (Larder & Kemp 1989, Richman et al. 1990, Larder et al. 1991, Richman 1991a).

Discussions of this problem characterize the possibility of increased resistance during the asymptomatic period as a theoretical cost and the postponement of symptoms as a documented benefit (Carpenter et al. 1990, Richman et al. 1990, Richman 1991b). For the majority of asymptomatic patients, however, the comparison is not between a demonstrated benefit and an untested theory. Rather it is between two theoretical arguments, which rely on different assumptions. If we accept the current guidelines for treatment of asymptomatically infected individuals, we are relying on the following assumption: The postponement of symptoms that occurs when treatment is begun a year or so before the normal onset of symptoms can be extrapolated to earlier time periods. Using this extrapolation, one can propose that symptoms will be postponed when treatment is begun several years prior to the normal onset of symptoms. If, however, treatment is restricted to people who are within a year or so of developing symptoms (i.e., only people for whom data show a statistically significant benefit), then we are relying instead on a different assumption: Treatment years before the normal onset of symptoms will decrease the usefulness of AZT against symptomatic HIV infection because the treated HIV will have become resistant.

Until additional data are obtained, the best we can do is to assess which of these assumptions is most consistent with our knowledge about both the biochemical mechanisms and the evolutionary processes involved. The first key issue is resistance to AZT. After a year or two of treatment, the HIV from asymptomatic patients tend to be partially resistant (Richman et al. 1990, Richman 1991a). Given that partial resistance is occurring in asymptomatically treated individuals, there is no reason to assume that selection for the additional mutations that increase resistance would fail to continue. Such an assumption would run counter to principles of natural selection.

The second key issue is whether treatment begun years prior to the normal onset of symptoms would delay that onset. The evidence demonstrating a delay of symptoms when treatment is begun toward the end of the asymptomatic period is not reliable evidence that a similar delay would occur if treatment were begun several years prior to the normal onset of symptoms. When treatment is begun within a year of the normal onset of symptoms, the density of HIV inside of the patient drops (Boucher et al. 1990). Because the density of HIV is associated with the depletion of T cells and the onset of symptoms, it is logical to conclude that this treatment-induced drop in HIV delays the onset of symptoms.

When treatment is begun earlier, however, the HIV the person are under evolutionary pressure to develop AZT resistance for a longer period of time. If resistance negates the value of AZT, it may also diminish any AZT-induced delay of symptoms in proportion to the earliness of asymptomatic treatment. One would expect the density of HIV to be reduced during the first year or so of treatment, but once resistance evolves, the HIV population may bounce back rapidly for two reasons. The first is that unregulated populations increase geometrically rather than arithmetically. So long as AZT is effective, the potential for geometric growth of HIV is kept in check. Once resistance evolves, the past reduction achieved by AZT treatment could be quickly offset by HIV's potential for geometric growth. Indeed, when AZT treatment is terminated, viral levels bounce back to or even above pretreatment levels within a matter of weeks (Spear et al. 1988, Reddy et al. 1989, Semple et al. 1991, Srugo et al. 1991, Piatak et al. 1993). Similarly, although indicators of virus density typically drop within the first few weeks after AZT treatment, they begin to rise again, often by the third month of treatment; the rise is particularly strong after AZT resistant strains are isolated (Reiss et al. 1988, Reddy et al. 1992, Tudor-Williams et al. 1992).

The second reason for a rapid rebound involves evolution of increased replication rates. During AZT therapy, HIV replication continues, free virus is often measurable in the blood, and viral abundance inside infected cells does not decrease detectably (Ho et al. 1989, Morrey et al. 1991, Oka et al. 1991, Semple et al. 1991, Uherová et al. 1991). Continued replication may occur partly because AZT cannot effectively penetrate the reservoirs of actively replicating HIV in lymphoid tissues (Langhoff et al. 1991, Spiegel et al. 1992, Embretson 1993b, Pantaleo et al. 1993). The reduction in HIV density long before the onset of symptoms, therefore, would not eliminate the selection within the host for steadily increasing replication rates. If so, once resistance evolves, the resistant strains should be replicating at rates that are higher than rates before AZT treatment. Insofar as the eventual progression to AIDS depends on HIV's replication rate, people who are treated years before their normal onset of symptoms may have little if any postponement of symptoms because of the rapid rebound, and little chance that severity of symptoms can be reduced by AZT once the symptoms occur because of increased AZT resistance.

These considerations indicate that early asymptomatic treatment may leave such individuals little, if any, better off than if AZT had never been discovered, and worse off than if AZT treatment had begun a few months before the onset of symptoms. The tragic irony is that those who accept early treatment may substantially increase their total financial costs—which may be as high as a quarter million dollars per year of life saved (Schulman et al. 1991)—while decreasing the overall effectiveness of treatment.

Any tendency for a slower development of resistance during asymptomatic treatment than during symptomatic treatment merely alters the tradeoff, thus advancing the appropriate time of treatment to an earlier date. But the possibility of slower development of resistance certainly does not warrant advancement of treatment to any time prior to symptoms so long as T4 counts are below

500/mm³. Until additional data are obtained, we must make our best educated assessment of how far treatment should be advanced prior to symptoms. The available data suggest that this time will be somewhere on the order of a few months to a year prior to the onset of symptoms. The lack of shortened survival among late-treated versus early-treated symptomatic patients (Hamilton et al. 1992) is particularly relevant because the processes implicated by this result (see above) are the same processes that would negate the value of early treatment of asymptomatic infections.

Some details of HIV infection have led some researchers to advocate antiviral treatment very early during an infection. One such detail concerns the timing of HIV replication during an infection. Even during the early years of an infection many HIV reproduce actively in lymphoid tissue, where viruses inside cells may be shielded from antiviral drugs by a mixture antibody and virus on the outside of cells. Very early treatment therefore has been suggested as a way to suppress early replication perhaps before a shielding effect develops (Fox & Cottler-Fox 1993, Macilwain 1993). The negative effect of resistance to one drug on the effectiveness of combination therapy has led other researchers to advocate very early treatment with combinations of antiviral drugs (Cox et al. 1993). These arguments in favor of very early treatment, however, do not incorporate early evolution of drug resistance or pre-existing resistance at the outset of infection. HIV's propensity for evolving resistance and for increasing its rate of replication during an infection, therefore, severely weaken these arguments for early treatment.

Very early treatment has been advocated on the basis of a mathematical model that attributes the development of AIDS to an overwhelming of the immune system's diversity (Nowak et al. 1991; see Chapter 8). The model, however, assigns new mutants a constant average replication rate rather than a steadily increasing replication rate. The evolutionary approach presented in this chapter implicates the continual increase in replication rate of new mutants as a key factor disfavoring the early treatment of asymptomatic patients.

Re-evolution of sensitivity

The usefulness of AZT prior to onset of symptoms will depends on whether resistant strains evolve toward sensitivity in the absence of AZT, and if so, how quickly. Bacteria that have evolved resistance to an antibiotic, will often rapidly evolve sensitivity once their exposure to the antibiotic has ended. But HIV's resistance to AZT differs from classic antibiotic resistance in bacteria. The return to sensitivity commonly occurs among bacteria because the resistant bacteria are at a competitive disadvantage when the antibiotic is absent (Eberhard 1990). They may, for example, produce enzymes that neutralize the antibiotics, but this production may consume resources that could otherwise be used to improve their competitive status.

The resistance of HIV to AZT is different. Mutations in the reverse transcriptase gene apparently change the structure of reverse transcriptase, reducing its interaction with AZT and thereby allowing it to transcribe the viral genes in the presence of AZT. If the AZT-resistant transcriptase is still highly competent at this task, HIV may suffer little if any competitive disadvantage when AZT is absent.

On the other hand, the mutations might alter the ability of transcriptase to function in the absence of AZT. Such mutations generally should reduce rather than increase transcriptase rate because the vast majority of mutations that alter enzyme function are detrimental to that function. Normally one might expect this reduction to result in a competitive inferiority in the absence of AZT, and hence a return to sensitivity if AZT use were curtailed. But because of HIV's great potential for generating genetic variability and the long durations of HIV infections, HIV apparently evolves rates of replication within hosts that eventually exceed the optimal rates for transmission to new hosts. Mutations that reduce transcriptase efficiency slightly may therefore delay the time at which replication rate rises above that most suitable for transmission, thus favoring rather than disfavoring transmission. The resistant HIV may therefore suffer little if any disadvantage relative to sensitive HIV over the entire cycle of infection and transmission.

Even if some AZT-resistant reverse transcriptases are less effective than the sensitive transcriptases at reverse transcription, there is no reason to believe that all AZT-resistant reverse transcriptases will be less effective. For those that are just as effective, withdrawal of exposure to AZT will not favor the susceptible over the resistant HIV. Boucher et al. (1992b) report a tendency for one of the resistance-conferring mutations (at codon 70) to be relatively unstable through time, but another (at codon 215) to be stable. In one patient, treatment was discontinued, yet the latter mutation persisted for up to one year. Albert et al. (1992) found a similarly slow and variable return to sensitivity among patients who were infected with an HIV strain that had multiple resistance-conferring mutations.

When viruses were compared in cell culture, the activity and infectiousness of some AZT-resistant strains did not differ significantly from sensitive strains (Rooke et al. 1990, Lacey et al. 1992, Wainberg et al. 1992). Drug-resistant strains often return to sensitivity slowly, if at all, when they are propagated in cell culture without AZT (Rooke et al. 1989, Wainberg et al. 1992).

These considerations suggest that at least some resistant mutants may tend to reevolve sensitivity sluggishly. If so, new infections may have a head start in the race to AZT resistance, and AZT resistance may increase progressively across transmission cycles. There is already some indication that AZT-resistant strains are present at the onset of AZT treatment (Land et al. 1990, Rooke et al. 1990, Mohri et al. 1992).

The earlier the initiation of AZT treatment, the greater the accumulation across the general population of the various mutations necessary for resistance. This accumulation may be particularly relevant to treatment during the asymptomatic period because asymptomatic and mildly symptomatic individuals should tend to be the most sexually active. When asymptomatic individuals are increasingly treated, the new infections will be increasingly generated from fully resistant or partially resistant viruses. Consequently, the window of time between onset of AZT treatment and evolution to any particular degree of AZT resistance will shrink. If an appropriate time to begin treatment is now six months before the onset of symptoms, in five years from now it may be three months. More generally, each cohort of AZT-treated individuals will experience a more transitory postponement of symptoms and reduced effectiveness of AZT when symptoms do finally arise.

On the bright side, two recent studies have provided some evidence for reversibility of AZT resistance. In one study, the HIV in five of 15 patients reevolved sensitivity within one year after cessation of AZT treatment (Land et al. 1991, 1992). The evolution to sensitivity was slower in those patients who had been taking AZT for a longer period of time (Land et al. 1991), suggesting that highly resistant HIV return to sensitivity more slowly than less resistant HIV. As the time since cessation of AZT treatment increased so did sensitivity, suggesting that at least in some patients a gradual return to sensitivity occurs over a period of about one year (Land et al. 1992). The partial reversion to sensitivity raises hopes that alternating treatments might make HIV reevolve sensitivity to one drug during the period of administration of a second.

The second study followed patients during such an alternation of treatment (St. Clair et al. 1991). When the condition of five AIDS patients treated with AZT for a year or more began to deteriorate, AZT treatment was replaced by treatment with another reverse transcriptase inhibitor: didanosine (= dideoxyinosine = ddI). The patients improved, suggesting that the AZT resistance was contributing to their deterioration. Over the following year, the HIV in these patients became more resistant to ddI but less resistant to AZT. A mutation that increased resistance to ddI reduced resistance to AZT (St. Clair et al. 1991). In the presence of ddI and absence of AZT, the AZT-resistant HIV were competitively inferior to the new ddI-resistant, AZT-sensitive mutants. The early data on the long-term control of HIV by ddI, however, mirror the results obtained from AZT treatment: HIV rebounds over the months during which resistance to ddI evolves and the patients deteriorate (St. Clair et al. 1991, Reddy et al. 1991, 1992).

The work to date indicates that many different combinations of mutations will influence resistance to AZT and ddI. As use of both antivirals increases, any mutations that increase resistance to one drug without reducing resistance to the other will have a competitive advantage. As these variants spread, the return to AZT sensitivity during ddI treatment will become increasingly sluggish.

Strains of HIV that are resistant to both AZT and ddI lend credence to this prediction (Japour et al. 1991), as does growth of HIV in cell culture. When exposed to increasing concentrations of both AZT and ddI, HIV rapidly developed resistance to both, and the resistant strains did not reevolve sensitivity when they were cultured without these antivirals for two months (Q. Gao et al. 1992a). Joint presentation of high initial concentrations of the two drugs, however, did not cause rapid evolution of resistance (Q. Gao et al. 1992b). This difference warrants concern because drug concentrations probably vary considerable among the different cells and tissues infected with HIV. Growth of HIV in people may therefore more closely resemble the experimental conditions under which HIV evolved resistance to both antivirals than those conditions under which sensitivity was prolonged.

HIV has demonstrated an ability to evolve resistance to virtually every drug that has been used against it, but resistance to one drug often does not automatically generate resistance to other promising drugs (Prasad et al. 1991, Richman et al. 1991ab, Rooke et al. 1991, Fitzgibbon et al. 1992, Mellors et al. 1992, Richman 1992, Sarver et al. 1992, Balzarini et al. 1993). These findings have led researchers to evaluate the simultaneous use of different antiviral drugs. If the HIV are sensitive to the drugs being used, joint administration can lead to synergistic suppression of the virus. As mentioned above, however, joint exposure to two-drug combinations, such as AZT and ddI, may eventually generate resistance to both. Moreover, if resistance to AZT has occurred, administration of AZT jointly with other drugs such as ddI may result in reduced effectiveness of the second drug (Cox et al, 1992). The inadequacies of two-drug strategies have led researchers to consider using three drugs. Simultaneous application of AZT, ddI, and another antiviral drug, called nevirapine, stopped replication of an HIV strain in the test tube (Chow et al. 1993). Although this discovery is encouraging, broad evolutionary considerations must dampen optimism about even this approach. If the triple combination could completely stop all replication of all the existing variants of HIV and all the variants that could be readily generated from the existing variants in all tissues, then we would have grounds for optimism. Using our knowledge about AZT resistance, however, we can expect that many different resistance-conferring mutations will be found for each antiviral drug, yielding many different permutations for drug-resistant HIV. If just one such permutation permits some reproduction in the presence of the triple combination, then this slightly resistant variant may form a population from which variants with improved replication abilities can be expected. Reiterations of this process should cause evolution of replication abilities toward that occurring in the absence of antivirals. Any difficulty that

HIV has in evolving resistance to triple combinations could, however, buy time. At the individual level, it may lengthen survival and improve the quality of life for individual patients who take the drug combinations. At the population level, joint treatment could slow the rate at which resistance to any one drug spreads through a region.

Restriction of asymptomatic treatment in practice

Until the uncertainties about reevolution of sensitivity can be clarified, the only conclusion that can be justified on the basis of hard data is to use AZT for asymptomatic patients who are within a year or so of becoming symptomatic. The clinical usefulness of this conclusion depends on our abilities to predict the progression of HIV infections to AIDS. Presently, the density of T4 cells is the major criterion used to determine whether an individual should be treated with AZT, but this criterion is only weakly associated with impending symptoms. Some individuals with T4 counts above 500 already present symptoms or are close to doing so, and many individuals with T4 counts below 500 are years away from developing AIDS (Osmond et al. 1991, Sheppard et al. 1991, Weiss et al. 1992). The analysis presented above suggests that other criteria need to be used in addition to T4 counts. Most other criteria by which HIV progression is measured (e.g., p24 antigen, $ß_2$-microglobulin, T4%, neopterin) provide only rough predictions when used individually. Use of these criteria in combination, however, may accurately predict the onset of symptoms (Osmond et al. 1991, Krämer et al. 1992, Lifson et al. 1992a). Additional indicators also show great promise for improving the accuracy of predictions and may extend predictions to a wide range of selected times prior to the onset of symptoms. These indicators involve quantification of HIV's genetic material (using polymerase chain reaction), the artificial stimulation and quantification of virus activity (using radiation-resistant HIV expression *ex vivo*), changes in the composition of white blood cells and blood chemistry, and direct assessments of viral characteristics that are associated with virulence (like replication rate and tendencies to cause fusion of infected with uninfected cells) (Mathez et al. 1990, Fauci et al. 1991, Schechter et al. 1991b, Levacher et al. 1992, Saah et al. 1992, Schellekens et al 1992, Natoli et al. 1993).

These conclusions drawn from consideration of evolutionary processes are more consistent with the European guidelines for treatment of asymptomatic infection than with the U.S. guidelines. The European guidelines restrict treatment to individuals whose T4 cells counts are less than 500/mm^3 and falling rapidly (Swart et al. 1990). Such individuals are especially likely to progress to AIDS or ARC within several months (Burcham et al. 1991). Incorporation of more accurate composite indicators (see above) should permit finer tuning in response to upcoming results, which may more precisely specify the benefits and costs of beginning treatment at various times before the onset of symptoms.

This reliance on predictors of disease progression is germane to a controversy that centers on short-range costs and benefits of AZT treatment. Early use of AZT has been questioned on the basis of the low proportions of people showing postponement of symptoms (Swart et al. 1990). AZT slowed the annual progression to symptoms from about 8% to 4% (Volberding et al. 1990). Indiscriminate treatment of 100 individuals with T4 counts below 500/mm^3 for one year would therefore postpone symptoms in only about four individuals. If, however, one could determine which infections would have become symptomatic within a year from the onset of the study and treat only those infections, the halving in progression rate would be translated into a benefit for approximately half of those treated. This greater protection per treated individual obviously offer a more substantial benefit to be measured against the negative side effects of treatment.

The long duration of HIV infections and the high rates at which genetic variation is generated make clinical concerns about resistance of HIV to antivirals different from traditional concerns about antibiotic resistance. A full antibiotic regimen generally has a negligible effect on the evolution of antibiotic resistance within the treated individual. Physicians may differ with regard to the point at which antibiotic treatment should be withheld to delay the generation of antibiotic resistance in the overall population, but wherever this point lies for individual physicians, it will generally be derived by weighing the benefit to the individual patient against the long-range cost to the population. HIV infections are different because of the high probability that the HIV within the treated patient will develop resistance to the prescribed antiviral. Treatment of asymptomatic patients during the year or so before symptoms may provide a benefit in terms of delaying the onset of symptoms, but withholding treatment may permit a greater treatment benefit once symptoms arise. These alternative benefits will inevitably be traded off against each other. Physician and patient will need to choose a longer symptom-free period and an increased severity of symptomatic disease when it eventually arises, or a shorter symptom-free period and a reduced severity of symptomatic disease.

The evolutionary analysis presented above indicates that if AZT treatment is begun earlier in the asymptomatic period, resistance of HIV to AZT will arise earlier, the postponement of symptoms will diminish, and AIDS will be less controllable. Because those people infected with partially resistant strains should tend to evolve fully resistant strains more quickly, they will pay a greater price from early treatment and should begin treatment later than they would have, had their HIV been fully sensitive. These conclusions are complicated by the variability in the relationship between duration of treatment and degree of AZT resistance after treatment (e.g., Tudor-Williams et al. 1992), a complication that will become increasingly important as AZT resistance becomes more prevalent at the outset of infection. To account for these concerns, assessments of AZT resistance will be needed early during infection and throughout treatment. Recent improvements in detecting the presence and degree of AZT resistance (e.g., Mayers et al. 1992) have made this monitoring more feasible.

Ideally such measurements should be compared with analogous measurements from placebo groups. Unfortunately for this goal (and perhaps also for the future of many of the individuals in placebo groups), the placebo group of the primary U.S. study was terminated by the board that was monitoring data and safety of the experiment. The board took this action when the evidence showed that the AZT treatment significantly postponed symptoms (Volberding et al. 1990). Besides hindering evaluation of the long-term usefulness of asymptomatic treatment, this decision draws attention to the need for a more detailed consideration of evolutionary processes when deciding whether to terminate experimental studies of HIV treatment. The ideas presented above indicate that termination of the placebo group had consequences for a large proportion of the placebo group that were opposite to the consequences envisioned by the monitoring board. That is, for the placebo patients who were several years away from developing symptoms, termination of placebo and initiation of AZT treatment probably reduced their chances of postponing AIDS with AZT and reduced their chances of receiving effective AZT treatment once they acquired AIDS.

Evolutionary considerations indicate that there is no basis for encouraging AZT use among patients who are two or more years away from AIDS symptoms. Ethical standards (e.g., Freedman 1992) therefore do not justify the board's action to terminate the placebo arm. Fortunately, the British-French counterpart of the U.S. study did not terminate its placebo arm. This investigation of about 1750 patients has been termed the "Concorde" study by analogy to the cooperative development of the Concorde aircraft by Britain and France. The Concorde study should eventually provide a more precise indication of the appropriate times to initiate treatment of asymptomatic individuals. The preliminary results support the argument developed above. After an average of about three years of treatment, the patients treated with AZT did not experience a longer AIDS-free period than the untreated patients, yet the results obtained at about one year of treatment were "not inconsistent" with results of the U.S. study (Aboulker & Swart 1993). These preliminary results are already leading some observers to predict that AZT will no longer be used to postpone the onset of AIDS (Maddox 1993). As described above, however, evolutionary considerations offer a more specific recommendation: AZT treatment should no longer be used to postpone the onset of AIDS when patients would otherwise be more than a year or so away from developing AIDS.

The Concorde study gave placebo participants the option of leaving the placebo group—that is, to begin taking AZT. The considerations presented in this chapter raise ethical concerns about such decisions as well. For placebo participants to make an informed decision about this option, they need to be advised that acceptance of AZT treatment might result in little, if any, postponement of AIDS, and a decreased ability to combat AIDS when it eventually arises.

Soon after the widespread acceptance of AZT treatment for asymptomatic infections, the State-of-the-Art Conference on AZT Therapy for Early HIV Infection concluded, "There is no laboratory marker other than T4 cell count that is necessary in deciding when to initiate AZT therapy" (Carpenter et al. 1990). This statement is a testament to the need for a more complete integration of evolutionary principles into policymaking and clinical practice.

OTHER STRATEGIES AGAINST AIDS

Vaccines

Perhaps the greatest hope in the fight against AIDS has centered on development of an effective vaccine. Immunodeficiency viruses cause infections in monkeys and cats that are very similar to HIV infections in humans, and experimental vaccines against these viruses have provided some protection (Gardner 1991, Gardner et al. 1992, Warren & Dolatshahi 1992). These results have raised the possibility of using similar vaccines to protect humans from HIV.

To be successful an AIDS vaccine must produce protection against at least some strains of HIV without adversely affecting the vaccinated individual. One obvious requirement is to avoid causing the disease. Vaccines against other diseases have contained benign mutants or weakened pathogens. Applying this approach to AIDS would be very dangerous because weakened or benign HIV could reevolve virulence, a likely prospect considering HIV's great potential for evolutionary change during the course of an infection. Reducing the virulence of HIV by selectively deleting virulence genes is risky because a given gene may have different effects in different viruses. Deleting the *nef* gene, for example, might reduce the virulence of some strains but increase the virulence of others (Haseltine 1991, Levy 1991; see chapter 8). Although deleted portions of a given virulence gene may be difficult for HIV to recreate (Daniel et al. 1992), natural selection should favor compensatory mutations in other genes to boost the vaccine virus towards its pre-deleted level of replication, and hence virulence. Long-term studies of many vaccinated animals will be necessary to evaluate this possibility, but the presumption that the risk of reversion to virulence is avoided by such deletions (Salomon 1993) is very shaky, given HIV's evolutionary versatility. Use of killed organisms poses lessened but similar dangers. Introduction of incompletely killed HIV might cause infection, and some components of killed HIV might interact with our immune systems to enhance infection by viable HIV (Berzofsky 1991). Several conventional approaches to vaccination therefore are dismissed or at least disfavored at the outset, approaches that have yielded substantial protection in experimental studies (Daniel et al. 1992, Warren & Dolatshahi 1992). Other approaches include inoculation with the protein components of HIV and genetic engineering of other viruses so that they contain HIV components. The hope is that our bodies will then generate immunity against these components of HIV, so that any HIV carrying them will be attacked when it enters the vaccinated person's body.

Once a successful vaccine is developed, the process must continue to guard against evolutionary end-runs by the pathogen around the defenses induced by the vaccine. Unfortunately, the available data suggest that a person's immunological defenses are a surmountable obstacle for HIV. The virus attaches to our cells using a molecule called gp120. Changes in just one of the hundreds of building blocks of gp120 can dramatically alter the ability of antibodies to attach to the molecule. This decreased attachment apparently allows the mutant HIV to escape the immune response generated against the parental viruses (Ivanoff et al. 1991, Wolfs et al. 1991). Such minor changes in building blocks need not occur at the site on gp120 that attaches to the host cells; changes in other parts of gp120 can change its shape, thereby making the virus resistant to antibody attack (Berzofsky 1991, Nara et al. 1991). The significance of variation in HIV is evident in the degree of success generated from the experimental vaccines. They generally protect against infection in about half of the recipients if the vaccine is made from viral components of the same strain that is subsequently introduced into the vaccinated animal (Kurth et al. 1991, Murphey-Corb et al. 1991, Warren & Dolatshahi 1992). Vaccines derived from different strains may protect against disease but generally do not prohibit infection (Kurth et al. 1991).

To appreciate the difficulty in generating an AIDS vaccine, consider the influenza virus, which has a mutation rate slightly less than that of HIV (Goodenow et al. 1989). Each new flu season holds the often-fulfilled promise of epidemic influenza against which recently used vaccines are ineffective. Because the dangers of killed influenza vaccines are relatively low, these new flu strains can be dealt with effectively if surveillance is diligent and resources are ready. One need only identify the epidemic type, grow it, kill it, and circulate it as a vaccine to combat the epidemic. For the safety reasons mentioned above, killed HIV vaccines would be dangerous. Moreover, HIV's longer duration of infection and the inadequate host immunity make a great deal of the existing variation present at one time; and this variation is generated without a lull. Unlike the influenza virus, HIV has no "AIDS season." Trying to control HIV's spread with a vaccine is like trying to control all of the flu epidemics of the next century at once with a single flu vaccine.

One way around this problem might be to engineer a vaccine to contain a smorgasbord of the various HIV proteins that can be recognized by our immune systems. An HIV strain need match only one of the proteins in the smorgasbord to be identified and eliminated by the immune system. This approach might reduce the proportion of HIV that could escape vaccination and the rate at which HIV could circumvent the vaccines, but probably would not fundamentally change the outcome: So long as it is possible for HIV to alter the structure of its proteins so that it cannot be recognized by the vaccine-stimulated immunity, it can escape detection and multiply.

Compounding all of the problems associated with HIV's variability is the fact that HIV can infect susceptible people, and susceptible cells within infected people, without leaving infected cells (Gust 1991). Nearly all of the studies that have demonstrated protection, challenged the vaccinated individuals with free virus rather than with virally infected cells. Vaccines that are effective against free virus may have little effect on the progression of disease because HIV apparently often infects people within the disguising cloak of our cellular membranes; and infected cells may be far more effective than free virus at spreading infection (Sato et al. 1992, Dimitrov et al. 1993). The few studies that have attempted to determine whether vaccines protect against viruses within cells have shown only partial protection. Inactivated SIV protected all eight rhesus monkeys against free SIV, but only half of the monkeys against SIV-infected cells (Heeney et al. 1992). An HIV-1 vaccine protected three chimpanzees against HIV-1-infected cells, but the protection was short lived (Fultz et al. 1992). The successes at vaccination are therefore only mildly encouraging (Sabin 1992, 1993).

The problem of membrane-cloaked viruses means that an effective vaccine must somehow activate the cells of our immune system that recognize and destroy infected cells, not just free virus. This task is feasible for some infected cells if the vaccine uses living viruses. Vaccination with living, benign measles virus, for example, provides effective protection against measles even though the measles virus, like HIV, can be transmitted directly from cell to cell (Gust 1991). Vaccination with living, benign SIV suggests some degree of similar protection (Daniel et al. 1992).

The destruction of infected cells involves internal processing of the virus by the cell and then transport of the processed viral fragments so that they are embedded in and protrude from the cell membrane in a very specific association with the compounds that allow our bodies to distinguish our own cells from foreign cells. Cells containing such protruding virus parts can then be recognized and destroyed by the immune system. But vaccination with live or inactivated HIV is dangerous, and getting the cell to take in and properly process parts of HIV will be a major trick (Berzofsky 1991). Even if this processing problem can be solved there remains the problem of cryptic infection: many of the infected cells in semen and blood may not be destroyed because their membranes do not contain any of the viral fragments that the destroying cells use to recognize infected cells (Sabin 1992). If all such novel challenges can be solved we will still be left with the great potential for viral evolution. Indeed the raw material evolution around this kind of control may already be present. The existing variation in HIV includes viruses that can circumvent this attack: the fragments of some viruses are not presented to or recognized by the cells that destroy infected cells (Berzofsky 1991, Phillips et al. 1991).

These considerations suggest that developing a safe and effective AIDS vaccine will be one of the most formidable challenges ever assigned to health sciences, and the foreseeable difficulties translate into millions of deaths from AIDS before a vaccine that is even moderately effective will be put into use.

The fake doorknob trick

Another strategy is to use compounds that seem essential for HIV to complete its life cycle. A molecule protruding from some of our white blood cells, called CD4, is a receptor for HIV, a doorknob that HIV grasps in order to enter our cells. (The 4 in T4, mentioned earlier in this chapter, refers to the presence of CD4 on the membrane of these T lymphocytes.) The hand that HIV uses to grasp CD4 is gp120. The hope is that creating a glut of fake doorknobs in the body will keep HIV busy grasping knobs that do not open any doors. In this vulnerable and distracted state outside of cells, the sidetracked HIV may then be destroyed by the immune system.

Not only do the tested strains of HIV and SIV ubiquitously use CD4 for entry, but they also use the same part of the CD4 molecule; and the part of the virus that grasps the CD4 molecule is very similar among different strains of HIV (Kang et al. 1991). This similarity suggests that a large variety of fake doorknobs might not be needed, and that HIV may have relatively few options for evolving a structure that would fail to grasp the fake doorknobs, yet still grasp the real ones that are attached to the outside of the cell.

Even if one assumes for the moment that HIV is entirely dependent on CD4 as a doorknob for entry into the cell, HIV may still be able to evolve its way around our efforts to use CD4 as a fake doorknob. The parts of CD4 exposed in the blood are not the same as the parts exposed when CD4 is embedded in our cell membranes. By varying the structure of their gp120 molecules, the virus might be able to distinguish between free and embedded CD4. The gp120 molecules could, for example, change in structure so that they need to interact with components of the cell membrane before binding to CD4, or they could reduce their binding to free CD4 by interacting with the part of free CD4 that is not exposed in membrane-bound CD4. By either means they could evolve to avoid binding to doorknobs that have no door. The great variability of gp120 (Hughes & Corrah 1990) lends credence to these possibilities.

Portions of the CD4 molecule have successfully blocked HIV infection in the test-tube, but attempts to control infection in humans have produced questionable results (Capon & Ward 1991). One problem is that the blocking ability decreases substantially as the density of normal CD4-bearing cells increases. Another problem stems from variability in gp120. Efforts have focused on producing compounds that bind to the part of gp120 that grasps CD4 because changes in this part of gp120 should be constrained: if this part changes too much, the virus will be unable to bind to CD4 and therefore unable to enter the cell. Any blocking of gp120 should be, in theory, a longer-term solution than interfering with other viral structures.

Unfortunately, recent evidence indicates that HIV can readily evolve its vulnerability to free CD4. Blockage of laboratory strains of HIV worked well in the test-tube, but the same blockage of freshly isolated strains required several hundred-fold increases in the concentrations of CD4 (Daar et al. 1990, Ashkenazi et al. 1991, Brighty et al. 1991, Layne et al. 1991). In one such insensitive strain, a mutation was documented precisely at the part of the HIV protein that grasps CD4 (Capon & Ward 1991). Such findings led researchers to suspect that growth outside of the host selected for an artificially high affinity for attachment to the CD4 molecule. But follow-up on this idea yielded a surprise: The binding sites of freshly isolated HIV bound to CD4 about as strongly as did the laboratory strains of HIV (Ashkenazi et al. 1991, Brighty et al. 1991). Viruses growing in the body apparently have other characteristics that reduce their tendency to be inhibited by free CD4.

The resolution to this paradox may be that the HIV living inside of our bodies have competing demands on their structure. They have to cope with antibodies, for example. Changes in gp120 may influence attachment to antibodies and to CD4 even when the attachment sites themselves are unchanged (Nara et al. 1991, Moore et al. 1992). HIV inside the body may therefore evolve a conformation that represents a tradeoff between getting into cells and avoiding attack by antibodies. The tradeoff might involve a difference between target cells in the body and target cells in the test tube; slight variations in a highly exposed portion of gp120, called the V3 loop, appear to influence the kind of cell that is attacked and the ability of CD4 to block the virus (Hwang et al. 1992). Alternatively, a floppy conformation of gp120 could protect against attack by the immune system, but in so doing cover the CD4 binding site until another part of gp120 (such as the V3 loop) attaches to the cell (see Callahan et al. 1991, Nara et al. 1991). This covering of the CD4 binding site may make entry into the cell somewhat lower, but the binding to free CD4 drastically lower. HIV grown in cell culture without exposure to antibodies would be selected only to get into cells efficiently and might therefore evolve a less floppy gp120 with a more exposed CD4 binding site. The constraints imposed on HIV by the immune system could thus make the fresh isolates less vulnerable than the laboratory strains to blockage by free CD4.

Although these explanations for the rapid change in vulnerability to free CD4 have not been adequately tested, the fundamental premise underlying an evolutionary explanation is well documented. By the time laboratory isolates of HIV are grown and tested, they typically deviate from the variants that comprise the majority within the source person (Meyerhans et al. 1989, Delassus et al. 1991). As the growth of the HIV outside of people continues, this rapid divergence continues.

Whatever the exact reason for the evolutionary change in vulnerability to free CD4, the existence of this change does not bode well for the evolutionary stability of CD4 therapy. Moderate concentrations of CD4 do not effectively block HIV inside the body (Daar & Ho 1991), but perhaps more importantly, the difference between fresh and older isolates demonstrates HIV's potential for evolving its vulnerability to blockage. In the short run, the blockage of recent isolates may be improved dramatically, for example, by booby-trapping the free CD4 with a toxin (Kennedy et al. 1993). In the long run, however, CD4 therapy will tend to create a population of HIVs that distinguishes the fake doorknobs from the real doorknobs on the cells. Recent studies show that mutant polio viruses can avoid binding to such doorknob decoys, but can still infect cells (Weiss 1990). If the more slowly mutating polio virus can evolve around this obstacle, it is likely that HIV will be able to do so as well.

There is another problem: HIV is not as dependent on CD4 to enter cells as was previously believed. HIV apparently can gain entry into neurons, some kinds of white blood cells (B lymphocytes), cancer cells, and the cells lining the intestinal tract even when CD4 is absent (Bhat et al. 1991, Fantini et al. 1991, Morrison et. al 1991, Stahmer et al. 1991, Brichacek et al. 1992, Yahi et al. 1992). As HIV already has the ability to enter cells without using CD4, it should be able to evolve less dependence on CD4 for entry.

Human ingenuity vs. HIV's versatility

The capacity of HIV to evolve its way around barriers is apparent in its track record of adapting to new cell types. In humans, HIV readily infects and propagates in white blood cells called monocytes. It cannot normally infect and propagate in monocytes isolated from the chimpanzee. But soon after HIV had been introduced into chimpanzees, it evolved the ability to infect chimpanzee monocytes (Watanabe et al. 1991). HIV's ability to grow in other white blood cells of the chimpanzee gave it a stepping-stone. By the trial-and-error procedure of mutation and natural selection, the population of HIV grown within chimpanzees soon came up with the right combination of instructions to break through the barriers that had previously prevented infection of monocytes. The precise nature of this barrier is not known, but it occurs early during the infection of a cell, and differences between chimpanzee and human CD4 molecules may play a role (Gendelman et al. 1991).

The preceding overview of options being pursued and the likely evolutionary responses of HIV to them leads me to conclude that if these and other approaches, such as antibody therapy, gene therapy, or blocking of the manufacture of HIV within cells (Mitsuya et al. 1990, 1991), yield effective treatment, the effectiveness will be short-lived. HIV will continue to evolve resistance to AZT and other antiviral compounds; it will evolve to recognize the difference between CD4 fragments and the CD4 molecules on living cells, and it will evolve around antibodies produced by vaccines, laboratories, or genetically engineered cells.

The basic problem is that HIV will evolve so that it no longer has the weak spot that is targeted by the anti-HIV strategy, so long as the weak spot is not essential to successful reproduction among all HIVs. The high mutation rate of HIV tilts the balance in its favor in this arms race. If we find a "magic bullet" against some HIVs, some other HIVs are bound to have, or will soon acquire, magic armor. The solutions that we are developing against HIV are therefore short-term solutions, much like the development of each new influenza vaccine.

Given this situation what are we to do? Pursuing the short-term solutions will undoubtedly provide important benefits. But we should also recognize that there may be long-term solutions that could eventually transform HIV into a more benign organism, thereby reducing the need to rely so heavily on the short-term solutions. As outlined in the previous chapter, investment in interventions that reduce the frequencies of sexual and needleborne transmission should provide such a long-term solution: an evolutionary transformation of HIV into a more benign pathogen.

CHAPTER 10

A Look Backward . . .

*He who has only once through his own efforts tried to trace
back the long path trod by his predecessors, who has felt how
clear and luminous his own knowledge becomes as he grows
aware of the historical circumstances out of which it has
arisen, and who discovers the basis of the errors by which
even genuine investigators have been misled, he who has
learned that a kernel of truth sticks in every error, will not
place himself with those who despise historical studies*

(Virchow 1877/1962)

It's pompous, I admit, but I think Virchow's point is well taken. Placing current
knowledge in historical perspective does give us a better idea of its value. Let
us look back to understand the insights that provided the basis for the union of
evolution and the health sciences that I offer in this book. The first major insight
was the recognition that other organisms, particularly those organisms invisible
to the naked eye, can cause disease by living inside our bodies. The second
involves the understanding of disease over spatial and temporal scales that are
larger than the scales associated with individual people. This insight involves the
spread of diseases among populations and the changes in diseases over time. The
third insight is that our activities can alter the effects of parasites across the entire
spectrum of temporal and spatial scales from the microscopic and chemical levels
through the level of the individual to the spread of disease across populations and
the change in disease characteristics over time.

INTERNAL PARASITES AS A CAUSE OF DISEASE

Worms in ancient civilizations

The ancient civilizations showed appreciable understanding of the relationships between parasitic worms and disease. Although therapy in Mesopotamia and ancient Egypt was based largely on religious activities, both cultures used effective drugs. Both cultures, for example, used hyoscyamus. In Egypt, it was used to treat "abdominal distress caused by roundworms or tapeworms and to expel 'magic' in the belly" (Slater 1965). Today the narcotic component of hyoscyamus is used to relieve tremors and control heart rate. A closely related drug, atropine, has been used in modern times to reduce gut motility in diarrhea; like some treatments used in ancient times, this use probably causes more harm than good because gut motility often appears to be a defense against pathogen invasion (see Chapter 2).

The Mesopotamians used a simple but effective surgical procedure to deal with a macroscopic internal parasite. For Mesopotamians, as for millions of people in recent years, one of life's painful inconveniences was the guinea worm, the nematode called *Dracunculus medinensis*. People become infected by inadvertently drinking water containing tiny aquatic crustaceans called cyclops, which have been infested with the *D. medinensis* larvae. An ingested female worm grows to a meter during a year-long anatomical itinerary. The trip starts in the stomach where it burrows out of the cyclops. Its next stop is the small intestine, where it detours through the intestinal wall and meanders through muscles and connective tissues, growing to its full length. It eventually makes its way to the tissues beneath the armpit, where it settles in for months of feeding and where females and males make their rendezvous. After several months, the female worm resumes her travels just below the skin, where her outline can be seen externally, as if a bulging meter-long vein in the forearm had embarked on a subdermal voyage. As its maternal duties draw near, the worm navigates to its final destination: the tissues just below the skin in a leg or foot. At this stage, the worm manipulates the person (*sensu* Chapter 2) to aid in its transmission: the worm coils and secretes a substance that produces an itching blister. The person relieves the fiery sensation by wading in water, which causes the blister to rupture. Within the crater of the ruptured blister is the reproductive opening of the female, which then sheds millions of baby worms. The jerky movements of the babies attract hungry cyclops which ingest the nematodes. The nematodes penetrate the gut wall of the cyclops and grow in its body cavity. The lethargic cyclops sinks to lower levels of the water column where people are most likely to gather their drinking water, starting the process over again.

The Mesopotamians put two and two together. Something was crawling around under the skin of people, who eventually developed a burning blister. If this thing could be pulled out, then the uncomfortable blister might be avoided.

The only problem was that if you cut through the skin, grabbed the worm, and tried to pull it out, you left a small part of a worm in your hand and a large part of a worm festering in your patient. The Mesopotamian physicians therefore withdrew the worm slowly so that the worm dried into a tough leathery tube that could be pulled without breaking. But to remove an entire worm this way takes a month, and it wouldn't do to have a foot or two of dried worm dangling from your patients for weeks. Besides being bad advertising, dried worms catching on objects might hinder further chances of successfully removing the worm. The solution was to roll up the worm on a stick. A carefully rolled worm could advertise technical know-how, something that may have been used as a symbol on the physician's place of practice.

This symbol may sound vaguely familiar. Biblical writings tell how the followers of Moses became discouraged by the harshness of the travel from Mount Hor.

> And the people spake against God and against Moses, Wherefore have ye brought us up out of Egypt to die in the wilderness? . . . And the Lord sent fiery serpents among the people, and they bit the people. . . . Therefore, the people came to Moses, and said, We have sinned, for we have spoken against the Lord, and against thee; pray unto the Lord, that he take away the serpents from us. And Moses prayed for the people. And the Lord said unto Moses, Make thee a fiery serpent, and set it upon a pole; and it shall come to pass that every one that is bitten, when he looketh upon it, shall live. And Moses made a serpent of brass and put it upon a pole . . . and it came to pass that if a serpent had bitten any man, when he beheld the serpent of brass, he lived. (Numbers 21:5-9)

Some medical scholars believe that the "fiery serpents" were *Dracunculus medinensis*. When bitten people saw the symbol of a serpent on a pole, they may well have become cured, especially if that symbol signified the presence of a physician qualified to remove the little dragons of Medina. The emblem of the ancient Greek physicians' society of Asclepius is a snake wrapped about a staff, and modern medicine uses two serpents coiled around a staff as its symbol. Although the modern symbol, the caduceus, is derived from the wand of Mercury, it, like the others, may have derived at least indirectly from an ancient symbol of expertise at extracting the little dragons of Medina.

The Egyptian physicians discovered that parasitic worms caused many diseases; then by extrapolation they attributed other ailments to invasions of worms. Although this extrapolation was largely incorrect, the logic behind it was similar to another logical argument that was to transform the study of disease: the germ theory. But this transformation was still three millennia in the future.

The Greeks carefully observed, described, and distinguished diseases, and then offered hypotheses to explain them. Building on Egyptian ideas they proposed that diseases represented imbalances of four fundamental elements: earth, water, fire, and air. But the first writings that hypothesized minute, invisible, self-replicating parasites as the cause of disease and epidemics came at the end of the Renaissance.

Contagia, miasma and the scale barrier

During the last century of the Renaissance, Girolamo Fracastoro gathered and interpreted information about the scourges of his day: smallpox, typhoid, leprosy, bubonic plague, syphilis, and typhus. In 1546, he published the idea that diseases were caused by disease-specific germs that could multiply within the body and be transmitted directly from person to person or indirectly on contaminated objects, even over long distances; moreover, he proposed that variations in the intensity of epidemics could be attributed to changes in the virulence of germs. In so doing, Fracastoro laid down the fundamental ideas of epidemiology and the application of evolutionary change to epidemiology three centuries before the existence of germs was documented and three centuries before Charles Darwin conceived evolutionary biology. But these ideas were largely overlooked, probably because of the paucity of knowledge about very small living things and very small building blocks of large living things. His ideas would be regenerated later, after this knowledge at the microscopic level had been gained.

Considering the spirit of scientific inquiry at the end of the Renaissance, it may seem surprising that it took three centuries to critically test whether germs were causes of disease. A microscope was invented by Galileo about 50 years after Fracastoro published his early version of the germ theory, and some parasites not visible to the naked eye would have been visible through his microscope. Perhaps the more important damper was the gap in knowledge between the spatial scale of human experience and the smaller scales of germs. From Fracastoro to Robert Koch, scientific probing into the nature of disease followed a progressive though haphazard course through the level of organ systems to organs to tissues to host cells and eventually to the interactions between these host cells and their smaller parasites.

By the seventeenth century, medical people were already thinking in terms of organ systems, thanks to anatomists like Andreas Vesalius. Vesalius's meticulous dissections and drawings of human anatomy redirected studies of human biology to directly observable evidence rather than untested hypotheses.

During the seventeenth and eighteenth centuries, a variety of new hypotheses of disease had their adherents. The English physician Thomas Sydenham promoted an ontological view: Diseases were specific entities that developed like an organism inside the host. He likened disease in an individual to a plant that springs from the earth, blooms, and dies. But Sydenham was interpreting disease at the level of the whole person. He was perplexed because he could understand only what distinguished one disease from another clinically, and not what the disease itself was.

Progress on this problem eventually came from Italy and France. Giovanni Morgagni and Marie Bichat merged Vesalius's tendency to look at the human body in terms of its component organ systems with Sydenham's penchant for classification. In 1761, Morgagni published a book that steered studies of disease away from the regions of the body such as the chest, head, or abdomen to the major macroscopic building blocks of the body: the organs. From hundreds of dissections he showed that different diseases affected different organs in a predictable way and proposed that the outward symptoms of disease resulted from these pathological changes in the organs. Bichat then honed understanding of disease to the tissues that make up the organs. He found that within a given organ a particular disease might typically affect one tissue, while another tissue of the same organ could be healthy. Another disease would affect organ tissues in a different way. Clearly a unified understanding of infectious disease would be found at or below the tissue level. Morgagni and Bichat moved the focus from the organism, through organ systems and organs, down to level of the damaged tissues.

Now the study of disease was ready for the microscope. In 1838, Schleiden and Schwann showed that cells were the building blocks of tissues. If the key to infectious disease lay below the tissue level, cells were the place to look. Johann Schoenlein used the microscope as a tool for understanding disease. In 1839, drawing insight from a recent discovery of a fungal parasite of silkworms, he discovered a microbial parasite of humans, a multicellular fungus now called *Trichophyton schoenleinii*, which causes a severe "ringworm" infection of the scalp. A year later, the German anatomist Jacob Henle regenerated the portions of Fracastoro's speculations that were consistent with the evidence accumulated during the intervening three centuries. Like Fracastoro, Henle reasoned that the microscopic agents of disease could multiply inside hosts. The evidence that accumulated since Fracastoro led some people to believe that some diseases like syphilis could be transmitted directly from person to person by contagia, whereas others like malaria were often acquired by miasma, some noxious substance emanating from the soil. Like Fracastoro, Henle realized that some diseases could be acquired both from direct contact and from some distance, and therefore reasoned that the contagia and miasma of a given disease were the same thing (Sigerist 1943).

In the early nineteenth century, most of the general ideas presented throughout the previous 3,000 years were still present in one form or another. Much of the populus still considered disease to be an act of divine punishment. Medical philosophy was splintered into different camps of ardent believers. The humoral and solidistic hypotheses of ancient Greece were still alive. Several versions of Sydenham's ontological viewpoint were represented, and there was an emerging physiological faction, which proposed that diseases were states of abnormal body function. Another camp, the vitalists, suggested that diseases could be understood according to the amount of vital force they contained.

But there was a promising feature infusing this philosophical confusion: some people in the various factions, like the vitalist Schoenlein, were using observations of disease and predictions to distinguish arguments. The advocates of solidistic causes of disease were proposing that pathological disruption would ultimately occur in the solid parts of the body; conversely, the humoristic advocates blamed the liquid parts (Rather 1962). The lack of evidence to distinguish between these competing beliefs stemmed from the scale of inquiry. It was not yet small enough. Even so, the integration of repeatable observation and classification was laying the groundwork for this finer scale of inquiry.

The microbial and submicrobial scales

By personally conducting tens of thousands of autopsies, the Austrian Karl von Rokitansky developed Morgagni's insights about organ pathology and disease into a classification system of disease. Rudolf Virchow guided thinking toward a philosophical resolution by reducing the spatiotemporal scale of infectious diseases down to the cellular and subcellular level. He built upon disease nomenclature developed by von Rokitansky, whom he called "the Linnaeus of pathological anatomy" (Nuland 1981). But in contrast to the pathological anatomists like von Rokitansky, Virchow proposed that neither anatomical nor histological changes need be present during disease. That is, disease could result from chemical alterations yielding physiological effects within host cells without having higher-order anatomical effects on tissues or organs. This reduction in temporal and spatial scale is clear from his 1854 article, "Specifiker und Specifisches." "Every anatomical change is a material one as well, but is every material change, therefore also anatomical: Can it not be molecular? . . . These finer molecular changes of matter are objects of physiology rather than anatomy; they are functional . . ." (Virchow 1877/1962). Virchow was also well aware of where his insights lay on this progression to an increasingly finer scale.

> One can have the greatest respect for anatomical, morphological, and histological studies, and one can regard them as the unavoidably necessary foundation for all further investigation—but must one proclaim them, therefore, the only ones to be pursued, the ones of exclusive significance? Many important phenomena in the body are of a purely functional kind, and when one attempts to explain these also with a mechanistic hypothesis, in terms of fine-molecular changes, it should never be forgotten that the methods for their observation and pursuit can never be anatomical. (Virchow 1877/1962)

Virchow's perspective negated the contradictions between the humoristic and solidistic factions. Because cells were both liquid and solid, cellular pathology would encompass both liquid and solid phases. Two centuries of medical meanderings carried Virchow well beyond Sydenham. At midcentury he could identify the manifestations of disease at the organ, tissue, and, at least hypothetically, at the cellular level. But like Sydenham he was perplexed; although he could distinguish one disease from another at these finer levels, he could not identify any substance of disease. Without this understanding, the physiological and ontological bases of diseases were still unclear.

As the last quarter of the nineteenth century began, the nagging problems about the substance of disease were soon to be solved by one of Henle's protégés. Building upon Pasteur's evidence for self-replicating microorganisms, Robert Koch identified the specific bacteria that caused anthrax. This discovery set in motion an avalanche of evidence that buried the other hypotheses of the day. An hypothesis very much like the one Fracastoro had proposed three centuries before, was finally confirmed.

The germ theory fundamentally changed the questions being asked about infectious disease. Before the germ theory, people asked, What is disease? After the germ theory was established, the questions were, Which germs cause which disease? How they do it? And, how can they be controlled? Investigation of the first two questions led quickly to the discovery of many bacterial pathogens. It also led to the search, during the twentieth century, for smaller pathogens such as rickettsiae, viruses, and viroids. This trend toward understanding how diseases develop on progressively smaller scales is now culminating in a deciphering of events that occur within molecules over tiny fractions of seconds. What portions of a DNA molecule code for the critical characteristics of host defense and parasite virulence? What controls the reading and use of this information? How does the activity of an antibody molecule depend on slight changes in the molecule's sequence of building blocks? Investigations of these questions have unified disease manifestations observable by the naked eye with characteristics of diseased organs, tissues, cells, and subcellular processes, down to interactions between portions of molecules. This unification has allowed the maturation of the two basic treatments of individuals to protect them against infectious diseases: antibiotic therapy and vaccination.

THE SUPERORGANISMAL SCALE

Fracastoro's emphasis on short-distance and long-distance transmission emphasized the need to understand disease in terms of spatial scales larger than the individual. His suggestion that virulence may change through time similarly emphasized the need to understand disease in terms of time scales longer than those of a patient's illness or an epidemic. But Fracastoro was too early.

The development and testing of ideas about transmission would have to wait until the mid-nineteenth century—until John Snow investigated the transmission of cholera by focusing on London's network of piped water. Even though the agent of cholera had not yet been discovered, Snow showed that cholera was sometimes waterborne. By making house-to-house records of cholera cases in a residential district of London, he showed that cholera occurred almost entirely among customers of a single water company, which obtained its water from a part of the Thames River that was heavily contaminated with raw sewage. Cholera rarely occurred when water was supplied by a competing company which used a pure source, even though the houses served by the two companies were intermixed (Snow 1855/1966). Snow showed that cholera could be transmitted by water, but he also showed that some of the cholera was not waterborne. By investigating the timing of these cases, Snow showed that cholera could sometimes be transmitted through contaminated food or direct contact.

While Snow was working on cholera in London, Ignaz Semmelweis was making strikingly similar analyses of data that he gathered from the hospitals of Vienna. By tabulating death rates of women after childbirth, he showed that high death rates occurred when doctors did not use precautionary treatment of hands and equipment. He deduced that the cause of childbed fever was transmitted on the hands of the doctors during their examinations (see Chapter 6).

These quantitative studies by Snow and Semmelweis, more than any others, gave birth to the field of epidemiology, the study of disease distribution and transmission in host populations. When Robert Koch identified the bacteria that caused cholera, tuberculosis and other infectious diseases a quarter century later, epidemiology matured rapidly. During the century since Koch's discoveries, studies have unified disease processes from the molecular level to the population level, and from milliseconds through ecological time scales. Unification of these interactions through the generally longer evolutionary time scales was less successful, however.

The germ theory led directly to a discovery that fundamentally changed scientists' large-scale views of infectious disease. People infected with the agents of such killers as cholera, diphtheria, typhoid fever, and dysentery sometimes showed no symptoms of disease. Yet pathogens transmitted from these asymptomatic infections could often give rise to lethal cases. With regard to large spatial scales this discovery suggested that to control an outbreak, more than just the overt cases had to be considered; mild and asymptomatic infections could also spread disease. The effect on our view of diseases over long time scales followed a more circuitous route. Prior to this time, the agents of diseases were thought of as antagonists to the host. The discovery of benign infections caused by potentially virulent agents suggested that given enough time any pathogens might have the option of not adversely affecting its host. To many biologists and health scientists, this option seemed the best of all possible worlds, not just for the host but for the parasite as well. The parasite could use just enough of the host resources to survive and be transmitted; its home and future food sources would remain intact.

Tracing this belief back to Pasteur, Rene Dubos (1960) wrote "The most efficient parasite . . . is the one that lives in harmony with its host, feeding upon it, of course, but not to the extent of depleting its vigor . . . Of interest to [Pasteur] were the phenomena associated with latent, dormant infectious processes, since these can be regarded as manifestations—even though temporary—of the ideal form of parasitism." As the germ theory emerged, van Beneden (1885), too, proposed that a parasite "profits by all the advantages enjoyed by the host on whom he thrusts his presence." During the early 1900s, parasitologists made similar brief references to benign coexistence as the logical evolutionary outcome (Woodcock 1909), but it was not until the 1930s that this view was clearly enunciated and accepted as dogma. Hans Zinsser (1935), N. H. Swellengrebel (1940), and especially Theobald Smith (1934) were avid purveyors of this idea. In the years that followed, some advocates tempered their generalizations by suggesting that some level of virulence might aid dissemination (Andrewes 1960); some others disagreed outright (Ball 1943, Cockburn 1963, Coatney et al. 1971), but none proposed an alternative evolutionary framework. Until just a decade ago, the supporters of commensalism as the ideal of parasitism held sway through charismatic writing. Lewis Thomas (1972), for example, wrote that "there is nothing to be gained, in an evolutionary sense by the capacity to cause illness or death. Pathogenicity may be something more frightening to them than to us." Dubos (1960) embraced this view in his introduction to H. J. Simon's book on the subject: "Infectious processes appear not as a form of warfare between a vicious parasite and a defensive host but rather as normal manifestations of the constant interplay between living things." He concludes that "given enough time a state of peaceful coexistence eventually becomes established between any host and parasite" (Dubos 1965). In this book I have argued that even if enough time is given, warfare between a vicious parasite and a defensive host may sometimes be a normal manifestation of the constant interplay between host and parasite.

CHAPTER 11

. . . And A Glimpse Forward
(Or WHO Needs Darwin)

EMERGING PATHOGENS

Insights without evolution

The AIDS pandemic has focused attention on "emerging" pathogens. If HIV can cause such devastation, what new viruses might be emerging from the existing pool of pathogens in humans and other organisms? In May 1989, for example, a meeting entitled "Emerging Viruses: The Evolution of Viruses and Viral Diseases" attracted considerable attention in the scientific media (Miller 1989, Weiss 1989a, Culliton 1990). The meeting helped to draw together insights from a broad range of disciplines. Yet, in spite of the title, the meeting emphasized proximate mechanisms of virulence and transmission, rather than applications of evolutionary principles. In this meeting and in recent writings from this perspective, the emergence of severe epidemic disease is attributed to the spread of pathogens from isolated populations of humans or other animals, and the presence of mutations, which by chance might transform a relatively friendly bug into a deadly bug (Kawaoka & Webster 1988, Culliton 1990, Kilbourne 1990, Ampel 1991, Morse 1991). But one question continues to surface, and continues to be left unanswered: Why have some organisms evolved to become so harmful while others have not? The discussions generally invoke mutations as the source of the increased lethality, but the presence of mutations is only part of the story.

Mutations explain how variation in virulence can be created, but not why the predominant viruses are virulent or benign. To address the problem fully, one must explain why the new, severe mutants have spread at a faster rate not only than the long-present competitors, which have had more time to finely tune themselves to the host, but also than the milder variants of the new mutants.

If the principles presented in this book are correct, evolutionary epidemiologists should be able to provide ultimate answers to specific questions about virulence—questions that have been asked but left unanswered by investigators approaching the problem from more proximate approaches. For example, one question involves a comparison between HIV and human herpes virus 6 (HHV-6), each of which infects T4 cells (Culliton 1990, Morse 1991). Why is one virus lethal while the other is not? One evolutionary answer is that HIV is remarkably variable and hence can evolve to increased virulence within a host, whereas HHV-6, being a DNA virus, is a much less variable. This lack of variability means that little, if any, evolutionary transformation toward a more virulent state would occur between the beginning and the end of an infection. Phrased another way, the higher degrees of genetic relatedness among the HHV-6 viruses inside of a host would favor greater "cooperation" for long-term transmission, and hence lower levels of reproduction inside the host (see also Chapters 1 and 8). The net effect is smaller increases in virulence for HHV-6 than for HIV during the years of evolution inside of a given host, and a lower level of virulence over the long run.

A lack of emphasis on fitness costs and benefits associated with virulence has led epidemiologists to emphasize the time over which each parasite species has been infecting humans. The presumption is that highly virulent parasites were recently transmitted to humans from some other species of host—much as the myxoma virus was highly lethal when first introduced into Australian rabbits and relatively benign in its natural host, a South American species of rabbit. One problem with this analogy is that the myxoma virus did not evolve to benignness (Chapter 3). The myxoma scenario has been applied to the emerging virus discussion to emphasize the costs that we would likely pay during the time period over which a new, lethal pathogen evolves toward benignness (W. H. McNeill, quoted by Weiss 1989a). But the myxoma virus was introduced into Australia as an agent for biological control; that is, it was chosen precisely because of its extraordinarily high virulence for Australian rabbits. Considering this history and the virus's vectorborne transmission, the myxoma scenario therefore seems a special case consistent with current evolutionary theory about virulence, rather than a representative example of host–parasite coevolution.

The most appropriate application of the myxoma virus story to humans would be to illustrate the introduction of an arthropodborne pathogen into a previously unexposed population of humans, under a very special set of circumstances. Specifically, if such a pathogen had transmission modes that favored the maintenance of a high level of virulence (e.g., if it were vectorborne and the vector were present in the new area), and if we by chance happened to select one of the most virulent pathogens from the spectrum of virulences, we might get something close to the myxoma situation. But my guess is that this kind of introduction would be rare relative to the frequency intimated by those promoting the myxoma analogy. The closest we have come is the bubonic plague; when it first visited European cities, it regularly cut their populations by half (Meiss 1978).

People writing about emerging viruses often conclude that the increased mobility of people in modern society creates a daunting challenge for controlling the spread of massive lethal epidemics. The logic I have presented raises the prospect of making this challenge more manageable. By using evolutionary insights we may be able to distinguish the many pathogens that we do not need to worry about from the few that we do. Our association with most emerging pathogens will not be highly lethal over long periods. But one of the important conclusions that can be drawn from this book is that some of the associations will remain severe, and we would be well advised to put some effort into figuring out how to distinguish these dangerous pathogens from the rest of the pack. This advice is particularly timely now that government administrators are considering funding of policies to intercept and arrest the pathogens of our future before they expand to pandemic proportions (Gibbons 1992).

Recent writings on the threat of emerging infectious diseases have included predictions about those diseases that could be problematic in the future (Kilbourne 1991, Morse 1991). Because principles of natural selection have not been woven into the analysis, however, these previous predictions have been inductive generalizations from past trends more than deductions from evolutionary principles. Pathogens that have caused localized, highly lethal outbreaks or large-scale, moderately lethal outbreaks are generally considered dangerous. Pathogens, such as newly recognized hepatitis and herpes viruses, which have become widely disseminated from relatively benign virus groups, are not considered major threats (Morse 1991).

The contribution of evolution

Applying the principles of natural selection should allow us to make long-term predictions that are more discriminating. I shall contrast these two approaches by rounding up the usual suspects. Application of the principles discussed in this book allows us to exonerate some and finger others. This application should give us an idea of the emerging pathogens on which we should focus our efforts and limited resources. In the paragraphs below, I evaluate the threat imposed by these usual suspects, beginning with those that we do not need to worry much about at least in terms of massive epidemics of lethal infections.

In August 1967, Marburg virus entered people apparently from laboratory monkeys. It killed a quarter of the 20 or so people who fell ill, but too few new infections were produced from existing infections to maintain the virus; after several transmission cycles the outbreak self-destructed (Howard 1984, Southwood 1987). Its ephemerality should be no surprise. It had a suicidal combination of attributes: it was directly transmitted and rapidly debilitating (Johnson 1989).

At about the same time that Marburg virus was causing problems in Europe, its cousin, called Ebola virus, killed about half of the 1000 or so people it infected in Zaire and Sudan (Howard 1984). The relatively large number of infections is attributable in part to transmission in hospitals through contaminated needles (Johnson 1989). This kind of attendant-borne transmission may favor pathogens of relatively high virulence, or, in this case, a delay in the extinction of an outbreak of pathogens that are too virulent to be stably maintained by normal routes of direct transmission (see Chapter 6). Lassa fever, which entered humans from the mouse, *Mastomys natalensis*, has a similar history of temporary outbreaks under hospital conditions. Argentine and Bolivian hemorrhagic fevers offer two more examples of suicidal pathogens transmitted directly from other mammals, but too immobilizing to be maintained by normal person-to-person transmission.

The dismissal of these pathogens requires a caveat. The preceding argument assumes that the pathogens are not durable in the external environment. If they are durable, the theoretical framework of this book proposes they could be stably maintained as a virulent pathogen in human populations (see Chapter 4). We therefore need more information on their durability to fully assess the danger they pose.

Legionnaires' disease represents only a slight variation on this theme. It acquired its name from the Legionnaires' convention in Philadelphia where, during the summer of 1976, it killed 29 of the 182 people who fell ill (Kilbourne 1991). The Legionnaires' bacterium lives independently of humans in aquatic environments, causing disease when it is wafted into the air, for example, by ventilation equipment, and inhaled. It can survive in the external environment for long periods of time, but it offers little potential for epidemic spread because it has little opportunity for continuous human-to-human cycling.

The pathogens mentioned above should burn themselves out or evolve to benignness so long as they rely on direct transmission between people and either do not have or do not evolve durability in the external environment. If these pathogens did acquire the ability to be transmitted from person to person efficiently enough to be maintained in humans, the framework of this book indicates that their virulence would decline to within the range of virulences found among other directly transmitted respiratory pathogens. For pathogens that are not particularly durable, this range is bounded by the typical strains of the influenza virus or measles on the virulent side and rhinovirus on the benign side.

If, however, their transmission involves a cultural vector, or if they are durable outside the host, we can expect a virulence bounded by more dangerous pathogens like the agents of smallpox, tuberculosis, or cholera. The key, then, is to establish surveillance not simply for new pathogens but also for biological characteristics of the pathogens (such as durability in the external environment and arthropodborne transmission) and cultural conditions (such as those permitting waterborne, needleborne, or attendant-borne transmission) that would favor increased virulence should an emerging pathogen rely on them for transmission.

HTLV as an emerging pathogen

HTLV infections. We need to keep a close watch on the human T cell lymphotropic viruses (HTLVs, also called human T cell leukemia/lymphoma viruses), which are in the same virus family as HIV (Retroviridae) but a different subfamily. Two kinds of HTLV have been discovered. HTLV-I was first isolated in 1978 and reported in 1980 (Poiesz et al. 1980), three years before the first report of HIV (Barre-Sinoussi et al. 1983), whereas HTLV-II was reported just one year before HIV (Kalyanaraman et al. 1982).

In about one out of 20 infected people, HTLV-I eventually triggers cancerous growth of white blood cells (leukemia and lymphoma) or damage to the brain and spinal cord with ensuing paralysis (Kondo et al. 1989; Blattner 1990; Kira et al. 1991). Evidence indicates that the cancers result from the activity of the HTLV inside the cancerous cells (Murphy & Blattner 1988, Yamaguchi et al. 1988, Alexandre & Verrier 1991, Berneman et al. 1992). An activating protein of HTLV, called tax, appears to be a nonessential stimulator of this growth, like HIV's activator, tat, is for Kaposi's sarcoma (Berneman et al. 1992, Duyao et al. 1992, Rosenblatt et al. 1992, Sakurai et al 1992, Yamaoka et al. 1992; stimulation by tat is described in Chapter 8). Tax also may be responsible for setting in motion the changes that lead to the neurological damage associated with HTLV-I infection (Sawada et al 1992). Because the cancers are generally fatal (Shimoyama 1991), they cause a mortality per HTLV-I infection that is comparable to the lethality of human pathogens like the tuberculosis bacterium. The time until death from HTLV, however, is longer—typically several decades after a person becomes infected.

As with HIV-1, the abundance of HTLV-I is typically 10- to 100-fold greater when disease is present than when infections are asymptomatic (Yoshida et al. 1989, Kira et al. 1991, Kubota et al. 1993). People who harbor large amounts of virus during early asymptomatic periods tend to have numerous abnormalities in their white-blood cells and progress to disease rapidly (Kira et al. 1991, Tachibana et al. 1992). In general, however, rates of multiplication and densities of HTLV in the blood are low, and free HTLV is rarely detectable in the blood

(Tokudome 1991). The low levels of replication appear to be controlled by a complex set of genetic instructions that suppress replication (Pavlakis et al. 1992). The rarity of free virus in the blood has led researchers to conclude that transmission occurs mainly by fusion of cells rather than invasion by free virus (Sugiyama et al. 1986, Murphy & Blattner 1988), even though free virus can infect cells (Fan et al. 1992).

This restricted replication of HTLV contrasts with replication by HIV-1. The latter is detectable throughout the infection; it reaches high densities in the blood during the first few months of infection before the still-intact immune system suppresses it, and then again during late stages when the crippled immune systems have lost their suppressive powers (Clark et al. 1991, Daar et al. 1991, Schnittman et al. 1991). HIV also produces more copies of the messages used for synthesizing viral proteins, particularly in the most virulent variants, and is lethal to cells more often than HTLV (Somasundaran & Robinson 1988, Gallo 1991, Kettman et al. 1991). The additional copies may provide one of the biochemical mechanisms through which HIV maintains a higher reproductive rate than HTLV. Although HIV reproduces more extensively than HTLV and is more transmissible (Blattner 1990), both groups of viruses appear to obtain a benefit from increased reproduction inside the host: Contact with susceptibles leads to infection more frequently as indicators of viral abundance increase (Sugiyama et al. 1986, Blattner 1990, Ho et al. 1991, Scarlatti et al. 1991). Although the numbers of HIV-infected cells are generally higher than the numbers of HTLV-infected cells, these numbers are comparable in severely affected people (Daar et al. 1991, Bagasra et al. 1992, Wattel et al. 1992, Embretson et al. 1993, Kubota et al. 1993).

HTLV-I, like HIV, activates production of compounds, called lymphokines, which normally control growth and differentiation of white blood cells, and which can eventually result in suppression of the immune system (Kuroda et al. 1991, Yu et al. 1991). In a minority of HTLV-I infections some kinds of white blood cells may eventually become decimated. This decimation is more severe as the number of HTLV in the blood increases (Yu et al. 1991) and can open the door for opportunistic infections with AIDS-causing organisms such as *Pneumocystis carinii* (Shearer & Clerici 1991). In accordance with the generally lower abundance of HTLV in an infected person, this immunosuppression is less severe, and the duration of time between initial infection and the onset of life-threatening symptoms is much longer for HTLV-I than for HIV-1 (Robert-Guroff et al. 1986, Tajima 1988).

The cancers triggered by HTLV-I sometimes bear an ominous similarity to cancers associated with HIV infections. A cancer called non-Hodgkin's lymphoma is the indicator of AIDS in about 3% of cases, and seems to be especially prevalent when the duration of infection is prolonged by AZT therapy (Pluda et al. 1990). That is, as the duration of HIV infection inches toward the duration of HTLV infection, its cancerous manifestations bear a closer similarity to HTLV. Although most of these cancers caused by HTLV-I involve cancerous T lymphocytes, a small percentage seem to involve cancers of the cell type (B lymphocytes) typical of the non-Hodgkin's lymphomas caused by HIV (Murphy & Blattner 1988). Reciprocally, some of the cancers caused by HIV involve T-cells and, like the T-cell cancers caused by HTLV-I, may be comprised of infected cells (Herndier et al 1992).

Geographical patterns of transmission and virulence. Could human activities inadvertently favor the development of especially productive HTLVs that have reduced intervals between infection and disease? The geographic pattern of HTLV disease and sexual transmission suggests that such a process may have already begun.

Studies over the past decade indicate that HTLVs are geographically widespread and have been infecting humans for millennia (Gessain et al. 1991, Maloney et al. 1992, Goubau et al 1992). In the United States, HTLV is about half as common as HIV among intravenous drug users and about one-tenth as common in the general population (Cantor et al. 1991, Lentino et al. 1991). HTLV-I infects about 1% to 10% of the general population in regions of Japan, Taiwan, Melanesia, the southeastern United States, the Caribbean, South America, Italy, and sub-Saharan Africa (Blayney et al. 1983, Merino et al. 1984, Levine et al. 1988, Cabrera et al. 1991, Delaporte et al. 1991b, Maloney et al. 1991, Vasquez et al. 1991, Yanagihara et al. 1991a, Trujillo et al. 1992). The isolates of HTLV-I from different geographic areas have consistent differences in structure (De et al. 1991, Gessain et al. 1991, Komurian et al. 1991, Komurian-Pradel et al. 1992, Sherman et al. 1992), although they and their monkey-infecting relatives are much less variable than HIV, probably because of lower rates of replication and mutation (Lal & Griffis 1991, Ehrlich et al. 1992). These geographic differences indicate that HTLV-I transmission between geographic areas has been more limited than HIV transmission over the past few decades.

HTLV-II has been found to infect about 5% of the Guaymi, a native people of Panama and up to one-third of remote aboriginal tribes in Brazil; it also occurs in Africa and among intravenous drug users in the United States and Europe (Blattner 1989, Ehrlich et al. 1989, Lee et al. 1989, Biggar et al. 1991, Delaporte et al. 1991a, De Rossi et al. 1991a, Maloney et al. 1992).

HTLV-I can be needleborne, sexually transmitted and transmitted from mother to baby at least partly through breast milk (Hino et al. 1985, Kajiyama et al. 1986, Robert-Guroff et al. 1986, Kusuhara et al. 1987, Nagamine et al. 1991, Ueda et al 1992, Kawase et al. 1992). Although HIV also can be transmitted from mother to child, the maternal transmission of HTLV may facilitate greater evolution toward benignness, because HTLV infection almost never leads to death before the person reaches reproductive age. (For a more general discussion of vertical transmission and evolution to benignness, see Chapter 3.)

The importance of the different routes of transmission varies geographically. The two most intensively studied areas are Japan and the Caribbean. The HTLV-I strains isolated from these areas arise from the same branch of the HTLV-I evolutionary tree, and probably diverged from an ancestral HTLV-I over the last few centuries (Saksena et al. 1993).

In Japan, rates of unprotected sexual contact are relatively low. Because access to birth control pills is restricted, birth control depends largely on condoms (Trager 1982, Carey et al. 1992, Miller et al. 1992). A survey completed during the 1970s showed that condoms were used by over 80% of all women using birth control, and over 90% of women in their early twenties; only 3% of women surveyed said that they would use birth control pills (Trager 1982). In the Caribbean, the percentages are reversed. Among Jamaican women, for example, less than 10% used condoms and about 70% used birth control pills (Schwartz et al. 1989). Condom use is also low in other areas of the Caribbean (Halsey et al. 1992).

The geographic clustering of HTLV in Japan indicates that transmission occurs primarily from mother to offspring (Hinuma et al. 1982, Tajima et al. 1982, Yamaguchi et al. 1983, Tajima 1988). Even in cities, HTLV infection has been associated more strongly with the person's geographic origin within Japan than with risky sexual contact (Tajima 1988). In the Caribbean, HTLV-I has the more uniform geographic distribution characteristic of sexual transmission, and it is especially prevalent among people who have many sexual partners (Clark et al. 1985, Murphy et al. 1989, Rodriguez et al. 1993). In Trinidad, for example, it is about six times as prevalent among male homosexuals as among the general population (Bartholomew et al. 1987).

Because venereal transmission of retroviruses tends to occur more readily from men to women than from women to men (Padian et al. 1991), sexually transmitted HTLV should show up in women sooner than in men. The age at which this female bias begins to appear is an indicator of sexually transmitted HTLV. A preponderance of active infections in women begins shortly after the age of 20 in Jamaica and Barbados, but after the age of 40 in Japan; it continues to rise with age in each of these areas (Tajima et al. 1982, Kajiyama et al. 1986, Riedel et al. 1989, Tajima & Ito 1990, Murphy et al. 1991).

The time period between infection and the onset of symptoms also varies geographically. In Japan, people who eventually develop HTLV-induced cancers tend to do so late in life, when about 60 years old on average (Tajima 1988, Shimoyama 1991). Although sexual transmission from men to women eventually creates a preponderance of infections among women, the frequency of cancers among women may be only slightly higher than that among men, and the frequency among infected women is lower than that among infected men (Sugiyama et al. 1986, Kondo et al. 1989). This difference between men and women and the lack of T cell cancers in people who did not acquire their infection from their parents suggest that cancers develop primarily and perhaps almost exclusively in infections acquired from parents (Sugiyama et al. 1986, Tajima & Ito 1990). The 60-year interval between birth and cancer therefore roughly reflects the time between infection and cancer.

In the Caribbean, infected people begin to develop cancers earlier, typically when in their early forties (Murphy & Blattner 1988). Cancer victims are predominantly women there, suggesting that cancerous infectious may be sexually transmitted. If so, the time between infection and cancer in the Caribbean is probably less than 40 years, about half as long as in Japan. The sketchy data from immigrant families suggest that British residents of Caribbean origin experience cancer at a similarly younger age than Hawaiian residents of Okinawan origin (Greaves et al. 1984, Blattner et al. 1986). The geographic differences therefore do not seem attributable to some environmental difference between the Caribbean and Japan.

These considerations indicate that both sexual partner rate and virulence of HTLV infections are greater in the Caribbean than in Japan. The current evidence draws attention to the need for studies designed to assess the extent to which this differences in virulence results from differences in the inherent harmfulness of the HTLVs as opposed to other influences on the course of infection.

Data from other geographic areas are more fragmentary, but the emerging trends are consistent with an association between sexual partner rates and HTLV virulence. In aboriginal people of Australia, the Solomon Islands, and Papua New Guinea, for example, genetically distinct groups of HTLV-I infect many people, but rarely cause cancers or neurological disease (Ajdukiewicz et al. 1989, Kirkland et al. 1991, Yanagihara et al. 1991ab, Saksena et al. 1992, Sherman et al. 1992). Accordingly, sociological study indicates that women in Papua New Guinea have limited opportunities for premarital sexual intercourse (Brabin et al. 1989). The patterns of infection in Papua New Guinea similarly suggest that the degree of sexual transmission is relatively low. The HTLV-I infections are clustered geographically and within family groups as in Japan, but prevalences of infections in males and females are similar, and the steady increases observed among women relative to men in Japan and Jamaica were not found in New Guinea (Kazura et al. 1987, Imai et al. 1990, Yanagihara et al. 1990). Only among women who migrated into endemic areas and had given birth to one or more children was there evidence of sexually transmitted infection (Brabin et al. 1989).

The data from Central and South America are even less complete, but the time until symptoms and potential for sexual transmission appear to be intermediate between Japan and the Caribbean (Cabrera et al. 1991, Trujillo et al. 1992, Wignall et al. 1992). In Panama, for example, both the proportion of infections progressing to cancer and the sexual partner rate appear to be lower than in Jamaica (Allman 1985, Reeves et al. 1988, Levine et al. 1989).

Future evolution of HTLV. The preceding comparisons suggest that geographic patterns of HTLV-I disease, like those for HIV, accord with predictions based on the frequencies of sexual transmission.   The recent entry of HTLV-I into Thailand, apparently from Japan (Hemachudha et al. 1992), presents an opportunity to track evolutionary increases in virulence. The rapid spread of HIV among Thai prostitutes suggests high sexual partner rates. If these rates do not diminish during the upcoming decades the virulence of the newly arrived HTLV-I should increase.

Current evidence indicates that HTLV-II can be transmitted by the same routes as HTLV-I: by needles and sex and from mother to offspring through breast feeding (Heneine et al. 1992).   Knowledge about geographic variation in transmission and the harmfulness of HTLV-II is just beginning to accumulate, but similar patterns may be occurring. HTLV-II infections among the Guaymi of Panama appear to be transmitted at very low rates; the precise modes are not certain, but some sexual and some parental transmission probably occur at low rates in the rural area that has been studied (Reeves et al. 1990). Accordingly, no disease has been detected in any of the 42 HTLV-II infected Guaymi who had been tested as of January 1992 (Reeves et al. 1990, F. Gracia, personal communication).

In the United States and Europe, needleborne transmission appears to be particularly important for both HTLVs (Feigal et al. 1991, Lentino et al. 1991, van den Hoek et al. 1991, Zanetti & Galli 1992). At greatest risk are individuals who have been using intravenous drugs for many years and those visiting shooting galleries (Feigal et al. 1991; Lentino et al. 1991). The prevalence of HTLV infection among these people increases more gradually and steadily than the prevalence of HIV infection (Lentino et al. 1991). This difference indicates that HTLV is less transmissible than HIV per needleborne contact, probably because HTLV is less abundant in the blood. HTLV has a lower prevalence than HIV in many European cities such as Amsterdam, where HIV has spread extensively through intravenous drug use (van den Hoek et al. 1991). This lower prevalence suggests that a dangerous potential exists for HTLV to spread, should it evolve the higher reproductive rates that would facilitate needleborne transmission.

Strains of HTLV circulating among intravenous drug users may have already moved partway down the evolutionary path toward increased virulence. In the United States, HTLV infections among intravenous drug users date back at least two decades (Biggar et al. 1991). Like HTLV-I and unlike HTLV-II among the Guaymi, HTLV-II in the United States is linked to unusual white-blood-cell cancers (Kalyanaraman et al. 1982, Ehrlich et al. 1989, Lee et al. 1989, Zucker-Franklin et al. 1992). Pathological changes in cells infected by HTLV-II provide some support for a cause–effect relationship (Miyamoto et al. 1991, Rosenblatt et al. 1992). In needleborne drug users, HTLV-II infections are also associated with neurological disease and with abnormal white-blood cell counts, but the available data are not yet sufficient to determine whether the HTLV-II infections caused these abnormalities (Biggar et al. 1991, Prince et al. 1992). Recently, HTLV-II infections in the United States have been linked to at least 10 cases of neurological disease that is similar to the disease caused by HTLV-I (Hjelle et al. 1992, Harrington et al. 1993, Murphy 1993). Most of these cases were found among native Americans. Although intravenous drug use provides a relatively common route of retroviral transmission in this ethnic group within the United States (Metler et al. 1991), links to intravenous drug use were not apparent among the native American cases; such links were apparent in some of the other cases (Hjelle et al. 1992, Harrington et al. 1993, Kaplan et al. 1993).

The gradual tendency for HTLV infection to increase with age and the lower prevalence of HTLV among long-exposed risk groups indicate that HTLV transmission has been slower than HIV transmission. But this difference may be diminishing. The rate of needleborne transmission and the prevalence of HTLV infection in San Francisco, for example, are comparable to those commonly found for HIV (Feigal et al. 1991).

Although incomplete, these details of HTLV distribution and infection indicate that HTLV is a threat, not because it might escape from a secluded source, but rather because it may evolve increased virulence in areas where environmental conditions favor this evolution. A lower mutation rate and a lower replication rate may have contributed to its relatively low virulence over the past century, but these characteristics can evolve. When HTLV enters areas with high levels of needleborne transmission and high rates of sexual transmission, it may follow an evolutionary course toward increased virulence, analogous to that proposed for its retroviral cousin, HIV-1. Reducing needleborne and sexual transmission should help keep this evolution from occurring and may reduce the harmfulness of those HTLV lineages that have already become particularly virulent.

Conversely, attempts to reduce mother-to-offspring transmission (e.g., see Sugiyama et al. 1986, Tajima & Ito 1990) could backfire. Transmission from mother to child should favor evolution toward benignness because mothers infected with benign viruses should have the most children and hence the greatest potential for parental transmission. The timing of illness in Japan supports this argument: HTLV rarely causes cancer until the mothers are past their reproductive years.

Evolutionary biologists will recognize this argument as an infectious version of the theory of senescence, whereby characteristics that provide an advantage before the end of the reproductive years will be favored even if they cause damage and death after the end of the normal reproductive years (Williams 1957, Hamilton 1966, Williams & Nesse 1991; see also Chapter 1). If this parental transmission is completely blocked, the benign strains that benefit from parental transmission will be disproportionately suppressed, leading to increased virulence. Moreover, parental transmission of HTLV may be slightly less important than previously thought, particularly in the Caribbean (Cruickshank et al. 1990, Ho et al. 1991). Investments in blocking parental transmission without blocking sexual transmission may therefore enhance HTLV's virulence, yielding a long-range cost with less short-range benefit than previously thought.

Emerging hepatitis viruses

The arguments about needleborne transmission of HTLV and HIV also apply to hepatitis viruses. Hepatitis B has been extensively needleborne for decades and is considered to be the most severe of the hepatitis viruses (Lee et al. 1989). Data from accidental punctures of hospital workers, for example, suggest that HIV-1 and hepatitis B impose comparable loss of life (Owens & Nease 1992, Schneiderman & Kaplan 1992).

The connection between replication of hepatitis B virus and tissue damage is largely indirect, as it is with HIV. Replication of hepatitis B stimulates the immune system to destroy liver cells (Tiollais & Buendia 1991). Because hepatitis B is transmitted largely from mother to offspring in much of the developing world (Tiollais & Buendia 1991), the evolutionary argument predicts geographic variation much like that predicted for HTLV: the virulence of the hepatitis B virus should be particularly high where needleborne and sexual transmission predominate and particularly low where maternal transmission predominates.

Hepatitis C has not been identified for long enough to determine its severity and whether it is a relatively new and spreading pathogen. It is especially worthy of scrutiny, however, because it appears to be especially needleborne (Wormser et al. 1991).

Pathogens emerging in institutions and among AIDS patients

As I mentioned in Chapter 6, the hospital environment is fertile ground for the entry of new pathogens into humans. Procedures such as surgery and catheterization can implant organisms directly into tissues, and the compromised defenses of hospitalized patients allow the implanted organisms to gain a foothold, even if they are not particularly well suited to using humans as hosts. This foothold may then allow the organisms to evolve improved abilities at a parasitism (Wallace 1989). Given the many pathogens that can cause serious hospital-acquired infections, one goal of the evolutionary epidemiologist is to distinguish those severe pathogens that are predisposed to cause a few isolated infections from those that have great potential for causing severe disease indefinitely—perhaps even by expanding into the uncompromised population if they can achieve a foothold.

Both attendant-borne transmission and sit-and-wait transmission (Chapters 4 and 6) are central to this problem. Attendant-borne transmission may favor increased virulence inside hospitals and similar institutions, but once these pathogens escape into the general population, they may often evolve toward lower virulence. But this generalization may not apply to sit-and-wait, hospital-acquired pathogens. Because sit-and-wait pathogens are, by definition, durable in the external environment, they may be especially prone to attendant-borne transmission. If they gain a foothold in humans, they may be virulent in hospitals because of attendant-borne transmission and maintain high virulence in the general public because they are durable in the external environment.

Consider *Pseudomonas aeruginosa*, one of the leading causes of hospital-acquired pneumonia (Leedom 1992). It can survive for six months in the external environment, a period comparable to the maximum persistence documented for sit-and-wait pathogens like the agents of tuberculosis or diphtheria (Mitscherlich & Marth 1984). It is commonly spread on hospital equipment and is lethal in about half of those having pneumonia or bloodstream infections, even with antibiotic therapy (Gallagher & Watanakunakorn 1989, Silver et al. 1992). *Pseudomonas aeruginosa* is inherently resistant to most antibiotics and can rapidly evolve resistance to others (Barton et al. 1986, Hamon-Poupinel et al. 1991, J. Fujita et al. 1992). This inherent resistance coupled with the extensive use of antibiotics seems to have fostered the spread of *P. aeruginosa* through inhibition its more benign competitors (Buisson et al. 1992). Should a group of *P. aeruginosa* evolve improved abilities at infecting healthy people, a most dangerous pathogen could be unleashed. We may already be in the midst of this process. Infections with *P. aeruginosa* were rare prior to the antibiotic era, but were recently found in about one out of every 1000 admissions; and they appear to be on the increase (Cross et al. 1983, Gallagher & Watanakunakorn 1989, Leedom 1992). One particular type of *P. aeruginosa*, referred to as 0:11, has been responsible for most of the damage (Morrison & Wenzel 1984).

If antibiotics always provided effective control, these issues would be of limited significance. Existing antibiotics, however, are often of little value against emerging hospital-acquired pathogens like *P. aeruginosa* (Gallagher & Watanakunakorn 1989, Greenough & Bennett 1990, Hamon-Poupinel et al. 1991, J. Fujita et al. 1992, Neu 1992); moreover, the rapid development of antibiotic resistance in hospitals (Gezon et al. 1973) raises the possibility that virulent strains may cause substantial mortality before appropriate antibiotics can be found. The high lethality of hospital-acquired *Staph. aureus* offers one worrisome illustration (Pavillard et al., 1982), but *M. tuberculosis* seems to be even more dangerous. The recent development of antibiotic resistance among *M. tuberculosis* strains appears to enhance their spread and lethality in institutional environments (Beck-Sagué et al 1992, Iseman 1992).

The AIDS pandemic may be similarly opening the door for new sit-and-wait pathogens of humans. Because AIDS patients frequently enter hospitals and medical care institutions, the effects of HIV, antibiotic resistance, and institutional environments such as hospitals are jointly enhancing the reemergence of lethal tuberculosis (Beck-Sagué et al 1992, Dooley et al. 1992ab, Fischl et al. 1992ab, Iseman 1992, Pearson et al. 1992).

Like many hospitalized patients, AIDS patients are particularly vulnerable to opportunistic pathogens. The members of the *Mycobacterium avium* group, for example, commonly infect AIDS patients in the United States and Europe (Gradon et al. 1992, Horsburgh 1992). These pathogens can survive for years outside of the host (Mitscherlich & Marth 1984) and are naturally resistant to anti-tuberculosis drugs (Wolinsky 1992). Luckily, they have shown little potential for transmission from person to person (Horsburgh 1992), but should they evolve an enhanced ability for transmission to uncompromised hosts, we may be confronting a particularly menacing adversary. The current incidence of *M. avium* pulmonary disease in the United States provides an indication of this danger: Excluding AIDS patients, one case occurs for every eight caused by *M. tuberculosis* (Wolinsky 1992). The incidence of such infections in Europe has increased to a similar level (Debrunner et al. 1992).

Emerging arthropodborne pathogens

We also need to pay special attention to emerging arthropodborne pathogens. When arthropod vectors are introduced into an area, vectorborne epidemics could begin by two routes. A vectorborne pathogen could enter the area from outside. Or it could arise endemically by being transferred to humans from some other local vertebrate host by an introduced vector. The first route has been the cause of some of the most severe epidemics in history. The devastation of medieval Europe by the bubonic plague and the periodic decimation of American and European cities by yellow fever during the colonial and early industrial periods are two examples.

Simultaneous introduction of vector and pathogen is feasible for many mosquito-borne viruses because they are often vertically transmitted from mother mosquito to offspring. Because vertically transmitted viruses tend to be benign (see Chapter 3 and Ewald & Schubert 1989), they allow infected mosquitoes a long life, which in turn increases the chances of introducing infected mosquitoes. Perhaps more importantly, vertical transmission allows the virus a second option for transmission. Besides infecting a human immediately through a mosquito bite, it can multiply and infect many mosquitoes, and broaden the window of time over which infective bites can occur.

In 1985, a mosquito known to have these kinds of associations with vectorborne viruses—the tiger mosquito, *Aedes albopictus*—arrived in the United States. Its aquatic larvae came across the Pacific as stowaways in the tiny pools of water in used tires brought to America for retreading. The mosquito has invaded broadly, from the southern United States into South America (Miller 1989, Morse 1991). Although it has not yet caused any extensive epidemics, it is the same genus as a major vector of yellow fever and is a vector of the dengue fever virus. The spread of the tiger mosquito also broadens the chances of transmission of other arthropodborne viruses into humans. The mosquito can be infected experimentally with viruses that can kill humans, such as the LaCrosse and San Angelo viruses. Recently, a dangerous encephalitis virus has been isolated from it in Florida (Mitchell et al. 1992). Although this virus has not been noticeably transmitted from person to person through mosquitoes, the possibilities of this occurrence might be just a few mutations away. If such viruses acquired these mutations, they could be especially difficult to control because they are often vertically transmitted from the mother mosquito to her young (Tesh 1980, Tesh & Shroyer 1980).

These dangers are particularly apparent in tropical areas where vectors may be abundant for a greater part of the year. For decades Rift Valley fever virus has been known as a severe disease of cattle and sheep in eastern and southern Africa. By 1977, the virus was spreading into Egypt, where it infected about 200,000 people and killed about 600 (House et al. 1992); it has continued to cause disease and death in Mauritania. Apparently, the still waters created by the Aswan dam on the Nile and the Diama dam on the Senegal River favored the development of these epidemics by fostering vast increases in the mosquito population. The extent of human–mosquito–human transmission is unclear. During the early outbreaks it was virtually nonexistent, but the large numbers of infected people during the later outbreaks are consistent with some human–mosquito–human transmission. So are the amounts of virus measured in infected people. They sometimes exceed 100 million viruses per milliliter of blood, certainly enough to infect human-biting mosquitoes (House et al. 1992).

This virus had passed several hurdles, permitting transfer to and rapid growth in humans. But more importantly, it is mosquito-borne. If the pathogen acquires mutations that facilitate the spread from person to mosquito to person, we could be dealing with a serious vectorborne disease of humans, a new yellow fever perhaps. Again, the process may have already begun. The severity of infections seems to have increased during this century; deaths were generally absent from the sporadic early outbreaks but present in the larger later ones (Howard 1984, Gear et al. 1987, Gonzalez et al. 1987, Niklasson et al. 1987).

At about the same time that the Rift Valley fever virus was emerging in Africa, a virus in the same virus family (the Bunyaviridae) was entering human populations across the Atlantic in the Amazon region. This oropouche virus normally is transmitted in a nonhuman cycle, probably involving birds (Pinheiro et al. 1976). But over the past few decades, it has caused about 200,000 cases of disease (Miller 1989), apparently by way of mosquito-like midges. The midges, like the mosquitoes transmitting Rift Valley fever, probably multiplied to great numbers because of human activities. In this case, expansion of cacao plantations increased the numbers of the minute midge breeding ponds that formed in discarded cacao shells. About 10% of oropouche infections developed a sufficient density of viruses in human blood to infect midges. Luckily, the life cycle of the midge seems to permit continuous transmission for only about six months. This narrow window of time limits the potential of oropouche virus to evolve as a vectorborne parasite of humans. If the vector of the virus had been an *Aedes* mosquito, the outcome might have been different. Oropouche virus can be transmitted albeit inefficiently by mosquitoes (Hoch et al. 1987). As with the Rift Valley fever virus, if oropouche virus generates mutations that permit continuous cycles of vectorborne transmission among humans, we may witness the evolutionary creation of a very dangerous virus.

If we divide our interception efforts equally among all emerging pathogens, we may be blocking many pathogens that would cause relatively little harm if they were introduced, and might miss an opportunity to control the worst killers by spreading resources too thin. If instead we focus on blocking pathogens that have a great potential for evolving and maintaining virulence, then fewer of the worst troublemakers should slip past our surveillance.

The dengue virus offers an illustration of just such a troublemaker. On average, the dengue virus is not as lethal as its cousin, the yellow fever virus, but like the yellow fever virus, dengue is transmitted by the mosquito *Aedes aegypti*. With control of *Aedes aegypti* in Mexico during the early 1960s, the dengue virus was driven to extinction there (Koopman et al. 1991). But it reinvaded during the late 1970s, and since then several types of dengue virus have been circulating (Koopman et al. 1991). This presence of several types is especially worrisome because dengue typically is most lethal when an individual has been infected with more than one type. With better funding of surveillance efforts, this reinvasion might have been blocked entirely or nipped in the bud.

These arguments lead to conclusions that are often very different from those offered by leading scientists who write on emerging pathogens from a proximate perspective. Conclusions generated without detailed consideration of natural selection dismiss, for example, pathogens such as HTLV and hepatitis as not particularly threatening because they are already widely disseminated (Morse 1991). And those pathogens that are recognized as threats by both approaches are recognized for different reasons. Rift Valley fever virus is recognized as a threat without consideration of natural selection because the virus is geographically localized and causes severe illness. The approach based on natural selection recognizes this virus as a threat because it is vectorborne and therefore should be favored by natural selection to maintain relatively high virulence. Detailed consideration of natural selection broadens the emphasis to include not just the movement of new pathogens into a virgin area, but also the characteristics of nature and our culture that favor the more virulent variants within a pathogen population. The long-present diseases account for a much greater proportion of death and suffering than do the transient though more lethal diseases associated with the introduction of a new pathogen into a previously isolated population. About 20 million people die each year from infectious diseases, and hundreds of millions more suffer severe illness, but the newness or oldness of pathogens in an area is not the major determinant of this damage. We need to understand enough about the evolution of virulence so that these numbers can be reduced, be they due to long present pathogens or newly introduced ones.

VACCINES AS EVOLUTIONARY TOOLS

The present efforts to control infectious diseases generally do not involve assessment of evolutionary stability. Rather, researchers focus on vulnerable aspects of a pathogen, such as biochemical components that can be used in a vaccine. The success of vaccines against smallpox, yellow fever, whooping cough, and measles raised hopes that all pathogens could be controlled by vaccines. But as it turns out, some of the conquered pathogens were particularly oafish adversaries. A smallpox virus, for example, carried antigens that were also carried by virtually all other smallpox viruses as well as its taxonomic relative, the vaccinia virus, which is the virus used in the smallpox vaccine. Once a population was widely inoculated with the vaccinia virus, immunity against vaccinia antigens protected against the smallpox viruses. It was like shooting down the "redcoats" during the American Revolution. If the individuals in a pathogen species always wore the same uniform, identifying and destroying them would be as easy as it was with smallpox. But most parasites practice guerrilla warfare. Their external appearances may be highly variable, and they may not wear recognizable uniforms at all. Some individual parasites, like those causing sleeping sickness, may change their coats regularly to avoid detection. Mobilizing the immune system to destroy pathogens wearing one coat is not terribly useful if parasites with different coats are continually being generated.

Assessing the potential for pathogens to evolve their way around future vaccines is, of course, speculative. But educated guesses can be made based on our knowledge of genetics, evolution, and outcomes of past confrontations. As mentioned in previous chapters, vaccines generated against sexually reproducing parasites like malaria, or mutation-prone viruses like HIV and influenza can be expected to provide partial and unstable solutions. Vaccination has already nullified easy adversaries. We are now left with the more wily ones, which probably will evade our vaccination efforts by changing their coats. They may do so facultatively, as do the protozoa that cause sleeping sickness; or evolutionarily, as do HIV and the influenza virus; or by both mechanisms, as do the protozoa that cause malaria.

To deal with pathogenic adversaries effectively over the long term, we shall need to use our knowledge about them to make them evolve into less dangerous organisms. Choosing the right vaccine can help us accomplish this control for pathogens that cannot be entirely eradicated. Molecular biology and immunology have given us many options for generation of new vaccines. To evaluate the long-term cost-effectiveness of these options, we must consider using vaccines as agents of selection against the most virulent strains. The virulence of some parasites is related to compounds that they release or carry on their surface. Generating a vaccine that triggers immunity against these compounds could tip the balance in favor of the more benign forms that lack these compounds. The vaccine would not in this case eliminate all individuals of a particular kind of parasite as did the smallpox vaccine. Rather it would alter the make-up of parasite populations—people will still become infected, but with a benign organism instead of a damaging one.

This point is best illustrated by diphtheria. Once a major killer, *Corynebacterium diphtheriae* now causes little, if any, disease in areas where vaccination programs have been fastidiously enacted. In the United States, for example, one case occurs annually for every 20 million people (Chen et al. 1985). This reduction is best attributed to the selective pressure exerted by the vaccine itself (Uchida et al. 1971, Pappenheimer & Gill 1973, Pappenheimer 1982). Classical diphtheria results from the effects of a toxin released by *C. diphtheriae*. To manufacture the toxin, *C. diphtheriae* must carry a viral toxin gene, which is switched on to produce toxin when *C. diphtheriae* has exploited the resources, particularly iron, in its immediate vicinity (Schmitt & Holmes 1991, Schmitt et al. 1992). The toxin shuts down the host's ability to make protein, causing cell death (Pappenheimer 1977, 1982), which apparently liberates nutrients for *C. diphtheriae*'s use. Accordingly, overt cases of diphtheria are more contagious than asymptomatic infections (Miller et al. 1972).

If, however, a person is immunized with detoxified diphtheria toxin, any *C. diphtheriae* that produce toxin are wasting valuable resources at times when nutrients are limited; 5% of total protein produced by these bacteria may be used to make the now impotent toxin (Pappenheimer & Gill 1973). Although both toxin-producing and toxinless *C. diphtheriae* can infect vaccinated hosts (Miller et al. 1972), the toxin-producers should be at a competitive disadvantage in a vaccinated population. Indeed, diphtheria has vanished from areas with extensive vaccination programs, while toxinless *C. diphtheriae* has been perpetuated (Pappenheimer 1982, Chen et al. 1985). The few outbreaks that occur annually in the United States, for example, typically are attributable to foreign travel or limited circulation among small groups of unvaccinated people who have compromised states of health, or live in poor, densely populated urban areas (Pappenheimer & Murphy 1983, Kallick et al. 1970, Harnisch et al. 1989). The potential for spread of diphtheria from these foci is apparently limited by vaccination and the natural immunity generated by toxinless infections.

This experience with *C. diphtheriae* provides a lesson for our vaccine development programs. Early in the process of vaccine development, researchers and funding agencies decide what parts of the pathogen or what manipulations of the whole pathogen should be considered for use as a vaccine. Later in the process, policymakers must choose which of the various alternative vaccines to use. Until now these decisions have considered characteristics such as degree of protection, ease of use and preparation, economic costs, and frequency of adverse reactions. The evolutionary approach provides an important addition to this list: the effect of the vaccination program on the evolution of the pathogen's virulence.

In particular, the evolutionary approach suggests that analogues of the compounds responsible for virulence should be preferentially incorporated into vaccines. The incorporation sometimes occurs if warranted by considerations of protection, cost and adverse reactions, but evolutionary consequences are left out of the equation. Current development of vaccines to protect against cholera, for example, involves field tests of killed *V. cholerae* supplemented by portions of the cholera toxin; when evaluated by traditional criteria these supplemented vaccines appear to be as effective as or more effective than unsupplemented vaccines (Sack et al. 1991). But the traditional criteria probably underestimate their effectiveness because the criteria do not include the evolutionary benefits. So long as the toxin-supplemented cholera vaccines prevent cholera toxin from causing disease, toxin production in vaccinated individuals becomes a liability for *V. cholerae*; toxin production no longer provides a benefit but still carries a cost. The mild variants that infect without toxin (Minami et al. 1991) may use the resources that would otherwise be wasted on toxin production to make compounds that increase their survival and reproduction. By raising the estimated effectiveness of such virulence-based vaccines, this consideration of the evolutionary benefits provides additional justification for their development.

The standard vaccine against whooping cough provides a similar example. It is a suspension of killed *Bordetella pertussis*, the bacterium that causes whooping cough. This vaccine occasionally causes severe damage to those it is supposed to protect, a flaw that has generated interest in developing safer alternative vaccines. Because the toxin produced by *B. pertussis* can trigger a protective immune response, it has been at the center of current efforts to develop a toxin-based vaccine (Burnette et al. 1992). In the mid-1980s a chemically inactivated pertussis toxin was used in a Swedish trial of about 3000 babies; it provided some protection, but four of the babies died (Storsaeter 1991). Although the deaths may have been unrelated to the vaccine, they generated a guarded response (Storsaeter 1991). The most recent toxin-based vaccines appear to provide greater protection than the standard vaccine with fewer dangerous side effects (Petersen et al. 1991, Podda et al. 1991, Feldman 1992, Pichichero et al. 1992). Particularly encouraging are the genetically engineered toxins (Podda et al. 1991, Burnette et al. 1992), which lack the dangerous parts of the toxin and have only slight alterations of the components that trigger immunity. The engineered toxins therefore will probably stimulate a stronger immunity more safely than the chemically inactivated toxins (Rappuoli et al. 1992).

Because the severe effects of whooping cough are attributable to this toxin, a safe vaccine generated from deactivated toxin might help control whooping cough by the same evolutionary process that apparently has caused the demise of diphtheria. Different strains of *B. pertussis* are differentially attacked by the immune response to the various vaccines (Blumberg et al. 1992), suggesting that a given vaccine will differentially disfavor certain variants of *B. pertussis*. If the toxoid vaccines prove to be as safe as or safer than the traditional vaccine, the evolutionary effects will provide an extra bonus: Virulent *B. pertussis* will be replaced with benign *B. pertussis*, which will naturally immunize people against any remaining virulent strains. If the toxoid vaccines prove to be less safe or less effective than the traditional vaccine, this evolutionary consideration should provide an impetus to invest in enough further research to make it as safe and effective as the traditional vaccine.

The evolutionary bonus may be lost, however, if the vaccine is made to protect against mild as well as virulent strains of *B. pertussis*. Researchers are now including additional nonpathogenic components from *B. pertussis* to improve the vaccine's effectiveness at inhibiting a broad spectrum of the existing variants (Podda et al. 1991). Similarly, researchers have suggested that cholera vaccines should include compounds that trigger immunity against the milder el tor *V. cholerae* but not against the more severe classical type (Osek et al 1992). Evolutionary considerations suggest that these additional compounds should not be chosen solely on the basis of their potency for triggering protection against a broader spectrum of organisms. Rather the vaccine components should be generated from disease-producing components, whenever possible, to tip the competitive advantage further in favor of mild variants.

The diphtheria model is feasible for many pathogens that are in less advanced stages of vaccine development. *Streptococcus pneumoniae*, for example, is a major cause of pneumonia, meningitis, and severe ear infections, killing about 40,000 people each year in the United States alone (Lee et al. 1991). It causes its negative effect largely through production of toxins called pneumolysins, which inhibit the attack of white blood cells and rupture cell membranes, thereby liberating nutrients for the bacterium and expanding the scope of infection (Rubins et al. 1992, Berry et al 1992). The similarity of the pneumolysins from different isolates of *Strep. pneumoniae* has led researchers to identify them as potentially useful additions to future vaccines (Lock et al 1992). The currently used vaccine, which is a collection of complex sugar chains found on the capsules enclosing the different strains of the bacterium, often yields only weak protection (Lee et al. 1991, Lock et al. 1992). Besides providing better protection over the short term, vaccines containing parts of the pneumolysin molecule should shift the competitive balance in favor of those *Strep. pneumoniae* without pneumolysins, thereby favoring evolution toward benignness. Evolutionary considerations therefore provide added incentive for rigorously pursuing the possibility of a pneumolysin-supplemented vaccine, and eventually a vaccine composed entirely of *Strep. pneumoniae*'s disease-producing constituents.

Once a safe and effective vaccine has been developed, the process of vaccine development is not over. Monitoring of strains must continue to detect any variants that may reevolve virulence by a mechanism that is not blocked by the vaccine. A few strains of *C. diphtheriae*, for example, can produce disease without producing a toxin (Kallick et al. 1970, Zuber et al. 1992). If the virulence of these variants is a consequence of some competitive superiority, then these variants will spread. Vaccine development needs to control this evolutionary process by determining ways to incorporate the analogues of the new virulence producing compounds into vaccines. It is important to note, however, that this kind of evolutionary control should be less difficult than the nonevolutionary control that has been the goal of conventional efforts. The evolutionary control requires that a pathogen evolve an entirely new mechanism virulence.

In addition to causing evolutionary decreases in virulence, virulence-based vaccines should provide more stable protection against resurgences of disease when vaccination efforts lapse. Unless the pathogen is, like the smallpox virus, driven to extinction, a vaccine based on components that are not disease-producing will leave a reservoir of pathogenic organisms. This reservoir can then spread when vaccination diminishes or when the pathogen evolves a side-run around the vaccine's defense.

Diphtheria vaccination illustrates the stability of control by virulence-based vaccines. In recent decades the proportion of people with protective immunity against diphtheria toxin has not been particularly high. In the United States it amounts to about three-quarters of children and one-quarter of adults (Chen et al. 1985). If the diphtheria vaccine protected equally against all strains of *C. diphtheriae*, the large numbers of unprotected people might have generated a resurgence in diphtheria, much like the resurgence of whooping cough that has occurred in areas where vaccination efforts have diminished (Hewlett 1990, Pinchichero et al. 1992). The real difference between diphtheria and whooping cough is probably even greater than the recognized difference because atypical, severe cases of whooping cough are often not properly reported (Heininger et al. 1992). By inhibiting just the toxin-producing strains, the diphtheria vaccine allows the mild strains to be present to protect against the severe strains should vaccination efforts lapse temporarily or miss a small percentage of a population.

Most of the major vaccination programs, such as those for measles, rubella, and mumps, parallel the whooping cough experience; they have been dealt setbacks from vaccine-caused disease or from outbreaks that spread among the unvaccinated (Hewlett 1990, Hilleman 1992, Pinchichero et al. 1992, Weiss 1992, Forsey et al. 1992). The control of disease by oral polio vaccine has been one of the most successful of these programs, especially if the cases of polio have been overestimated through misdiagnosis (de Quadros 1992, Sabin 1992). The evolutionary mechanisms involved in widespread oral polio vaccination, however, are very much like those indirect effects of diphtheria vaccination mentioned above. A propagating mild strain protects against infection by the severe strains. In the case of polio vaccination, however, the mild strains are administered in the vaccine rather than being selected for by the vaccine. The major evolutionary uncertainty about the live polio vaccine is whether the competition between mild strains will eventually lead to a reversion to virulence. Because the neurological damage is probably a side effect (*sensu* Chapter 2) that does not benefit the poliovirus, prospects for long-term control are good so long as vaccines are not made from viral strains that have a predilection for neurons. If strains with neurological predilections are used, competition between the vaccine strains could lead to increased replication rates and increased neurological damage as an indirect effect.

These considerations emphasize the need to integrate evolutionary considerations of vaccination policies with evolutionary considerations of virulence. Live vaccines tend to work better than dead vaccines, but if live vaccines are to be used, we had better understand the environmental variables that cause benign pathogens to evolve increased severity. If we fail to do so, our vaccination efforts may backfire. We may be introducing large numbers of benign organisms into environments that will favor their evolutionary transformation into dangerous organisms. The danger of live vaccines would depend on the rate at which variation is generated and the virulence to which the parasite tends to evolve. Live HIV vaccines, for example, would be near the most dangerous end of this danger continuum, and live rhinovirus vaccines would be near the least dangerous end.

THE EMERGENCE OF EVOLUTIONARY EPIDEMIOLOGY AND DARWINIAN MEDICINE

A union of disciplines

Ecologists studying parasitism have stressed the importance of evolutionary approaches (Price 1980, Levin & Pimentel 1981, Anderson & May 1982, Ewald 1983, May and Anderson 1983), but human epidemiology traditionally has focused on ecological rather than evolutionary time scales. Evolutionary epidemiology broadens the focus of epidemiology to encompass the evolutionary changes in pathogen and host characteristics such as virulence, resistance, and the adaptive significance of disease manifestations.

The field of epidemiology is, in essence, the ecology of disease. Since the time of Charles Darwin, ecology and evolutionary biology have been tightly interwoven. At first glance it may therefore seem surprising that so little evolutionary thinking has been incorporated into epidemiology. Consideration of the goals of medicine and epidemiology, however, yields an explanation for this paucity. The primary goals of medicine and epidemiology are to assist individual patients and control the spread of diseases. The few introductions of evolutionary thinking into human epidemiology during the first three-quarters of the 20th century tended to occur when evolutionary changes interfered directly with these goals. The attention given to the evolution of antibiotic resistance is the classic example (see Chapter 6). The ideas presented in this book broaden the application of evolution to other aspects of epidemiology directly relevant to health care: the evolution of virulence and, more generally, the manifestations of disease.

When extended to medical issues beyond parasitism (Williams & Nesse 1991) and parasitic diseases of organisms other than humans, the evolutionary approach offers another dimension to our understanding of disease in general. One practical benefit of this dimension concerns economic investments. If the cultural vectors hypothesis, for example, is correct, the cost of interventions to eliminate cultural vectors (e.g., providing water purification systems, improving hygienic standards of attendants in hospitals, or sterilizing agricultural equipment) must be weighed against two positive effects. The first is the short-term benefit traditionally recognized by epidemiologists: the reduction of disease transmission. The second is a long-term benefit specified by evolutionary epidemiology: an evolutionary reduction in the parasite's virulence.

Evolutionary biology, ecology, and epidemiology are among the most interdisciplinary of disciplines. Development of evolutionary epidemiology and Darwinian medicine will undoubtedly draw in still other disciplines. The future investigations advocated in this book will require integration of insights from sociology, psychology, and anthropology, because one needs to know not only how transmission occurs but also whether the relevant social settings permit transmission, say, from immobilized infected people or from people receiving alternative symptomatic treatments.

Is and ought

As we shift attention from what has happened in the past to what we can do to shape the future, we inevitably encounter the *is* versus *ought* dichotomy. To address the consequences of current and future policies, we take our knowledge of what is and has been to assess what will be. When we use these assessments to decide which future polices we are to pursue, we move from *is* to *ought*. Because *ought* depends on our values, people with different values will inevitably disagree about what policies we *ought* to pursue. But knowledge about what *is* does affect our decisions about what we *ought* to do, because it allows us to assess better how alternative courses of action fit with our values.

One practical benefit from the evolutionary approach to disease stems from the tendency for superstition to fill the vacuum left by incomplete knowledge. Curiosity can be readily explained from an evolutionary perspective: Curiosity leads to increased knowledge, and increased knowledge can increase survival and reproduction. Curiosity, however, does not stop at the question, How does it work? Curiosity also makes us ask, Why are things the way they are? Why, for example, are human beings now being plagued with AIDS? Without an evolutionary approach, scientists can provide the public with no firmly grounded answer to this question. And if scientists cannot offer a solid answer, religious extremists who believe that HIV was sent to punish homosexuals, prostitutes, and drug addicts may have a relatively stronger influence on public policy and public sentiment. The end result of improved knowledge about the evolutionary origins of AIDS may therefore be less victimization of people who do not have sufficient socioeconomic and political power to defend themselves against the condemnations that come from nonscientific circles.

In discussing future options I am not attempting to prescribe what we *ought* to do socially. Rather, I am trying to understand and explain relationships among natural processes, social practices, and the evolution of disease. I believe that resolution of these *is*-type problems will help us make better informed choices about *ought*-type options, but the particular choices we make individually and collectively will depend on the particular social values we accept or reject individually and collectively.

Many of my leaps from *is* to *ought* in this book are to advocate the need for scientific study of a particular area. I have advocated social interventions to find out whether certain cultural changes can reduce virulence. I suggest that we ought to invest regionally in mosquito-proof housing to determine whether this intervention would make vectorborne pathogens like *Plasmodium falciparum* and dengue evolve toward lower levels of virulence. I suggest that we ought to make massive regional investments in water purification to determine whether the diarrheal organisms in such areas evolve to a lower level of virulence than the organisms in areas where such purification has not been made. I suggest that when we try to develop vaccines, we ought to target the compounds responsible for virulence, so that we stand a better chance of driving the problematic pathogens to a lower state of virulence. And I suggest that we ought to invest more heavily in programs that reduce sexual transmission and needleborne transmission of HIV to determine whether these changes will drive HIV to a more benign state.

These interventions will cost a great deal of money. What will we get in return? If my hypotheses are incorrect, most of these interventions will have improved the lives of many people aesthetically and reduced the much illness and death. If my hypotheses are correct, we will have done this and more. We shall have found a new way to deal with our diseases, by getting evolution to work *for* us instead of *against* us. In the past, our efforts have been focused on protecting individuals from pathogens that are imminently threatening, by using an armamentarium of antibiotics and vaccines. By using evolutionary tactics, we should be able to change the pathogens so that they will not be the terrible enemies that they once were, so that we will not need to invest so heavily in the "arms races" to deter them just before they attack us or to destroy them just after they have attacked. We shall, in a sense, domesticate them so that they can live with us in a less damaging way than they have throughout our history.

Glossary

adaptive Refers to a characteristic of an organism favored by natural selection.

AIDS Abbreviation for acquired immune deficiency syndrome, which is an umbrella term for a variety of life-threatening diseases associated with HIV-induced decimation of the immune system.

amino acids Building blocks of proteins. Each amino acid is encoded by a triplet of ribonucleotides called a codon.

analgesic A drug that reduces pain.

antibodies Protein molecules that are released from B lymphocytes and bind to antigens, which may protrude from the surfaces of pathogens. This binding facilitates recognition and destruction of the pathogens by other cells in the immune system.

antigens Compounds that trigger the production of antibodies by the host and bind to the antibodies produced.

ARC Abbreviation for AIDS related complex, which is a collection of signs and symptoms that often appear as HIV infections progress from an asymptomatic state to AIDS.

arthropodborne Refers to transmission by a member of the phylum Arthropoda. Insofar as parasitic diseases of terrestrial vertebrates are concerned, the most significant arthropods are mosquitoes, midges, tsetse flies, sandflies, reduviid bugs (i.e., kissing bugs), blackflies, ticks, lice, fleas, and mites.

asymptomatic Refers to an infection that does not generate symptoms.

AZT (azidodideoxythymidine = zidovudine) A molecule formed from two molecules of a modified building block of nucleic acids (thymine). AZT inhibits HIV by interfering with HIV's reverse transcriptase.

benignness A state of parasitism in which little harm is caused to the hosts, which show either no symptoms or mild symptoms.

CD4 A receptor on some T lymphocytes that allows the lymphocytes to bind to and hence influence the activity of other white blood cells. The gp120 molecule of HIV can bind to the CD4 receptor, thus allowing entry of HIV into the lymphocyte.

cell cultures Cells growing on artificial nutrient media under laboratory conditions. Researchers infect cell cultures in order to study pathogens and their interactions with host cells.

codon A triplet of RNA building blocks (ribonucleotides) that codes for an amino acid or for a signal to start or stop protein synthesis. The sequence of codons in RNA determines the sequence of amino acids and the length of the protein and, hence, the size, shape, and activity of the protein.

colonization The living of an organism on the surface of another organism without causing any detectable damage to the host organism.

commensalism A symbiotic relationship in which one member benefits without harming or helping the other. The categorization of a symbiosis as commensalism reflects the inaccuracy with which fitness benefits and costs are estimated. Symbiotic organisms are bound to have at least some slight effects on each other. If one could measure these effects accurately, virtually all of the relationships categorized as commensalistic would be either slightly parasitic or slightly mutualistic, and commensalism would represent a theoretical dividing line between mutualism and parasitism rather than a discrete category of symbiotic relationships.

cultural vector Refers to a set of characteristics that allow transmission from immobilized hosts to susceptibles, when at least one of the characteristics is some aspect of human culture.

cytotoxic T cells Lymphocytes that attack and destroy infected cells by recognizing antigens on the surface of infected cells.

defense Short-hand term that refers to a manifestation of a disease that increases the evolutionary fitness of the individual expressing the manifestation.

diarrhea Stools released from the body in a liquid or semi-liquid form.

DNA (deoxyribonucleic acid) A long-chain molecule that encodes information by variations in the sequences of the four different building blocks (deoxyribonucleotides) used along its length. In most organisms the DNA sequences comprise the genes, the primary library of information that is necessary for the development and maintenance of the organism.

dysentery Bloody diarrhea.

envelope proteins Proteins that protrude from the surface of a virus that generally participate in the binding of the virus to host cells.

epidemic A disease outbreak that spreads sufficiently to affect simultaneously the different local groups in a geographic region. Narrowly defined, "epidemic" refers to outbreaks in human populations and "epizootic" to outbreaks in populations of other animals. In this book I use the term "epidemic" broadly, to encompass diseases of human and nonhuman hosts.

epidemiology A scientific discipline that investigates the prevalence and spread of diseases within and among populations of hosts. Epidemiology encompasses any aspect of the environment, the host, or the parasite that is relevant to the prevalence or spread of disease.

fever An increase in body temperature above that normally maintained in healthy organisms.

fitness The measure of the evolutionary success of an organism relative to that of competitors within the same species. Darwin envisioned this success in terms of improved fit between the organism and its environment that results from differential success of competing individuals. Modern evolutionary biologists envision this success in terms of the relative frequencies of alternative genetic instructions.

genotype The particular set of genes within the organism.

gp120 (glycoprotein 120) A proteinaceous molecule that extends from the surface of HIV, and binds to the CD4 receptor, allowing entrance of HIV into a cell.

group selection The favoring of a characteristic as a consequence of the differential success of groups of organisms. Group selection is typically weak relative to the differences between the success of individuals within the group, but if groups are small and mix regularly, and if the individuals in groups are genetically related, group selection may be important. These conditions seem especially applicable to groups of parasites inside of individual hosts. Use of the term is a source of argument among evolutionary biologists because the term was used during midcentury to identify infeasible scenarios based on group benefits. When feasible, group selection are often identical or very similar to kin selection.

HIV Abbreviation for the human immunodeficiency virus.

HTLV Abbreviation for a retrovirus that is commonly known by several names—human T-cell lymphotropic virus, human T-cell leukemia virus, or human T-cell leukemia/lymphoma virus.

hybridization In molecular biology, the joining of one side of a nucleic acid chain to a complementary half. When the two halves are from two different organisms, the strength of this joining provides an indication of the similarity of the two nucleotide sequences and hence the evolutionary relatedness of the organisms.

immune system The cells of the body that protect against infection by generalized responses such as inflammation, and by specific responses such as the attachment of antibodies to antigens and the destruction of infected cells through recognition of foreign antigens presented on the cell surface.

incidence The number of people that become infected over a given period of time relative to the total size of the population.

inclusive fitness The effect of a characteristic on the passing on of genetic instructions for the characteristic. The term was originally introduced to emphasize that the evolutionary success of genetic instructions must include the passing on of the instructions through relatives as well as through the individual's own offspring. Evolutionary biologists often use the term "fitness" broadly to refer to inclusive fitness, even though a narrow definition of fitness refers only to the success achieved through the individual's own reproductive activity.

infectious disease A disease caused by a pathogen.

infection The invasion of a organism by a pathogen, which completes at least part of its life cycle in the host organism.

infestation Parasitism by multicellular parasites. (For brevity in theoretical arguments, I have used "infection" broadly to include infestations.)

inflammatory response A reaction of the lymphatic system and local tissues elicited by parasites or other irritants and characterized by swelling and a reddening as blood collects in dilated vessels and lymphatic fluids accumulate in the tissues. Pathogen-destroying white blood cells move from the blood into the tissues during the response.

kin selection The favoring of a characteristic as a consequence the effects of the characteristic on relatives, which share the genetic instructions for the characteristic. In other words, kin selection pertains to the components of inclusive fitness that are accrued through genetically related individuals.

latency A quiescent state of infection in which a pathogen is not reproducing or reproducing very sluggishly.

lymphocyte A heterogeneous category of white blood cells with specialized immunological functions. B lymphocytes give rise to antibody-producing cells. T lymphocytes respond to antigen-presenting cells by proliferating and activating other white blood cells (like B lymphocytes) or killing infected cells directly.

manipulation Short-hand term that refers to a symptom that increases the evolutionary fitness of the pathogens that cause the symptom.

mutualism A symbiotic relationship that provides fitness benefits to both species.

mutation A change in the sequence of the building blocks (nucleotides) that comprise the genes.

natural selection The process of differential survival and reproduction that results in changes in gene frequencies and in the characteristics that the genes encode.

nef An HIV-encoded protein originally thought to be the negative regulatory factor that suppresses HIV replication. Current evidence indicates that different versions of nef exist, some suppress HIV replication, others enhance replication, and still others have no discernable effect.

neonate A newborn infant.

nucleic acid Chainlike molecules that are composed of nucleotides and encode genetic information.

nucleotide Building blocks of nucleic acids. Each nucleotide consists of a sugar attached to a phosphoric acid and one of four different nitrogen-containing ringed molecules. In DNA, these molecules are adenine, thymine, cytosine, and guanine. In RNA, uracil is used in place of thymine, the sugar is a ribose (instead of deoxyribose), and the nucleotide is called a ribonucleotide. In both RNA and DNA, it is the sequence of the four molecules that encodes information.

pandemic A disease outbreak that spreads continentally or worldwide.

parasite An individual that lives in or on another individual, and lowers the host individual's fitness. I use "parasite" broadly to encompass pathogens as well as multicellular parasites.

parasitism A symbiotic association in which one member benefits at the expense of the other.

pathogen A parasite whose organization is at or below the level of the individual cell. The category includes protozoal, bacterial, and viral parasites.

pathogenesis The process by which disease organisms generate disease.

plasmid A loop of DNA that can occur in bacteria and can be transferred between bacteria. Plasmids can contain genes that code for toxin production, antibiotic resistance, and abilities to invade host cells.

plasmodia (singular: **plasmodium**) The protozoal agents of malaria.

prevalence The extent to which a host population is infected with a parasite.

protein A molecule composed of long chains of amino acids. The associations of different parts of protein chains gives proteins a three dimensional structure that allows them to act as building blocks for organisms and regulate biological processes.

proximate Refers to explanations that deal with the mechanics of life processes: how living things function (cf. ultimate).

retrovirus A member of a family of viruses that uses RNA as genetic information and transcribes this information into DNA using reverse transcriptase. The family Retroviridae includes HIV, which is in the subfamily Lentivirinae; and HTLV, which is in the subfamily Oncovirinae.

reverse transcriptase An enzyme found in HIV and other viruses that use RNA to encode their genetic information. Reverse transcriptase uses the virus's RNA as a template to form a complementary strand of DNA, and then replaces the original RNA strand with a DNA strand that is complementary to the first DNA strand.

RNA (ribonucleic acid) A long-chain molecule that encodes information by variations in the sequences of the four different building blocks (ribonucleotides) used along its length. In some viruses (like human immunodeficiency viruses, hepatitis viruses, and influenza viruses), RNA and the information it encodes comprise the genes—the library of viral information that is necessary for viral invasion and replication. For most organisms RNA serves as a messenger carrying the information encoded by DNA to the sites of protein synthesis, where it then interacts with other kinds of RNA to link together amino acids to form proteins.

serum The fluid portion of the blood.

seroconversion The process by which a host develops an immune response, detectable in the serum, to an infecting organism.

seropositive The state of having an immune response that is detectable in the serum.

sexual partner rate A term I use to refer to the potential for sexual transmission of HIV. Sexual partner rate reflects the rate at which sexual contact with new partners occurs weighted by the amount of unprotected sexual contact per partner.

simian A monkey or non-human ape.

SIV Abbreviation for simian immunodeficiency virus. SIVs are lentiviruses isolated from simian hosts.

strain Formally, an isolate of pathogen that is propagated in the laboratory. I use the term somewhat more loosely to refer to pathogens that are recently derived from a common lineage and are very similar or identical genetically.

symbiosis The intimate living together of two different species. The term is sometimes used more restrictively as a synonym of *mutualism*—relationships that yield a net fitness benefit for both species. I use "symbiosis" broadly to include mutualism, commensalism, and parasitism.

symptom A perceptible change in the host that indicates disease. In medical circles, *symptoms* often are defined as subjective manifestations of disease, whereas *signs* are defined as objective manifestations; in this book I use "symptoms" more broadly to encompass both objective and subjective manifestations.

tat The transactivating protein that transforms HIV from a latent or sluggishly replicating state to an actively replicating state.

T4 cells A class of lymphocytes that influence the activity of other white blood cells, and are characterized by the presence of CD4 molecules as receptors protruding from their outer membranes.

transmission The process by which a parasite moves from one host to another.

trematodes Parasitic flatworms in the class Trematoda and phylum Platyhelminthes, commonly referred to as flukes. They have complex life cycles which typically involve a vertebrate host and an arthropod host. The most notable human disease caused by a trematode is schistosomiasis.

trypanosomes Protozoal parasites responsible diseases such as sleeping sickness.

ultimate Refers to explanations that deal with evolutionary origins: why organisms have the characteristics they have.

vertebrates Animals with backbones: mammals, birds, reptiles, amphibians, and fishes.

vertical transmission Transmission of a parasite from a host to the host's offspring.

virulence I use the term broadly to reflect the magnitude of the negative effect of a parasite on its host.

virus A parasitic organism composed of a protein coat, nucleic acids enclosed by the coat, and sometimes a few enclosed proteins that facilitate infection of host cells.

white blood cells (leukocytes) The cells of the immune system, which circulate in blood, lymph and body tissues, and directly or indirectly destroy invading organisms and infected or damaged cells.

References

Aber, R. C., Allen, N., Howell, J. T., Wilkenson, H. W., & Facklam, R. R. 1976. Nosocomial transmission of group B streptococci. *Pediatrics 58*, 346–53.

Aboulker, J. P., & Swart, A. M. 1993. Preliminary analysis of the Concorde trial. *Lancet 341*, 889–90.

Abrams, D. I. 1991. Acquired immunodeficiency syndrome and related malignancies: A topical overview. *Semin. Oncol. 18*, 41–5.

Acton, H. W., & Knowles, R. 1928. *On the dysenteries of India.* Calcutta: Thacker, Spink.

Adib, S. M., Joseph, J. G., Ostrow, D. G., Tal, M., & Schwartz, S. A. 1991. Relapse in sexual behavior among homosexual men: A 2-year follow-up from the Chicago MACS/CCS. *AIDS 5*, 757–60.

Agarwal, S. K., Goel, M., Das, R., & Kumar, A. 1984. Transmissible antibiotic resistance among *Shigella* species. *Indian J. Med. Res. 80*, 402–8.

Agut, H., Rabanel, B., Remy, G., Tabary, T., Chamaret, S., Dauguet, C., Candotti, D., Huraux, J. M., Ingrand, D., Chippaux, C., Guetard, D., & Montagnier, L. 1992. Isolation of atypical HIV-1-related retrovirus from AIDS patient. *Lancet 340*, 681–2.

Ahmad, N., & Venkatesan, S. 1988. Nef protein of HIV-1 is a transcriptional repressor of HIV-1 LTR. *Science 241*, 1481–4.

Ajdukiewicz, A., Yanagihara, R., Garruto, R. M., Gajdusek, D. C., & Alexander, S. S. 1989. HTLV-I myeloneuropathy in the Solomon Islands. *N. Engl. J. Med. 321*, 615–16.

Akari, H., Sakuragi, J., Takebe, Y., Tomonaga, K., Kawamura, M., Fukasawa, M., Miura, T., Shinjo, T., & Hayami, M. 1992. Biological characterization of human immunodeficiency virus type 1 and type 2 mutants in human peripheral blood mononuclear cells. *Arch. Virol. 123*, 157–67.

Albert, J., Abrahamsson, B., Nagy, K., Aurelius, E., Gaines, H., Nyström, G., & Fenyö, E. M. 1990. Rapid development of isolate-specific neutralizing antibodies after primary HIV-1 infection and consequent emergence of virus variants which resist neutralization by autologous sera. *AIDS 4*, 107–12.

Albert, J., Böttiger, B., Biberfeld, G., & Fenyö, E. M. 1989. Replicative and cytopathic characteristics of HIV-2 and severity of infection. *Lancet i*, 852–3.

Albert, J., Bredberg, U., Chiodi, F., Böttiger, B., Fenyö, E. M., Norrby, E., & Biberfeld, G. 1987. A new human retrovirus isolate of west African origin (SBL-6669) and its relationship to HTLV-IV, LAV-II, and HTLV-IIIB. *AIDS Res. Hum. Retroviruses 3*, 3–10.

Albert, J., Wahlberg, J., Lundeberg, J., Cox, S., Sandström, E., Wahren, B., & Uhlen, M. 1992. Persistence of azidothymidine-resistant human immunodeficiency virus type 1 RNA genotypes in posttreatment sera. *J. Virol. 66*, 5627–30.

Albert, M. J., Siddique, A. K., Islam, M. S., Faruque, A. S. G., Ansaruzzaman, M., Faruque, S. M., & Sack, R. B. 1993. Large outbreak of clinical cholera due to *Vibrio cholerae* non-01 in Bangladesh. *Lancet 341*, 704.

Alexandre, C., & Verrier, B. 1991. Four regulatory elements in the human c-*fos* promoter mediate transactivation by HTLV-I tax protein. *Oncogene 6*, 543–51.

Allan, J. S., Short, M., Taylor, M. E., Su, S., Hirsch, V. M., Johnson, P. R., Shaw, G. M., & Hahn, B. H. 1991. Species-specific diversity among simian immunodeficiency viruses from African green monkeys. *J. Virol. 65*, 2816–28.

Allen, S., Tice, J., Vandeperre, P., Serufilira, A., Hudes, E., Nsengumuremyi, F., Bogaerts, J., Lindan, C., & Hulley, S. 1992. Effect of serotesting with counselling on condom use and seroconversion among HIV discordant couples in Africa. *Br. Med. J. 304*, 1605–9.

Allman, J. 1985. Conjugal unions in rural and urban Haiti. *Soc. Econ. Studies 34*, 27–57.

Ameisen, J. C., Guy, B., Chamaret, S., Loche, M., Mouton, Y., Neyrinck, J. L., Khalife, J., Leprevost, C., Beaucaire, G., Boutillon, C., Gras-Masse, H., Maniez, M., Kieny, M. P., Laustriat, D., Berthier, A., Mach, B., Montagnier, L., Lecocq, J. P., & Capron, A. 1989. Antibodies to the nef protein and to nef peptides in HIV-1-infected seronegative individuals. *AIDS Res. Hum. Retroviruses 5*, 279–91.

Ampel, N. M. 1991. Plagues—what's past is present: Thoughts on the origin and history of new infectious diseases. *Rev. Infect. Dis. 13*, 658–65.

Ancelle, R., Bletry, O., Baglin, A. C., Brun-Vezinet, F., Rey, M. A., & Godeam, P. 1987. Long incubation period for HIV-2 infection. *Lancet i*, 688–9.

Anderson, C. 1991. Cholera epidemic traced to risk miscalculation. *Nature 354*, 255.

Anderson, D. J., Obrien, T. R., Politch, J. A., Martinez, A., Seage, G. R., Padian, N., Horsburgh, C. R., & Mayer, K. H. 1992. Effects of disease stage and zidovudine therapy on the detection of human immunodeficiency virus type-1 in semen. *JAMA 267*, 2769– 74.

Anderson, M. G., & Clements, J. E. 1992. Two strains of SIV(mac) show differential transactivation mediated by sequences in the promoter. *Virology 191*, 559–68.

Anderson, R. M., & May, R. M. 1982. Coevolution of hosts and parasites. *Parasitology 85*, 411–26.

Andre, D. A., Weiser, H. H., & Malaney, G. W. 1967. Survival of bacterial enteric pathogens in farm pond water. *J. Am. Water Works Assoc. 59*, 503–8.

Andrewes, C. H. 1960. The effect on virulence of changes in parasite and host. In *Virus virulence and pathogenicity*, ed. G. E. W. Wolstenholme & C. M. O'Connor, pp. 34–9. Boston: Little, Brown.

Anonymous. 1989a. An Aussie fungus among us. *Sci. News 136*, 46.

Anonymous. 1989b. Clinical trials of zidovudine in HIV infection. *Lancet ii*, 483–4.

Anonymous. 1992. Yellow fever: the global situation. *Bull. WHO 70*, 667–9.

Aoki, Y. 1968. Serological groups of *Shigella* in Japan and neighboring countries. A review. *Trop. Med. 10*, 116–26.

Arendrup, M., Nielsen, C., Hansen, J. E. S., Pedersen, C., Mathiesen, L., & Nielsen, J. O. 1992. Autologous HIV-1 neutralizing antibodies: emergence of neutralization-resistant escape virus and subsequent development of escape virus neutralizing antibodies. *J. Acquired Immune Defic. Syndr. 5*, 303– 7.

Arora, D. R., Midha, N. K., Ichhpujani, R. L., & Chugh, T. D. 1982. Drug resistant shigellosis in North India. *Indian J. Med. Res. 76*, 74–9.

Ascher, M. S., Sheppard, H. W., Arnon, J. M., & Lang, W. 1991. Viral burden in HIV disease. *J. Acquired Immune Defic. Syndr. 4*, 824–5.

Ashkenazi, A., Smith, D. H., Marsters, S. A., Riddle, L., Gregory, T. J., Ho, D. D., & Capon, D. J. 1991. Resistance of primary isolates of human immunodeficiency virus type 1 to soluble CD4 is independent of CD4-rgp120 binding affinity. *Proc. Natl. Acad. Sci. USA 88*, 7056–60.

Askew, R. R. 1971. *Parasitic insects*. London: Heinemen.

Axelrod, R., & Hamilton, W. D. 1981. The evolution of cooperation. *Science 211*, 1390–7.

Aye, D. T., Sack, D. A., Wachsmuth, I. K., Kyi, D. T., & Thwe, S. M. 1991. Neonatal diarrhea at a maternity hospital in Rangoon. *Am. J. Public Hlth. 81*, 480–1.

Aytay, S., & Schulze, I. T. 1991. Single amino acid substitutions in the hemagglutinin can alter the host range and receptor binding properties of H1-strains of influenza-A virus. *J. Virol. 65*, 3022–8.

Azevedo, M., Prater, G., & Dwight, M. 1989. The status of women in Cameroon and Chad. In *Cameroon and Chad in historical and contemporary perspectives.*, ed. M. Azevedo, pp. 155–75. Lewiston: Edwin Mellen.

Åsjö, B., Morfeldt-Manson, L., Albert, J., Biberfeld, G., Karlsson, A., Lidman, K., & Fenyö, E. M. 1986. Replicative capacity of human immunodeficiency virus from patients with varying severity of HIV infection. *Lancet ii*, 660–2.

Babiker, H. A., Creasey, A. M., Fenton, B., Bayoumi, R. A. L., Arnot, D. E., & Walliker, D. 1991. Genetic diversity of *Plasmodium falciparum* in a village in eastern Sudan. 1. Diversity of enzymes, 2D-PAGE proteins and antigens. *Trans. Roy. Soc. Trop. Med. Hyg. 85*, 572–7.

Babu, P. G., Saraswathi, N. K., Devapriya, F., & John, T. J. 1993. The detection of HIV-2 infection in southern India. *Indian J. Med. Res., Sect. A 97*, 49–52.

Bacchetti, P., & Moss, A. R. 1989. Incubation period of AIDS in San Francisco. *Nature 338*, 251–3.

Bachelerie, F., Alcami, J., Hazan, U., Israel, N., Goud, B., Arenzana-Seisdedos, F., & Virelizier, J. L. 1990. Constitutive expression of human immunodeficiency virus (HIV) nef protein in human astrocytes does not influence basal or induced HIV long terminal repeat activity. *J. Virol. 64*, 3059–62.

Bagasra, O., Hauptman, S. P., Lischner, H. W., Sachs, M., & Pomerantz, R. J. 1992. Detection of human immunodeficiency virus type 1 provirus in mononuclear cells by *in situ* polymerase chain reaction. *N. Engl. J. Med. 326*, 1385–91.

Baker, C. J. 1977. Summary of the workshop on perinatal infections due to group B *Streptococcus. J. Infect. Dis. 136*, 137.

Baker, C. J. 1979. Group B streptococcal infections in neonates. *Pediatr. Rev. 1*, 5–15.

Baker, D. H., & Wood, R. J. 1992. Cellular antioxidant status and human immunodeficiency virus replication. *Nutr. Rev. 50*, 15–18.

Bakhanashvili, M., & Hizi, A. 1992. Fidelity of the reverse transcriptase of human immunodeficiency virus type 2. *FEBS Let. 306*, 151–156.

Bakhanashvili, M., & Hizi, A. 1992. Fidelity of the RNA-dependent DNA synthesis exhibited by the reverse transcriptases of human immunodeficiency virus type 1 and type 2 and of murine leukemia virus: mispair extension frequencies. *Biochemistry 31*, 9393–9398.

Bakhanashvili, M., & Hizi, A. 1993. The fidelity of the reverse transcriptases of human immunodeficiency viruses and murine leukemia virus, exhibited by the mispair extension frequencies, is sequence dependent and enzyme related. *FEBS Let. 319*, 201–5.

Balashov, Y. Z. 1984. Interaction between blood-sucking arthropods and their hosts, and its influence on vector potential. *Annu. Rev. Entomol. 29*, 137–56.

Ball, G. H. 1943. Parasitism and evolution. *Am. Nat. 77*, 345–64.

Balzarini, J., Karlsson, A., Perez-Perez, M. J., Vrang, L., Walbers, J., Zhang, H., Öberg, B., Vandamme, A. M., Camarasa, M. J., & De Clercq, E. 1993. HIV-1-specific reverse transcriptase inhibitors show differential activity against HIV-1 mutant strains containing different amino acid substitutions in the reverse transcriptase. *Virology 192*, 246–53.

Banet, M. 1986. Fever in mammals: Is it beneficial? *Yale J. Biol. Med. 59*, 117–24.

Banks, T. A., & Rouse, B. T. 1992. Herpesviruses—immune escape artists. *Clin. Infect. Dis. 14*, 933–41.

Barillari, G., Buonaguro, L., Fiorelli, V., Hoffman, J., Michaels, F., Gallo, R. C., & Ensoli, B. 1992. Effects of cytokines from activated immune cells on vascular cell growth and HIV-1 gene expression: implications for AIDS-Kaposi's sarcoma pathogenesis. *Journal of Immunology 149*, 3727–34.

Barin, F., Denis, F., Baillou, A., Leonard, G., Mounier, M., M'Boup, S., Gershy-Damet, G., Sangare, A., Kanki, P., & Essex, M. 1987. A STLV-III related human retrovirus, HTLV-IV: Analysis of cross-reactivity with the human immunodeficiency virus (HIV). *J. Virol. Methods 17*, 55–61.

Barre-Sinoussi, F., Chermann, J. C., Rey, F., Nugeyre, M. T., Chamaret, S., Gruest, J., Dauget, C., Axler-Blin, C., Brun-Vezinet, F., Rousioux, C., Rozenbaum, W., & Montagnier, L. 1983. Isolation of a T-lymphotropic retrovirus from a patient at risk for AIDS. *Science 220*, 868-70.

Bartholomew, C., Saxinger, W. C., Clark, J. W., Gail, M., Dudgeon, A., Mahabir, B., Hull-Drysdale, B., Cleghorn, F., Gallo, R. C., & Blattner, W. A. 1987. Transmission of HTLV I and HIV among homosexual men in Trinidad. *JAMA 257*, 2604-8.

Barthwell, A., Seney, E., Marks, R., & White, R. 1989. Patients successfully maintained with methadone escaped human immunodeficiency virus infection. *Arch. Gen. Psychiatry 46*, 957.

Bartlett, J. G., O'Keefe, P., Tally, F. P., Louie, T. J., & Gorbach, S. L. 1986. Bacteriology of hospital-acquired pneumonia. *Arch. Intern. Med. 146*, 868-71.

Barton, L. L., Lustig, R. H., Fong, C., & Walentik, C. A. 1986. Neonatal septicemia due to *Pseudomonas aeruginosa. Am. Family Physician 33*, 147-51.

Barua, D. 1970. Survival of cholera vibrios in food, water and fomites. In *Principles and practice of cholera control* Geneva: World Health Organization.

Baselski, V. S., Medina, R. A., & Parker, C. D. 1979. *In vivo* and *in vitro* characterization of virulence deficient mutants of *Vibrio cholerae. Infect. Immun. 24*, 111-16.

Baselski, V. S., Medina, R. A., & Parker, C. D. 1978. Survival and multiplication of *Vibrio cholerae* in the upper bowel of infant mice. *Infect. Immun. 22*, 435-40.

Basu, S., Bhattacharya, P., & Mukerjee, S. 1966. Interaction of *Vibrio cholerae* and *Vibrio* el tor. *Bull. WHO 34*, 371-8.

Beardsley, E. 1788. History of a dysentery in the 22nd regiment of the late continental army. In Proceedings of the New Haven Medical Society, pp. 68-71. New Haven, Connecticut: New Haven County Medical Society.

Beck-Sagué, C., Dooley, S. W., Hutton, M. D., Otten, J., Breeden, A., Crawford, J. T., Pitchenik, A. E., Woodley, C., Cauthen, G., & Jarvis, W. R. 1992. Hospital outbreak of multidrug-resistant *Mycobacterium tuberculosis* infections. Factors in transmission to staff and HIV-infected patients. *JAMA 268*, 1280-6.

Belitsky, V. 1989. Children infect mothers in AIDS outbreak at a Soviet hospital. *Nature 337*, 493.

Belnap, D., & O'Donnell, J. J. 1955. Epidemic gastroenteritis due to *Escherichia coli* 0:111. *J. Pediat. 47*, 178-93.

Bender, B. S., Laughon, B. E., Gaydos, C., Forman, M. S., & Bennett, R. 1986. Is *Clostridium difficile* endemic in chronic-care facilities? *Lancet ii*, 11-13.

Benenson, A. S. 1990. *Control of communicable diseases in man*, 15th edition. Washington, D.C.: American Public Health Association.

Benoit, S. N., Gershy-Damet, G. M., Coulibaly, A., Koffi, K., Sangare, V. S., Koffi, D., Houdier, R., Josseran, R., Guelain, J., Aoussi, E., Odehouri, K., Ehouman, A., & Coulibaly, N. 1990. Seroprevalence of HIV infection in the general population of the Côte d'Ivoire west Africa. *J. Acquired Immune Defic. Syndr. 3*, 1193-6.

Bentley, D. W. 1990. Clostridium difficile-associated disease in long-term care facilities. *Infect. Control Hosp. Epidemiol. 11*, 432-8.

Beral, V. 1991. Epidemiology of Kaposi's sarcoma. *Cancer Surv. 10*, 5-22.

Beral, V., Bull, D., Darby, S., Weller, I., Carne, C., Beecham, M., & Jaffe, H. 1992. Risk of Kaposi's sarcoma and sexual practices associated with faecal contact in homosexual or bisexual men with AIDS. *Lancet 339*, 632-5.

Beral, V., Jaffe, H., & Weiss, R. 1991. Overview: cancer, HIV and AIDS. *Cancer Surv. 10*, 1-3.

Berlin, B. S. 1980. Influenza. In *The biologic and clinical basis of infectious diseases*, 2nd edition, ed. G. P. Youmans, P. Y. Paterson, & H. M. Sommers, pp. 353-66. Philadelphia: W. B. Saunders.

Bermejo, A., & Veeken, H. 1992. Insecticide-impregnated bed nets for malaria control: A review of the field trials. *Bull. WHO 70*, 293-6.

Berneman, Z. N., Gartenhaus, R. B., Reitz, M. S., Blattner, W. A., Manns, A., Hanchard, B., Ikehara, O., Gallo, R. C., & Klotman, M. E. 1992. Expression of alternatively spliced human T-lymphotropic virus type I pX mRNA in infected cell lines and in primary uncultured cells from patients with adult T-cell leukemia/lymphoma and healthy carriers. *Proc. Natl. Acad. Sci. USA 89*, 3005-9.

Berry, A. M., Paton, J. C., & Hansman, D. 1992. Effect of insertional inactivation of the genes encoding pneumolysin and autolysin on the virulence of *Streptococcus pneumoniae* type 3. *Microb. Pathog. 12*, 87-93.

Berzofsky, J. A. 1991. Approaches and issues in the development of vaccines against HIV. *J. Acquired Immune Defic. Syndr. 4*, 451-9.

Bhat, S., Spitalnik, S. L., Gonzalezscarano, F., & Silberberg, D. H. 1991. Galactosyl ceramide or a derivative is an essential component of the neural receptor for human immunodeficiency virus type 1 envelope glycoprotein gp120. *Proc. Natl. Acad. Sci. USA 88*, 7131-4.

Biggar, R. J. 1990. AIDS incubation in 1891 HIV seroconverters from different exposure groups. *AIDS 4*, 1059-66.

Biggar, R. J. 1986 . The AIDS problem in Africa. *Lancet i*, 79-83.

Biggar, R. J. 1988. Overview Africa, AIDS, and epidemiology. In *AIDS in Africa. The social and policy impact. Studies in African Health and Medicine. Vol. 10.*, ed. N. Miller & R. C. Rockwell, pp. 1-8. Lewiston/Queenston: The Edwin Mellen Press.

Biggar, R. J., Buskell-Bales, Z., Yakshe, P. N., Caussy, D., Gridley, G., & Seeff, L. 1991. Antibody to human retroviruses among drug users in three East Coast American cities, 1972-1976. *J. Infect. Dis. 163*, 41-6.

Björkman, A., & Phillips-Howard, P. A. 1991. Adverse reactions to sulfa drugs: Implications for malaria chemotherapy. *Bull. WHO 69*, 297–304.

Black, R. E., Levine, M. M., Clements, M. L., Angle, P., & Robins-Browne, R. 1981. Proliferation of enteropathogens in oral rehydration solutions prepared with river water from Honduras and Surinam. *J. Trop. Med. Hyg. 84*, 195–8.

Blaser, M. J., La Force, F. M., Wilson, N. A., & Wang, W. L. L. 1980. Reservoirs for human campylobacteriosis. *J. Infect. Dis. 141*, 665–9.

Blatteis, C. M. 1986. Fever: Is it beneficial? *Yale J. Biol. Med. 59*, 107–16.

Blattner W A, Nomura A, Clark J W, Ho G Y F, Nakao Y, Gallo R, & Robert-Guroff M. 1986. Modes of transmission and evidence for viral latency from studies of human T-cell lymphotrophic virus type I in Japanese migrant populations in Hawaii. *Proc. Natl. Acad. Sci. USA 83*, 4895–8.

Blattner, W. A. 1990. Epidemiology of HTLV-I and associated diseases. In *Human Retrovirology: HTLV*, ed. W. A. Blattner, pp. 251–65. New York: Raven Press.

Blattner, W. A. 1991. HIV epidemiology: past, present, and future. *FASEB J. 5*, 2340–8.

Blattner, W. A. 1989. Retroviruses. In *Viral infections of humans*, ed. A. S. Evans, pp. 545–92. New York: Plenum.

Blayney, D. W., Blattner, W. A., Robert-Gurdoff, M., Jaffe, E. S., Fisher, R. I., Bunn, P. A., Patton, M. G., Rarick, H. R., & Gallo, R. C. 1983. The human T-cell leukemia-lymphoma virus in the southeastern United States. *JAMA 250*, 1048.

Block, N. B., & Ferguson, W. 1940. An outbreak of Shiga dysentery in Michigan. *Am. J. Public Hlth. 30*, 43–52.

Blumberg, B. M., Epstein, L. G., Saito, Y., Chen, D., Sharer, L. R., & Anand, R. 1992. Human immunodeficiency virus type-1 *nef* quasispecies in pathological tissue. *J. Virol. 66*, 5256–64.

Bohnhoff, M., Miller, C. P., & Martin, W. R. 1964. Resistance of the mouse's intestinal tract to experimental *Salmonella* infection. I. Factors which interfere with the initiation of infection by oral inoculation. II. Factors responsible for its loss following streptomycin treatment. *J. Exp. Med. 120*, 805–828.

Bøjlen, K. 1934. *Dysentery in Denmark*. Copenhagen: Bianco Lunos Bogtrykkeri.

Boorstein, S. M., & Ewald, P. W. 1987. Costs and benefits of behavioral fever in *Melanoplus sanguinipes* infected with *Nosema acridophagus*. *Physiol. Zool. 60*, 586–95.

Boucher, C. A. B. 1992. Clinical significance of zidovudine-resistant human immunodeficiency viruses. *Res. Virol. 143*, 134–6.

Boucher, C. A. B., Lange, J. M. A., Miedema, F. F., Weverling, G. J., Koot, M., Mulder, J. W., Goudsmit, J., Kellam, P., Larder, B. A., & Tersmette, M. 1992. HIV-1 biological phenotype and the development of zidovudine resistance in relation to disease progression in asymptomatic individuals during treatment. *AIDS 6*, 1259–64.

Boucher, C. A. B., & Lange, J. M. A. 1992. HIV-1 sensitivity to zidovudine and clinical outcome. *Lancet 339*, 626.

Boucher, C. A. B., O'Sullivan, E., Mulder, J. W., Ramautarsing, C., Kellam, P., Darby, G., Lange, J. M. A., Goudsmit, J., & Larder, B. A. 1992. Ordered appearance of zidovudine resistance mutations during treatment of 18 human immunodeficiency virus-positive subjects. *J. Infect. Dis. 165*, 105–10.

Boucher, C. A. B., Tersmette, M., Lange, J. M. A., Kellam, P., DeGoede, R. E. Y., Mulder, J. W., Darby, G., Goudsmit, J., & Larder, B. A. 1990. Zidovudine sensitivity of human immunodeficiency viruses from high-risk, symptom-free individuals during therapy. *Lancet 336*, 585–90.

Boudart, D., Lucas, J. C., Muller, J. Y., Besnier, M., & Courouce, A. M. 1992. Serological evidence of successive HIV-2 and HIV-1 infections in a bisexual man. *AIDS 6*, 593.

Bouma, J. E., & Lenski, R. E. 1988. Evolution of a bacteria/plasmid association. *Nature 335*, 351–2.

Bowerman, G. E. 1983. *The compensations of war. The diary of an ambulance driver during the great war*. Austin, Tex.: University of Texas Press.

Bowes, G. K. 1938. Outbreak of Sonne dysentery due to consumption of milk. *Br. Med. J. ii*, 1092–4.

Boyd, J. S. K. 1940. Laboratory diagnosis of bacillary dysentery. *Trans. Roy. Soc. Trop. Med. Hyg. 33*, 553–71.

Boyer, K. M., Petersen, N. J., Farzaneh, I., Pattison, C. P., Hart, M. C., & Maynard, J. E. 1975. An outbreak of gastroenteritis due to *E. coli* 0142 in a neonatal nursery. *J. Pediat. 86*, 919–27.

Böttiger, B., Palme, I. B., daCosta, J. L., Dias, L. F., & Biberfeld, G. 1988. Prevalence of HIV-1 and HIV-2/HTLV-4 infections in Luanda and Cabinda, Angola. *J. Acquired Immune Defic. Syndr. 1*, 8–12.

Brabin, L., Brabin, B. J., Doherty, R. R., Gust, I. D., Alpers, M. P., Fujino, R., Imai, J., & Hinuma, Y. 1989. Patterns of migration indicate sexual transmission of HTLV-I infection in non-pregnant women in Papua New Guinea. *Int. J. Cancer 44*, 59–62.

Brichacek, B., Derderian, C., Chermann, J. C., & Hirsch, I. 1992. HIV-1 infectivity of human carcinoma cell lines lacking CD4 receptors. *Cancer Lett. 63*, 23–31.

Brighty, D. W., Rosenberg, M., Chen, I. S. Y., & Iveyhoyle, M. 1991. Envelope proteins from clinical isolates of human immunodeficiency virus type-1 that are refractory to neutralization by soluble CD4 possess high affinity for the CD4 receptor. *Proc. Natl. Acad. Sci. USA 88*, 7802–5.

Brodeur, J., & McNeil, J. N. 1989. Seasonal microhabitat selection by an endoparasitoid through adaptive modification of host behavior. *Science 244*, 226–8.

Brooks, D. R., & McLennan, D. A. 1992. The evolutionary origin of *Plasmodium falciparum*. *J. Parasitol. 78*, 564–6.

Brown, C. R., & Brown, M. B. 1990. The great egg scramble. *Nat. Hist. 2*, 34–40.

Brown, P. B. 1992. Who cares about malaria? *New Sci. 136*, 37–41.

Bruce-Chwatt, L. J., & de Zulueta, J. 1980. *The rise and fall of malaria in Europe. An historico-epidemiological study*. Oxford: Oxford University Press.

Bryceson, A., Tomkins, A., Ridley, D., Warhurst, D., Goldstone, A., Bayliss, G., Toswill, J., & Parry, J. 1988. HIV-2-associated AIDS in the 1970s. *Lancet ii*, 221.

Buisson, Y., Nizou, J. Y., Talarmin, A., & Meyran, M. 1992. Nosocomial spread of a *Pseudomonas aeruginosa* phenotype producing a betalactamase strongly induced by clavulanic acid *in vitro*. *Pathol. Biol. 40*, 566–72.

Bukrinsky, M. I., Stanwick, T. L., Dempsey, M. P., & Stevenson, M. 1991. Quiescent T lymphocytes as an inducible virus reservoir in HIV-1 infection. *Science 254*, 423–7.

Bull, J. J., & Molineux, I. J. 1992. Molecular genetics of adaptation in an experimental model of cooperation. *Evolution 46*, 882–95.

Bull, J. J., Molineux, I. J., & Rice W R. 1991. Selection of benevolence in a host-parasite system. *Evolution 45*, 875–82.

Buonaguro, L., Barillari, G., Chang, H. K., Bohan, C. A., Kao, V., Morgan, R., Gallo, R. C., & Ensoli, B. 1992. Effects of the human immunodeficiency virus type 1 tat protein on the expression of inflammatory cytokines. *J. Virol. 66*, 7159–67.

Burcham, J., Marmor, M., Dubin, N., Tindall, B., Cooper, D. A., Berry, G., & Penny, R. 1991. CD4% is the best predictor of development of AIDS in a cohort of HIV-infected homosexual men. *AIDS 5*, 365–72.

Burgdorfer, W., & Brinton, L. P. 1975. Mechanisms of transovarial infection of spotted fever rickettsiae in ticks. *Ann. N.Y. Acad. Sci. 266*, 61–72.

Burnet, F. M., & Clark, E. 1942. *Influenza: A survey of the last 50 years in the light of modern work on the virus of epidemic influenza*. Melbourne: Macmillan.

Burnet, F. M., & White, D. O. 1972. *Natural history of infectious disease*, 4th edition. Cambridge: Cambridge University Press.

Burnet, J. 1869. *History of the water supply to Glasgow, from the commencement of the present century*. Glasgow: Bell and Bain.

Burnette, W. N., Mar, V. L., Whiteley, D. W., & Bartley, T. D. 1992. Progress with a recombinant whooping cough vaccine: A review. *J. Roy. Soc. Med. 85*, 285–7.

Cabrera, M. E., Gray, A. M., Cartier, L., Araya, F., Hirsh, T., Ford, A. M., & Greaves, M. F. 1991. Simultaneous adult T-cell leukemia/lymphoma and sub-acute polyneuropathy in a patient from Chile. *Leukemia 5*, 350–3.

Callahan, L. N., Phelan, M., Mallinson, M., & Norcross, M. A. 1991. Dextran sulfate blocks antibody binding to the principal neutralizing domain of human immunodeficiency virus type 1 without interfering with gp120-CD4 interactions. *J. Virol. 65*, 1543–50.

Calsyn, D. A., Saxon, A. J., Freeman, G., & Whittaker, S. 1991. Needle-use practices among intravenous drug users in an area where needle purchase is legal. *AIDS 5*, 187–93.

Cantor, K. P., Weiss, S. H., Goedert, J. J., & Battjes, R. J. 1991. HTLV-I/II seroprevalence and HIV/HTLV coinfection among United States intravenous drug users. *J. Acquired Immune Defic. Syndr. 4*, 460–7.

Capon, D. J., & Ward, R. H. R. 1991. The CD4-GP120 interaction and AIDS pathogenesis. *Annu. Rev. Immunol. 9*, 649–78.

Carael, M., Van De Perre, P. H., Lepage, P. H., Allen, S., Nsengumuremyi, F., Van Goethem, C., Ntahorutaba, M., Nzaramba, D., & Clumeck, N. 1988. Human immunodeficiency virus transmission among heterosexual couples in central Africa. *AIDS 2*, 201–5.

Carey, R. F., Herman, W. A., Retta, S. M., Rinaldi, J. E., Herman, B. A., & Athey, T. W. 1992. Effectiveness of latex condoms as a barrier to human immunodeficiency virus-sized particles under conditions of simulated use. *Sex. Transm. Dis. 19*, 230–4.

Cargnel, A., Orlando, G., Zehender, G., & Zanetti, A. R. 1991. Drug addiction and AIDS. *Biomedical and social developments in AIDS and associated tumors*, ed. G. Giraldo, M. Salvatore, M. Piazza, D. Zarrilli, & E. Bethgiraldo, pp. 45–54. Basel, Switz.: Karger.

Carpenter, C. C. J., Brookmeyer, R., Couch, R. B., Fischl, M. A., Frazer-Howze, D., Friedland, G., Kidd, P. G., Lagakos, S. W., Mayer, C., Osborn, J. E., Richman, D. D., Saag, M. S., Sande, M. A., Sanford, J. P., Sherer, R., Schram, N. R., Thompson, M. A., Volberding, P. A., & Wolff, S. M. 1990. State-of-the-art conference on azidothymidine therapy for early HIV infection. *Am. J. Med. 89*, 335–44.

Carruthers, R. I., Larkin, T. S., Firstencel, H., & Feng, Z. 1992. Influence of thermal ecology on the mycosis of a rangeland grasshopper. *Ecology 73*, 190–204.

Carstensen, H., Henrichsen, J., & Jepsen, O. B. 1985. A national survey of severe group B streptococcal infections in neonates and young infants in Denmark, 1978–83. *Acta Paediatr. Scand. 74*, 934– 41.

Castro, K. G., Dooley, S. W., & Curran, J. W. 1992. Transmission of HIV-associated tuberculosis to health-care workers. *Lancet 340*, 1043–4.

Catania, J. A., Coates, T. J., Kegeles, S., Fullilove, M. T., Peterson, J., Marin, B., Siegel, D., & Hulley, S. 1992. Condom use in multi-ethnic neighborhoods of San Francisco: The population-based AMEN (AIDS in Multi-Ethnic Neighborhoods) study. *Am. J. Public Hlth. 82*, 284–7.

Catania, J. A., Coates, T. J., Stall, R., Turner, H., Peterson, J., Hearst, N., Dolcini, M. M., Hudes, E., Gagnon, J., Wiley, J., & Groves, R. 1992. Prevalence of AIDS-related risk factors and condom use in the United States. *Science 258*, 1101–6.

Cate, T. R. 1972. True myxoviruses. In *Zinsser microbiology* 15th edition, ed. W. K. Joklik & D. T. Smith, pp. 897–904. New York: Appleton-Century-Crofts.

Centers for Disease Control. 1989. Coordinated community programs for HIV prevention among intravenous-drug users—California, Massachusetts. *Morbid. Mortal. Weekly Rep. 38*, 369–74.

Centers for Disease Control. 1991. Nosocomial transmission of multidrug-resistant tuberculosis among HIV-infected persons—Florida and New York, 1988–1991. *Morbid. Mortal. Weekly Rep. 40*, 585–91.

Certa, V., Rotmann, D., Matile, H., & Reber-Liske, R. 1987. A naturally occurring gene encoding the major surface antigen precursor p190 of *Plasmodium falciparum*. *EMBO J. 6*, 4137–42.

Chen, F., Evins, G. M., Cook, W. L., Almeida, R., Hargrettbean, N., & Wachsmuth, K. 1991. Genetic diversity among toxigenic and nontoxigenic *Vibrio cholerae* 01 isolated from the Western hemisphere. *Epidemiol. Infect. 107*, 225–33.

Chen, R. T., Broome, C. V., Weinstein, R. A., Weaver, R., & Tsai, T. F. 1985. Diphtheria in the United States, 1971–81. *Am. J. Public Hlth. 75*, 1393–7.

Cheng-Mayer, C., Iannello, P., Shaw, K., Luciw, P. A., & Levy, J. A. 1989. Differential effects of nef on HIV replication: Implications for viral pathogenesis in the host. *Science 246*, 1629–32.

Cheng-Mayer, C., Seto, D., Tateno, M., & Levy, J. A. 1988. Biologic features of HIV-1 that correlate with virulence in the host. *Science 240*, 80–2.

Chequer, P., Hearst, N., Hudes, E. S., Castilho, E., Rutherford, G., Loures, L., & Rodrigues, L. 1992. Determinants of survival in adult brazilian AIDS patients, 1982–1989. *AIDS 6*, 483–7.

Cherfas, J. 1990. Mad cow disease: Uncertainty rules. *Science 249*, 1492–3.

Chester, K. S. 1942. *The nature and prevention of plant diseases*. Philadelphia: Blakiston.

Chin, W., Contacos, P. G., Collins, W. E., Jeter, M. H., & Albert, E. 1968. Experimental mosquito transmission of *Plasmodium knowlesi* to man and monkey. *Am. J. Trop. Med. Hyg. 17*, 355–8.

Chow, Y. K., Hirsch, M. S., Merrill, D. P., Bechtel, L. J., Eron, J. J., Kaplan, J. C., & Daquila, R. T. 1993. Use of evolutionary limitations of HIV-1 multidrug resistance to optimize therapy. *Nature 361*, 650–4.

Chowdhury, M. I. H., Koyanagi, Y., Suzuki, M., Kobayashi, S., Yamaguchi, K., & Yamamoto, N. 1992. Increased production of human immunodeficiency virus (HIV) in HIV-induced syncytia formation: an efficient infection process. *Virus Genes 6*, 63–78.

Chu, A. B., Nerurkar, L. S., Witzel, N., Andresen, B. D., Alexander, M., Kang, E. S., Brouwers, P., Fedio, P., Lee, Y. J., & Sever, J. L. 1986. Reye's syndrome: Salicylate metabolism, viral antibody levels, and other factors in surviving patients and unaffected family members. *Am. J. Dis. Child. 140*, 1009–12.

Clark, J., Saxinger, C., Gibbs, W. N., Lofters, W., Lagranade, L., Deceulaer, K., Ensroth, A., Robert-Guroff, M., Gallo, R. C., & Blattner, W. A. 1985. Seroepidemiologic studies of human T-cell leukemia/lymphoma virus type I in Jamaica. *Int. J. Cancer 36*, 37–41.

Clark, S. J., Saag, M. S., Decker, W. D., Campbell-Hill, S., Roberson, J. L., Veldkamp, P. J., Kappes, J. C., Hahn, B. H., & Shaw, G. M. 1991. High titers of cytopathic virus in plasma of patients with symptomatic primary HIV-1 infection. *N. Engl. J. Med. 324*, 954–60.

Clements, A. 1992. Thailand stifles AIDS campaign. *Br. Med. J. 304*, 1264.

Cloney, D. L., & Donowitz, L. G. 1986. Overgown use for infection control in nurseries and neonatal intensive care units. *Am. J. Dis. Child. 140*, 680–3.

Clumeck, N. 1989. AIDS in Africa. In *AIDS: Pathogenesis and treatment*, ed. J. A. Levy, pp. 37–63. New York: Marcel Dekker.

Coatney, G. R. 1976. Relapse in malaria—an enigma. *J. Parasitol. 62*, 3–9.

Coatney, G. R., Collins, W. E., McWilson, W., & Contacos, P. G. 1971. *The primate malarias*. Washington, D.C.: U.S. Government Printing Office.

Coatney, G. R., Cooper, W. C., & Young, M. D. 1950. Studies in human malaria. XXX. A summary of 204 sporozoite-induced infections with the chesson strain of *Plasmodium vivax*. *J. Natl. Malaria Soc. 9*, 381–96.

Cockburn, A. 1963. *The evolution and eradication of infectious diseases*. Baltimore: Johns Hopkins University Press.

Coffin, J. M. 1990. Genetic variation in retroviruses. In *Applied virology research, volume 2. Virus variability, epidemiology and control*, ed. E. Kurstak, R. G. Marusyk, F. A. Murphy, & M. J. V. van Regenmortel, pp. 11–31. New York: Plenum.

Cogswell, F. B., Collins, W. E., Krotoski, W. A., & Lowrie, R. C. 1991. Hypnozoites of *Plasmodium simiovale*. *Am. J. Trop. Med. Hyg. 45*, 211–13.

Cohen, J. B., & Wofsy, C. B. 1989. Heterosexual transmission of AIDS. In *AIDS: pathogenesis and treatment*, ed. J. A. Levy, pp. 135–57. New York: Marcel Dekker.

Colebunders, R., Ryder, R., Francis, H., Nekwei, W., Bahwe, Y., Lebughe, I., Ndilu, M., Vercauteren, G., Nseka, K., Perriens, J., Van der Stuyft, P., Quinn, T. C., & Piot, P. 1991. Seroconversion rate, mortality, and clinical manifestations associated with the receipt of a human immunodeficiency virus-infected blood transfusion in Kinshasa, Zaire. *J. Infect. Dis. 164*, 450–6.

Collins, F. H., Sakai, R. K., Vernick, K. D., Paskewitz, S., Seeley, D. C., Miller, L. H., Collins, W. E., Campbell, C. C., & Gwadz, R. W. 1986. Genetic selection of a *Plasmodium*-refractory strain of the malaria vector *Anopheles gambiae*. *Science 234*, 610–2.

Colwell, R. R., Seidler, R. J., Kaper, J., Joseph, S. W., Garges, S., Lockman, H., Maneval, D., Bradford, H., Roberts, N., Rommers, E., Huq, I., & Huq, A. 1981. Occurrence of *Vibrio cholerae* serotype 01 in Maryland and Louisiana estuaries. *Appl. Environ. Microbiol. 41*, 555–8.

Concia, E., Marone, P., Marino, L., Riccardi, A., & Sciarra, E. 1985. Group B streptococcal colonization among hospital personnel. *Boll. Inst. Sieroter. Milan 64*, 165–6.

Connor, R. I., Mohri, H., Cao, Y. Z., & Ho, D. D. 1993. Increased viral burden and cytopathicity correlate temporally with CD4+ T lymphocyte decline and clinical progression in human immunodeficiency virus type 1-infected individuals. *J. Virol. 67*, 1772–7.

Contacos, P. G., Elder, H. A., Coatney, G. R., & Genther, C. 1962. Man to man transfer of two strains of *Plasmodium cynomolgi* by mosquito bite. *Am. J. Trop. Med. Hyg. 11*, 186–94.

Conway, D. J., Greenwood, B. M., & McBride, J. S. 1991. The epidemiology of multiple-clone *Plasmodium falciparum* infections in Gambian patients. *Parasitology 103*, 1–6.

Conway, D. J., & McBride, J. S. 1991. Genetic evidence for the importance of interrupted feeding by mosquitoes in the transmission of malaria. *Trans. Roy. Soc. Trop. Med. Hyg. 85*, 454–6.

Coombs, R. W., Krieger, J. N., Collier, A. C., Ross, S. O., Chaloupka, K., Murphy, V. L., Cummings, D. K., & Corey, L. 1990. Plasma viremia and recovery of HIV from semen: Implications for transmission/therapy. *Arch. AIDS Res. 4*, 280–1.

Cooper, M. L., Keller, H. M., Walters, W. W., Partin, J. C., & Boye, D. E. 1959. Isolation of enteropathogenic *Escherichia coli* from mothers and newborn infants. *Am. J. Dis. Child.* 97, 255–66.

Cooper, M. L., Walters, E. W., Keller, H. M., Sutherland, J. M., & Wiseman, H. J. 1955. Epidemic diarrhea among infants associated with the isolation of a new serotype of *Escherichia coli* 0127:B8. *Pediatrics* 16, 215–27.

Cooperstock, M. 1987. Indigenous flora in pathogenesis. *Textbook of pediatric infectious diseases*, 2nd edition, ed. R. D. Feigin & J. D. Cherry, pp. 106–33. Philadelphia: W. B. Saunders.

Corbitt, G., Bailey, A. S., & Williams, G. 1990. HIV infection in Manchester, 1959. *Lancet 336*, 51.

Corey, L., & Fleming, T. R. 1992. Treatment of HIV infection—progress in perspective. *N. Engl. J. Med. 326*, 484–5.

Costanzo-Nordin, M. R., Reap, E. A., O'Connell, J. B., Robinson, J. A., & Scanlon, P. J. 1985. A nonsteroid anti-inflammatory drug exacerbates coxsackie B3 murine myocarditis. *J. Am. Coll. Cardiol. 6*, 1078–82.

Coudron, P. E., Mayhall, C. G., Facklam, R. R., Spadora, A. C., Lamb, V. A., Lybrand, M. R., & Dalton, H. P. 1984. *Streptococcus faecium* outbreak in a neonatal intensive care unit. *J. Clin. Microbiol. 20*, 1044–8.

Cowen, R. 1991. Fighting the mite: May the best bee win. *Sci. News 139*, 5.

Craun, G. F., & McCabe, L. J. 1973. Review of the causes of water-borne disease outbreaks. *J. Am. Water Works Assoc. 65*, 74– 84.

Craven, D. E., Reed, C., Kollisch, N., DeMaria, A., Lichtenberg, D., Shen, K., & McCabe, W. R. 1981. A large outbreak of infections caused by a strain of *Staphylococcus aureus* resistant to oxacillin and aminoglycosides. *Am. J. Med. 71*, 53–8.

Crosby, A. W. 1976. *Epidemic and peace, 1918*. Westport, Conn.: Greenwood Press.

Cross, A., Allen, J. R., Burke, J., Ducel, G., Harris, A., John, J., Johnson, D., Lew, M., MacMillan, B., Meers, P., Skalova, R., Wenzel, R., & Tenney, J. 1983. Nosocomial infections due to *Pseudomonas aeruginosa*: Review of recent trends. *Rev. Infect. Dis. 5 (Suppl. 5)*, S837–45.

Crossley, K., Loesch, D., Landesman, B., Mead, K., Chern, M., & Strate, R. 1979. An outbreak of infections caused by strains of *Staphylococcus aureus* resistant to methicillin and aminoglycosides. I. Clinical studies. *J. Infect. Dis. 139*, 273– 9.

Cruickshank, J. K., Richardson, J. H., Morgan, O. S. C., Porter, J., Klenerman, P., Knight, J., Newell, A. L., Rudge, P., & Dalgleish, A. G. 1990. Screening for prolonged incubatin of HTLV-I infection in British and Jamaican relatives of British patients with tropical spastic paraparesis. *Br. Med. J. 300*, 300–4.

Cruickshank, R. 1941. Infected dust. *Lancet 240*, 493.

Cruickshank, R., & Swyer, R. 1940. An outbreak of Sonne dysentery. *Lancet 241*, 803–5.

Cullen, B. R., & Garrett, E. D. 1992. A comparison of regulatory features in primate lentiviruses. *AIDS Res. Hum. Retroviruses 8*, 387–93.

Culliton, B. J. 1990. Emerging viruses, emerging threat. *Science 247*, 279–80.

Curran, J. W., Jaffe, H. W., Hardy, A. M., Morgan, W. M., & Selik, R. 1988. Epidemiology of HIV infection and AIDS in the USA. *Science 239*, 610–16.

da Graça, J. V., & Mason, T. E. 1983. Detection of avocado sunblotch viroid in flower buds by polyacrylamide gel electrophoresis. *Phytopathol. Z. 108*, 262–6.

da Graça, J. V., van Vuuren, S. P., van Lelyveld, L. J., & Martin, M. M. 1981. Latest advances in avocado sunblotch research. *Citr. Trop. Fruit J. 572*, 20–3.

Daar, E. S., & Ho, D. D. 1991. Relative resistance of primary HIV-1 isolates to neutralization by soluble CD4. *Am. J. Med. 90*, S22–6.

Daar, E. S., Li, X. L., Moudgil, T., & Ho, D. D. 1990. High concentrations of recombinant soluble CD4 are required to neutralize primary human immunodeficiency virus type 1 infection. *Proc. Natl. Acad. Sci. USA 87*, 6574–8.

Daar, E. S., Moudgil, T., Meyer, R. D., & Ho, D. D. 1991. Transient high levels of viremia in patients with primary human immunodeficiency virus type 1 infection. *N. Engl. J. Med. 324*, 961–4.

Dadaglio, G., Michel, F., Langlade-Demoyen, P., Sansonetti, P., Chevrier, D., Vuillier, F., Plata, F., & Hoffenbach, A. 1992. Enhancement of HIV-specific cytotoxic T lymphocyte responses by zidovudine (AZT) treatment. *Clin. Exp. Immunol. 87*, 7–14.

Dales, G. F. 1964. The mythical massacre at Mohenjo Daro. *Expedition 6*, 36–43.

Daley, C. L., Small, P. M., Schecter, G. F., Schoolnik, G. K., Mcadam, R. A., Jacobs, W. R., & Hopewell, P. C. 1992. An outbreak of tuberculosis with accelerated progression among persons infected with the human immunodeficiency virus—an analysis using restriction-fragment length polymorphisms. *N. Engl. J. Med. 326*, 231–5.

Darby, G., & Larder, B. A. 1992. The clinical significance of antiviral drug resistance. *Res. Virol. 143*, 116–20.

Davidson, P. T., & Le, H. Q. 1992. Drug treatment of tuberculosis: 1992. *Drugs 43*, 651–73.

Davis, D. L., & Buffler, P. 1992. Reduction of deaths after drug labelling for risk of Reye's syndrome. *Lancet 340*, 1042.

Davis, L. E., Cole, L. L., Lockwood, S. J., & Kornfeld, M. 1983. Experimental influenza B virus toxicity in mice: A possible model for Reye's syndrome. *Lab. Invest. 48*, 140–7.

Davis, L. E., Green, C. L., & Wallace, J. M. 1985. Influenza B virus model of Reye's syndrome in mice: The effect of aspirin. *Ann. Neurol. 18*, 556–9.

Dawson, M. H. 1988. AIDS in Africa: Historical roots. In *AIDS in Africa. The social and policy impact. Studies in African health and medicine.* Vol. 10, ed. N. Miller & R. C. Rockwell, pp. 57–69. Lewiston/Queenston: The Edwin Mellen Press.

Day, J. F., Ebert, K. M., & Edman, J. D. 1983. Feeding patterns of mosquitoes (*Diptera*: *Culicidae*) simultaneously exposed to malarious and healthy mice, including a method for separating blood meals from conspecific hosts. *J. Med. Entomol. 20*, 120–7.

Day, J. F., & Edman, J. D. 1983. Malaria renders mice susceptible to mosquito feeding when gametocytes are most infective. *J. Parasitol. 69*, 163–70.

De, B. K., Lairmore, M. D., Griffis, K., Williams, L. J., Villinger, F., Quinn, T. C., Brown, C., Nzilambi, N., Sugimoto, M., Araki, S., & Folks, T. M. 1991. Comparative analysis of nucleotide sequences of the partial envelope gene (5′ domain) among human T lymphotropic virus type I (HTLV-I) isolates. *Virology 182*, 413–19.

De, S. N. 1961. *Cholera: Its pathology and pathogenesis.* Edinburgh:Oliver & Boyd.

De, S. P., Sen, R., Ghosh, A. K., & Shrivastava, D. L. 1965. Some observations on *Vibrio cholerae* strains isolated during the controlled field trial of cholera vaccines in Calcutta in 1964. *Indian J. Med. Res. 53*, 614–22.

De, S. P., Sinha, R., & Deb, B. C. 1969. Patterns of *V. cholerae* infection in endemic areas. *J. Indian Med. Assoc. 52*, 458–9.

De Cock, K. M., Barrere, B., Diaby, L., Lafontaine, M., Gnaore, E., Porter, A., Pantobe, D., Lafontant, G. C., Dago-Akribi, A., Ette, M., Odehouri, K., & Heyward, W. l. 1990a. AIDS—the leading cause of adult death in the west African city of Abidjan, Ivory Coast. *Science 249*, 793–6.

De Cock, K. M., Barrere, B., Lafontaine, M. F., Diaby, L., Gnaore, E., Pantobe, D., & Odehouri, K. 1991. Mortality trends in Abidjan, Côte d'Ivoire, 1983–1988. *AIDS 5*, 393–8.

De Cock, K. M., Odehouri, K., Colebunders, R. L., Adjorlolo, G., Lafontaine, M. F., Porter, A., Gnaore, E., Diaby, L., Moreau, J., Heyward, W. L., Kadio, A., Heroin, P., Kanga, J. M., Beda, B., Niamkey, E., Achi, Y., Coulibaly, N., Attia, Y., Giordano, C., Rayfield, M., & Schochetman. 1990b. A comparison of HIV-1 and HIV-2 infections in hospitalized patients in Abidjan, Côte d'Ivoire. *AIDS 4*, 443–8.

De Jong, J., De Ronde, A., Keulen, W., Tersmette, M., & Goudsmit, J. 1992. Minimal requirements for the human immunodeficiency virus type 1 V3 domain to support the syncytium-inducing phenotype: analysis by single amino acid substitution. *J. Virol. 66*, 6777–80.

De Leys, R., Vanderborght, B., Haeseveldt, M. V., Heyndrickx, L., van Geel, A., Wauters, C., Bernaerts, R., Saman, E., Nijs, P., Willems, B., Taelman, H., van der Groen, G., Piot, P., Tersmette, T., Huisman, J. G., & van Heuverswyn, H. 1990. Isolation and partial characterization of an unusual human immunodeficiency retrovirus from two persons of west-central African origin. *J. Virol. 64*, 1207–16.

De Meis, C., De Vasconcellos, A. C. P., Linhares, D., & Andrada-Serpa, M. J. 1991. HIV-1 infection among prostitutes in Rio de Janeiro, Brazil. *AIDS 5*, 236–7.

de Quadros, C., Olive, J., Carrasco, P., Silveira, C., Fitzsimmons, J., & Pinheiro, F. 1992. Update: eradication of paralytic poliomyelitis. *JAMA 268*, 1650.

De Ronde, A., Klaver, B., Keulen, W., Smit, L., & Goudsmit, J. 1992. Natural HIV-1 Nef accelerates virus replication in primary human lymphocytes. *Virology 188*, 391–5.

De Rossi, A., Mammano, F., Del Mistro, A., & Chieco-Bianchi, L. 1991a. Serological and molecular evidence of infection by human T-cell lymphotropic virus type II in Italian drug addicts by use of synthetic peptides and polymerase chain reaction. *Eur. J. Cancer 27*, 835–8.

De Rossi, A., Pasti, M., Mammano, F., Ometto, L., Giaquinto, C., & Chiecobianchi, L. 1991b. Perinatal infection by human immunodeficiency virus type 1 (HIV-1): relationship between proviral copy number *in vivo*, viral properties *in vitro*, and clinical outcome. *J. Med. Virol. 35*, 283–9.

de Vincenzi, I., Ancelle-Park, R. A., Brunet, J. B., Costigliola, P., Ricchi, E., Chiodo, F., Roumeliotou, A., Papaevengelou, G., Coutinho, R. A., Vanhaastrecht, H. J. A., Brettle, R., Robertson, R., Kraus, M., Heckmann, W., Saracco, A., Johnson, A. M., Vandenbruaene, M., Goeman, J., Cardoso, J., Sobel, A., Gonzalez-Lahoz, J., Andres-Medina, R., Casabona, J., & Tor, J. 1992. Comparison of female to male and male to female transmission of HIV in 563 stable couples. *Br. Med. J. 304*, 809–13.

de Zoysa, I., & Feachem, R. G. 1985. Interventions for the control of diarrhoeal diseases among young children: Rotavirus and cholera immunization. *Bull. WHO 63*, 569–83.

Dearruda, E., Mifflin, T. E., Gwaltney, J. M., Winther, B., & Hayden, F. G. 1991. Localization of rhinovirus replication *in vitro* with *in situ* hybridization. *J. Med. Virol.* *34*, 38–44.

Debrunner, M., Salfinger, M., Brandli, O., & Vongraevenitz, A. 1992. Epidemiology and clinical significance of nontuberculous mycobacteria in patients negative for human immunodeficiency virus in Switzerland. *Clin. Infect. Dis. 15*, 330–45.

DeFoliart, G. R., Grimstad, P. R., & Watts, D. M. 1987. Advances in mosquito-borne arbovirus/vector research. *Annu. Rev. Entomol. 32*, 479–505.

Del Mistro, A., Chotard, J., Hall, A. J., Whittle, H., Derossi, A., & Chiecobianchi, L. 1992. HIV-1 and HIV-2 seroprevalence rates in mother-child pairs living in the Gambia (west Africa). *J. Acquired Immune Defic. Syndr. 5*, 19–24.

Delaporte, E., Louwagie, J., Peeters, M., Montplaisir, N., d'Auriol, L., Ville, Y., Bedjabaga, L., Larouze, B., Van der Groen, G., & Piot, P. 1991a. Evidence of HTLV-II infection in central Africa. *AIDS 5*, 771–2.

Delaporte, E., Monplaisir, N., Louwagie, J., Peeters, M., Martin-Prevel, Y., Louis, J. P., Trebucq, A., Bedjabaga, L., Ossari, S., Honore, C., Larouze, B., d'Auriol, L., Van der Groen, G., & Piot, P. 1991b. Prevalence of HTLV-I and HTLV-II infection in Gabon, Africa: Comparison of the serological and PCR results. *Int. J. Cancer 49*, 373–6.

Delassus, S., Cheynier, R., & Wain-Hobson, S. 1991. Evolution of human immunodeficiency virus type 1 nef and long terminal repeat sequences over 4 years *in vivo* and *in vitro*. *J. Virol. 65*, 225– 31.

Deloron, P., & Chougnet, C. 1992. Is immunity to malaria really short-lived? *Parasitol. Today 8*, 375–8.

Deom, C. J., Caton, A. J., & Schulze, I. T. 1986. Host cell-mediated selection of a mutant influenza A-virus that has lost a complex oligosaccharide from the tip of the hemagglutinin. *Proc. Natl. Acad. Sci. USA 83*, 3771–5.

Deshmukh, D. R. 1985. Animal models of Reye's syndrome. *Rev. Infect. Dis. 7*, 31–40.

Desjardins, P. R., Drake, R. J., Atkins, E. L., & Bergh, B. O. 1979. Pollen transmission of avocado sunblotch virus experimentally demonstrated. *Calif. Agric. 33*, 14–15.

Desjardins, P. R., Drake, R. J., Sasaki, P. J., Atkins, E. L., & Bergh, B. O. 1984. Pollen transmission of avocado sunblotch viroid and the fate of the pollen recipient tree. *Phytopathology 74*, 845.

DesJarlais, D. C., & Friedman, S. R. 1988. HIV infection among persons who inject illicit drugs: problems and prospects. *J. Acquired Immune Defic. Syndr. 1*, 267–73.

DesJarlais, D. C., & Friedman, S. R. 1989. AIDS and IV drug use. *Science 245*, 578–9.

Desser, S. S., Fallis, A. M., & Garnham, P. C. C. 1968. Relapse in ducks chronically infected with *Leucocytozoon simondi* and *Parahaemoproteus nettionis*. *Can. J. Zool. 46*, 281–5.

DeWolf, F., Lange, J. M. A., Goudsmit, J., Cload, P., DeGans, J., Schellekens, P. T. A., Coutinho, R. A., Fiddian, A. P., & Van Der Noordaa, J. 1988. Effect of zidovudine on serum human immunodeficiency virus antigen levels in symptom-free subjects. *Lancet i*, 373–6.

Diallo, M. O., Ackah, A. N., Lafontaine, M. F., Doorly, R., Roux, R., Kanga, J. M., Heroin, P., & De Cock, K. M. 1992. HIV-1 and HIV-2 infections in men attending sexually transmitted disease clinics in Abidjan, Côte d'Ivoire. *AIDS 6*, 581–5.

Dietrich, U., Adamski, M., Kreutz, R., Seipp, A., Kühnel, H., & Rübsamen-Waigmann, H. 1989. A highly divergent HIV-2-related isolate. *Nature 342*, 948–50.

Dietrich, U., Grez, M., von Briesen, H., Panhans, B., Geißendörfer, M., Kühnel, H., Maniar, J., Mahambre, G., Becker, W. B., Becker, M. L. B., & Rübsamen-Waigmann, H. 1993. HIV-1 strains from India are highly divergent from prototypic African and United States/European strains, but are linked to a South African isolate. *AIDS 7*, 23–7.

Dimitrov, D. S., Willey, R. L., Sato, H., Chang, L. J., Blumenthal, R., & Martin, M. A. 1993. Quantitation of human immunodeficiency virus type 1 infection kinetics. *J. Virol. 67*, 2182–90.

Diperri, G., Cazzadori, A., Concia, E., & Bassetti, D. 1992. Transmission of HIV-associated tuberculosis to health-care workers. *Lancet 340*, 1412.

Dixon, R. E. 1978. Effect of infections on hospital care. *Ann. Intern. Med. 89*, 749–53.

Dizon, J. J. 1965. Carriers of cholera El Tor in the Philippines. In *Proceedings of the Cholera Research Symposium*, ed. O. A. Bushnell & C. S. Brookhyser, pp. 322–6. Washington, D.C.: U. S. Government Printing Office.

Dizon, J. J., Tukumi, H., Barua, D., Valera, J., Jamyme, F., Gomez, F., Yamamoto, S. I., Wake, A., Gomez, C. Z., Takahira, Y., Paraan, A., Rolda, L., Alvero, M., Abou-Gareeb, A. H., Kobari, K., & Azurin, J. C. 1967. Studies on cholera carriers. *Bull. WHO 37*, 737–43.

Domenico, P., Landolphi, D. R., & Cunha, B. A. 1991. Reduction of capsular polysaccharide and potentiation of aminoglycoside inhibition in gram-negative bacteria by bismuth subsalicylate. *J. Antimicrob. Chemother. 28*, 801–10.

Dooley, S. W., Jarvis, W. R., Martone, W. J., & Snider, D. E. 1992a. Multidrug-resistant tuberculosis. *Ann. Intern. Med. 117*, 257–9.

Dooley, S. W., Villarino, M. E., Lawrence, M., Salinas, L., Amil, S., Rullan, J. V., Jarvis, W. R., Bloch, A. B., & Cauthen, G. M. 1992b. Nosocomial transmission of tuberculosis in a hospital unit for HIV-infected patients. *JAMA 267*, 2632–4.

Doolittle, R. F. 1989. The simian-human connection. *Nature 339*, 338–9.

Doran, T. F., De Angelis, C., Baumgardner, R. A., & Mellits, E. D. 1989. Acetaminophen: More harm than good for chickenpox? *Pediatr. Pharmacol. Ther. 114*, 1045–8.

Doyle, R. J., & Lee, N. C. 1986. Microbes, warfare, religion, and human institutions. *Can. J. Microbiol. 32*, 193–200.

Drew, W. L. 1986. Is cytomegalovirus a cofactor in the pathogenesis of AIDS and Kaposi's sarcoma? *Mount Sinai J. Med. 53*, 622–6.

Dubos, R. 1960. Forward. to *Attenuated infection* Philadelphia: J. B. Lippincott.

Dubos, R. 1965. *Man adapting*. New Haven, Conn.: Yale University Press.

Dudgeon, L. S., Urguhart, A. L., Logan, W. R., Taylor, J. F., Wilken, A., Ryrie, B. J., & Banforth, J. 1919. Study of bacillary dysentery occurring in the British forces in Macedonia. In *British Medical Research Committee Special Report Series No. 40*, ed. L. S. Dudgeon, pp. 5–83. London: British Medical Research Council.

Dufoort, G., Courouce, A. M., Ancelle-Park, R., & Bletry, O. 1988. No clinical signs 14 years after HIV-2 transmission via blood transfusion. *Lancet ii*, 510.

Duggan, J. M., Oldfield, G. S., & Ghosh, H. K. 1985. Septicaemia as a hospital hazard. *J. Hosp. Infect. 6*, 406–12.

Dunkle, L. M., Naqvi, S. H., McCallum, R., & Lofgren, J. P. 1981. Eradication of epidemic methicillin-gentamicin-resistant *Staphylococcus aureus* in an intensive care nursery. *Am. J. Med. 70*, 455–8.

DuPont, H. L. 1979. *Shigella* species (bacillary dysentery). In *Principles and practice of infectious disease* ed. G. L. Mandell, R. G. Douglas, & J. E. Bennett, pp. 1751–72. New York: Wiley.

DuPont, H. L., & Hornick, R. B. 1973. Adverse effect of Lomotil therapy in shigellosis. *JAMA 226*, 1525–8.

DuPont, H. L., Hornick, R. B., Snyder, L. J. P., Formal, S. B., & Gangarosa, E. J. 1972. Immunity in shigellosis. II. Protection induced by oral live vaccine or primary infection. *J. Infect. Dis. 125*, 12–16.

DuPont, H. L., Sullivan, P., Pickering, L. K., Haynes, G., & Ackerman, P. B. 1977. Symptomatic treatment of diarrhea with bismuth subsalicylate among students attending a Mexican university. *Gastroenterology 73*, 715–18.

Duyao, M. P., Kessler, D. J., Spicer, D. B., & Sonenshein, G. E. 1992. Transactivation of the murine c-myc gene by HTLV-I tax is mediated by NFkB. *AIDS Res. Hum. Retroviruses 8*, 752–4.

Dwyer, G., Levin, S. A., & Buttel, L. 1990. A simulation model of the population dynamics and evolution of myxomatosis. *Ecol. Monogr. 60*, 423–47.

Dyson, R. H. 1982. Paradigm changes in the study of the Indus civilization. In *Harappan civilization*, ed. G. Possehl, pp. 417– 27. Warminster, U.K.: Artis & Philips.

Easmon, C. S. F., Hastings, M. J. G., Clare, A. J., Bloxham, B., Marwood, R., & Rivers, R. P. A. 1981. Nosocomial transmission of group B streptococci. *Br. Med. J. 283*, 459–61.

Eberhardt, K. E. W., Thimm, B. M., Spring, A., & Maskos, W. R. 1992. Dose-dependent rate of nosocomial pulmonary infection in mechanically ventilated patients with brain oedema receiving barbiturates: A prospective case study. *Infection 20*, 12–18.

Eberhard, W. G. 1990. Evolution in bacterial plasmids and levels of selection. *Q. Rev. Biol. 65*, 3–22.

Ede, R. J., & Williams, R. 1988. Reye's syndrome in adults. *Br. Med. J. 296*, 517–18.

Edelman, R., & Pierce, N. F. 1984. Summary of the 19th United States–Japan joint cholera conference. *J. Infect. Dis. 149*, 1014–17.

Edlin, B. R., Tokars, J. I., Grieco, M. H., Crawford, J. T., Williams, J., Sordillo, E. M., Ong, K. R., Kilburn, J. O., Dooley, S. W., Castro, K. G., Jarvis, W. R., & Holmberg, S. D. 1992. An outbreak of multidrug-resistant tuberculosis among hospitalized patients with the acquired immunodeficiency syndrome. *N. Engl. J. Med. 326*, 1514–21.

Edwards, R. L. 1960. Relationship between grasshopper abundance and weather conditions in Saskatchewan, 1930–1958. *Can. Entomol. 92*, 619–24.

Effros, R. B., Walford, R. L., Weindruch, R., & Mitcheltree, C. 1991. Influences of dietary restriction on immunity to influenza in aged mice. *J. Gerontol.:Biol. Sci. 46*, B142–7.

Ehrlich, G. D., Andrews, J., Sherman, M. P., Greenberg, S. J., & Poiesz, B. J. 1992. DNA sequence analysis of the gene encoding the HTLV-I P21E transmembrane protein reveals inter- and intraisolate genetic heterogeneity. *Virology 186*, 619–27.

Ehrlich, G. D., Glaser, J. B., LaVigne, K., Quan, D., Mildvan, D., Sninsky, J. J., Kwok, S., Papsidero, L., & Poiesz, B. J. 1989. Prevalence of human T-cell leukemia/lymphoma virus (HTLV) type II infection among high-risk individuals: Type-specific identification of HTLVs by polymerase chain reaction. *Blood 74*, 1658–64.

Eigen, M., & Nieselt-Struwe, K. 1990. How old is the immunodeficiency virus? *AIDS 4 (Suppl. 1)*, S85–93.

Elford, J., Tindall, B., & Sharkey, T. 1992. Kaposi's sarcoma and insertive rimming. *Lancet 339*, 938.

Embretson, J., Zupancic, M., Beneke, J., Till, M., Wolinsky, S., Ribas, J. L., Burke, A., & Haase, A. T. 1993a. Analysis of human immunodeficiency virus-infected tissues by amplification and *in situ* hybridization reveals latent and permissive infections at single-cell resolution. *Proc. Natl. Acad. Sci. USA 90*, 357–61.

Embretson, J., Zupancic, M., Ribas, J. L., Burke, A., Racz, P., Tenner-Racz, K., & Haase, A. T. 1993b. Massive covert infection of helper T lymphocytes and macrophages by HIV during the incubation period of AIDS. *Nature 362*, 359–62.

Ensoli, B., Barillari, G., Salahuddin, S. Z., Gallo, R. C., & Wong-Staal, F. 1990. Tat protein of HIV-1 stimulates growth of cells derived from Kaposi's sarcoma lesions of AIDS patients. *Nature 345*, 84–6.

Ensoli, B., Buonaguro, L., Barillari, G., Fiorelli, V., Gendelman, R., Morgan, R. A., Wingfield, P., & Gallo, R. C. 1993. Release, uptake, and effects of extracellular human immunodeficiency virus type-1 tat protein on cell growth and viral transactivation. *J. Virol. 67*, 277–87.

Epstein, P. R. 1992. Cholera and the environment: An introduction to climate change. *Physic. Soc. Respons. Q. 2*, 146-60.

Ericsson, C. D., DuPont, H. L., & Johnson, P. C. 1986. Nonantibiotic therapy for traveler's diarrhea. *Rev. Infect. Dis. 8 (Suppl. 12)*, S202–6.

Esrey, S. A., Feachem, R. G., & Hughes, J. M. 1985. Interventions for the control of diarrhoeal diseases in young children: Improving water supply and excreta disposal facilities. *Bull. WHO 63*, 757–72.

Esrey, S. A., Potash, J. B., Roberts, L., & Shiff, C. 1991. Effects of improved water supply and sanitation on ascariasis, diarrhoea, dracunculiasis, hookworm infection, schistosomiasis, and trachoma. *Bull. WHO 69*, 609–21.

Essex, M., & Kanki, P. J. 1988. The origins of the AIDS virus. *Sci. Am. 259(10)*, 64–71.

Evans, L. A., Moreau, J., Odehouri, K., Legg, H., Barboza, A., Cheng-Mayer, C., & Levy, J. A. 1988. Characterization of a noncytopathic HIV-2 strain with unusual effects on CD4 expression. *Science 240*, 1522–4.

Ewald, P. W. 1988. Cultural vectors, virulence, and the emergence of evolutionary epidemiology. *Oxford Surv. Evol. Biol. 5*, 215–45.

Ewald, P. W. 1980. Evolutionary biology and the treatment of signs and symptoms of infectious disease. *J. Theor. Biol 86*, 169–76.

Ewald, P. W. 1983. Host–parasite relations, vectors, and the evolution of disease severity. *Annu. Rev. Ecol. Syst. 14*, 465–85.

Ewald, P. W. 1987b. Pathogen-induced cycling of outbreak insect populations. In *Insect outbreaks*, ed. P. Barbosa & J. C. Schultz, pp. 269–86. San Diego: Academic Press.

Ewald, P. W. 1987a. Transmission modes and evolution of the parasitism–mutualism continuum. *Ann. N.Y. Acad. Sci. 503*, 295– 306.

Ewald, P. W. 1991b. Transmission modes and the evolution of virulence, with special reference to cholera, influenza and AIDS. *Human Nature 2*, 1–30.

Ewald, P. W. 1991a. Waterborne transmission and the evolution of virulence among gastrointestinal bacteria. *Epidemiol. Infect. 106*, 83–119.

Ewald, P. W., & Schubert, J. 1989. Vertical and vector-borne transmission of insect endocytobionts, and the evolution of benignness. In *CRC handbook of insect endocytobiosis: Morphology, physiology, genetics and evolution*, ed. W. Schwemmler, pp. 21–35. Boca Raton, Fla.: CRC Press.

Fabio, G., Scorza, R., Lazzarin, A., Marchini, M., Zarantonello, M., Darminio, A., Marchisio, P., Plebani, A., Luzzati, R., & Costigliola, P. 1992. HLA-associated susceptibility to HIV-1 infection. *Clin. Exp. Immunol. 87*, 20–3.

Fackelmann, K. A. 1992. No survival bonus from early AZT. *Sci. News 141*, 100.

Fahey, J. L., Taylor, J. M. G., Korns, E., & Nishanian, P. 1986. Diagnostic and prognistic factors in AIDS. *Mount Sinai J. Med. 53*, 657–63.

Fan, N., Gavalchin, J., Paul, B., Wells, K. H., Lane, M. J., & Poiesz, B. J. 1992. Infection of peripheral blood mononuclear cells and cell lines by cell-free human T-cell lymphoma/leukemia virus type I. *J. Clin. Microbiol. 30*, 905–10.

Fandeur, T., Gysin, J., & Mercereau-Puijalon, O. 1992. Protection of squirrel monkeys against virulent *Plasmodium falciparum* infections by use of attenuated parasites. *Infect. Immun. 60*, 1390–6.

Fantini, J., Yahi, N., & Chermann, J. C. 1991. Human immunodeficiency virus can infect the apical and basolateral surfaces of human colonic epithelial cells. *Proc. Natl. Acad. Sci. USA 88*, 9297–301.

Fauci, A. S., Schnittman, S. M., Poli, G., Koenig, S., & Pantaleo, G. 1991. Immunopathogenic mechanisms in human immunodeficiency virus (HIV) infection. *Ann. Intern. Med. 114*, 678–93.

Feachem, R. 1981. Environmental aspects of cholera epidemiology. I. a review of selected reports of endemic and epidemic situations. *Trop. Dis. Bull. 78*, 675–98.

Feachem, R. 1982. Environmental aspects of cholera epidemiology. III. Transmission and control. *Trop. Dis. Bull. 79*, 1–47.

Feachem, R. 1986. Preventing diarrhea: What are the policy options? *Health Policy Plan. 1*, 109–17.

Feigal, E., Murphy, E., Vranizan, K., Bacchetti, P., Chaisson, R., Drummond, J. E., Blattner, W., McGrath, M., Greenspan, J., & Moss, A. 1991. Human T cell lymphotropic virus types I and II in intravenous drug users in San Francisco: Risk factors associated with seropositivity. *J. Infect. Dis. 164*, 36–42.

Feldman, R. A., Ghat, P., & Kamath, K. R. 1970. Infection and disease in a group of South Indian families IV: Bacteriological methods and a report on the frequency of enterobacterial infections in preschool children. *Am. J. Epidemiol. 92*, 367–75.

Feldman, S., Perry, C. S., Andrew, M., Jones, L., Moffitt, J. E., Abney, R., Carlyle, W., Freeman, E. E., Hendrick, J., Hopper, S., Ray, M., Sistrunk, W., Smith, W. H., Stone, L., Welch, P., Womack, N., Miller, J., Thompson, R. H., Simmons, L., Sherwood, J. A., Denney, S. J., Shaak, C., Cooke, D. T., & McCaslin, L. 1992. Comparison of acellular (B type) and whole-cell pertussis-component diphtheria-tetanus-pertussis vaccines as the first booster immunization in 15-to 24-month-old children. *Journal of Pediatrics 121*, 857–61.

Felsen, J. 1945. *Dysentery, colitis and enteritis*. Philadelphia: W. B. Saunders.

Felsenfeld, O. 1963. Some observations on the cholera (El Tor) epidemic in 1961–1962. *Bull. WHO 28*, 289–96.

Fenner, F., & Myers, K. 1978. Myxoma virus and myxomatosis in retrospect: The first quarter century of a new disease. In *Viruses and Environment*, ed. E. Kurstak & K. Maramorosh, pp. 539–70. New York: Academic Press.

Fenyö, E. M., Albert, J., & Åsjö, B. 1989. Replicative capacity, cytopathic effects and cell tropism of HIV. *AIDS 3*, S5–12.

Ferguson, W. W. 1956. Experimental diarrheal disease of human volunteers due to *Escherichia coli. Ann. NY Acad. Sci. 66*, 71–7.

Fernandez-Larsson, R., Srivastava, K. K., Lu, S., & Robinson, H. L. 1992. Replication of patient isolates of human immunodeficiency virus type-1 in T-cells—a spectrum of rates and efficiencies of entry. *Proc. Natl. Acad. Sci. USA 89*, 2223–6.

Ferro, A., Ghidinelli, M., Mane, I., Dusi, S., Gomes, P., Andrian, C., Perra, A., Frongia, O., Sechi, M. A., Tambe, A. M., Sabbatani, S., Cao, Y. J., Lillo, F., & Varnier, O. E. 1992. Epidemiology and transmission of HIV-2 in west Africa. In *AIDS and human reproduction*, ed. F. Melica, pp. 24–8. Basel, Switz.: Karger.

Finck, A. D., & Katz, R. L. 1972. Prevention of cholera-induced intestinal secretion in the cat by aspirin. *Nature 238*, 273–4.

Fine, P. E. F. 1975. Vectors and vertical transmission: An epidemiological perspective. *Ann. N.Y. Acad. Sci. 266*, 173–94.

Finkelstein, R. A. 1973. Cholera. *CRC Critical Reviews in Microbiology 2*, 553–623.

Fischl, M. A., Daikos, G. L., Uttamchandani, R. B., Poblete, R. B., Moreno, J. N., Reyes, R. R., Boota, A. M., Thompson, L. M., Cleary, T. J., Oldham, S. A., Saldana, M. J., & Lai, S. H. 1992a. Clinical presentation and outcome of patients with HIV infection and tuberculosis caused by multiple-drug-resistant bacilli. *Ann. Intern. Med. 117*, 184–90.

Fischl, M. A., Richman, D. D., Grieco, M. H., Gottlieb, M. S., Volberding, P. A., Laskin, O. L., Leedom, J. M., Groopman, J. E., Mildvan, D., Schooley, R. T., Jackson, G. G., Durack, D. T., King, D., & AZT Collaborative Working Group. 1987. The efficacy of azidothymidine (AZT) in the treatment of patients with AIDS and AIDS-related complex. *N. Engl. J. Med. 317*, 185–91.

Fischl, M. A., Richman, D. D., Hansen, N., Collier, A. C., Carey, J. T., Para, M. F., Hardy, D. W., Dolin, R., Powderly, W. G., Allan, J. D., Wong, B., Merigan, T. C., McAuliffe, V. J., Hyslop, N. E., Rhame, F. S., Bahour, H. H., Spector, S. A., Volberding, P., Pettinelli, C., Anderson, J., & AIDS Clinical Trials Group. 1990. The safety and efficacy of zidovudine (AZT) in the treatment of subjects with mildly symptomatic human immunodeficiency virus type 1 (HIV) infection: A double-blind, placebo-controlled trial. *Ann Intern Med. 112*, 727–37.

Fischl, M. A., Uttamchandani, R. B., Daikos, G. L., Poblete, R. B., Moreno, J. N., Reyes, R. R., Boota, A. M., Thompson, L. M., Cleary, T. J., & Lai, S. H. 1992b. An outbreak of tuberculosis caused by multiple-drug-resistant tubercle bacilli among patients with HIV infection. *Ann. Intern. Med. 117*, 177–83.

Fisher, J. D., & Fisher, W. A. 1992. Changing AIDS-risk behavior. *Psychol. Bull. 111*, 455–74.

Fisher, R. A. 1930. *The genetical theory of natural selection*. Oxford: Clarendon.

FitzGerald, J. M., Grzybowski, S., & Allen, E. A. 1991. The impact of human immunodeficiency virus infection on tuberculosis and its control. *Chest 100*, 191–200.

Fitzgibbon, J. E., Howell, R. M., Haberzettl, C. A., Sperber, S. J., Gocke, D. J., & Dubin, D. T. 1992. Human immunodeficiency virus type 1 *pol* gene mutations which cause decreased susceptibility to 2′,3′-dideoxycytidine. *Antimicrob. Agents Chemother. 36*, 153–7.

Florman, A. L., & Holzman, R. S. 1980. Nosocomial scalded skin syndrome. *Am. J. Dis. Child. 134*, 1043–5.

Food and Drug Administration 1991. *FDA Antiviral Drugs Advisory Committee reviews new AZT data. Talk paper T91-6.* Washington, D.C.: FDA.

Formal, S. B., Oaks, E. V., Olsen, R. E., Wingfield-Eggleston, M., Snoy, P. J., & Cogan, J. P. 1991. Effect of prior infection with virulent *Shigella flexneri* 2a on the resistance of monkeys to subsequent infection with *Shigella sonnei*. *J. Infect. Dis. 164*, 533–7.

Forsey, T., Bentley, M. L., Minor, P. D., & Begg, N. 1992. Mumps vaccines and meningitis. *Lancet 340*, 980.

Fouchier, R. A. M., Groenink, M., Kootstra, N. A., Tersmette, M., Huisman, H. G., Miedema, F., & Schuitemaker, H. 1992. Phenotype-associated sequence variation in the third variable domain of the human immunodeficiency virus type 1 gp120 molecule. *J. Virol. 66*, 3183–7.

Fox, C. H. 1992. Possible origins of AIDS. *Science 256*, 1259–60.

Fox, C. H., & Cottler-Fox, M. 1992. The pathobiology of HIV infection. *Immunol. Today 13*, 353–6.

Frant, S., & Abramson, H. 1938. Epidemic diarrhea of the new-born. III. Epidemiology of outbreaks of highly fatal diarrhea among new-born babies in hospital nurseries. *Am. J. Public Hlth. 28*, 36–43.

Fraser, A. M., & Smith, J. 1930. Endemic bacillary dysentery in Aberdeen. *Q. J. Med. 23*, 245–59.

Freedman, B. 1992. Suspended judgment. AIDS and the ethics of clinical trials: Learning the right lessons. *Controlled Clin. Trials 13*, 1–5.

Fricke, W., Augustyniak, L., Lawrence, D., Brownstein, A., Kramer, A., & Evatt, B. 1992. Human immunodeficiency virus infection due to clotting factor concentrates: results of the seroconversion surveillance project. *Transfusion 32*, 707–9.

Friedland, G. H. 1990. Early treatment for HIV. *N. Engl. J. Med. 322*, 1000–2.

Froland, S. S., Jenum, P., Lindboe, C. F., Wefring, K. W., Linnestad, P. J., & Böhmer, T. 1988. HIV-1 infection in Norwegian family before 1970. *Lancet i*, 1344–5.

Fuertes, J. H. 1897. *Water and public health: The relative purity of waters from different sources.* New York: Wiley.

Fujita, J., Negayama, K., Takigawa, K., Yamagishi, Y., Kubo, A., Yamaji, Y., & Takahara, J. 1992a. Activity of antibiotics against resistant *Pseudomonas aeruginosa*. *J. Antimicrob. Chemother. 29*, 539–46.

Fujita, K., Silver, J., & Peden, K. 1992b. Changes in both gp120 and gp41 can account for increased growth potential and expanded host range of human immunodeficiency virus type-1. *J. Virol. 66*, 4445–51.

Fultz, P. N., Nara, P., Barre-Sinoussi, F., Chaput, A., Greenberg, M. L., Muchmore, E., Kieny, M. P., & Girard, M. 1992. Vaccine protection of chimpanzees against challenge with HIV-1 infected peripheral blood mononuclear cells. *Science 256*, 1687–90.

Futaki, K. 1926. The dysentery bacilli in Japan and their classification. *Transactions of the 6th Congress of Far Eastern Association of Tropical Medicine* pp. 395–403. Kagomachi, Koishikawa-Ku: Waibunsha Printing Co.

Gage, S. H., & Mukerji, M. K. 1977. A perspective of grasshopper population distribution in Saskatchewan and interrelationship with weather. *Env. Entomol. 6*, 469–79.

Gallagher, P. G., & Watanakunakorn, C. 1985. Group B streptococcal bacteremia in a community teaching hospital. *Am. J. Med. 78*, 795–800.

Gallagher, P. G., & Watanakunakorn, C. 1989. Pseudomonas bacteremia in a community-teaching hospital. *Rev. Infect. Dis. 11*, 846–52.

Gallo, R. C. 1991. Human retroviruses: A decade of discovery and link with human disease. *J. Infect. Dis. 164*, 235–43.

Gama Sosa, M. A., DeGasperi, R., Kim, Y. S., Fazely, F., Sharma, P., & Ruprecht, R. M. 1991. Serine phosphorylation-independent downregulation of cell-surface CD4 by nef. *AIDS Res. Hum. Retroviruses 7*, 859–60.

Gamagemendis, A. C., Carter, R., Mendis, C., Dezoysa, A. P. K., Herath, P. R. J., & Mendis, K. N. 1991. Clustering of malaria infections within an endemic population: Risk of malaria associated with the type of housing construction. *Am. J. Trop. Med. Hyg. 45*, 77–85.

Gangarosa, E. J., & Mosley, W. H. 1974. Epidemiology and surveillance of cholera. In *Cholera*, ed. D. Barua & W. Burrows, pp. 381–403. Philadelphia: W. B. Saunders.

Gao, F., Yue, L., White, A. T., Pappas, P. G., Barchue, J., Hanson, A. P., Greene, B. M., Sharp, P. M., Shaw, G. M., & Hahn, B. H. 1992. Human infection by genetically diverse SIV$_{sm}$-related HIV-2 in west Africa. *Nature 358*, 495–9.

Gao, Q., Gu, Z. X., Parniak, M. A., Li, X. G., & Wainberg, M. A. 1992a. *In vitro* selection of variants of human immunodeficiency virus type-1 resistant to 3′-azido-3′-deoxythymidine and 2′,3′-dideoxyinosine. *J. Virol. 66*, 12–19.

Gao, Q., Parniak, M. A., Wainberg, M. A., & Gu, Z. X. 1992b. Generation of nucleoside-resistant variants of HIV-1 by *in vitro* selection in the presence of AZT or DDI but not by combinations. *Leukemia 6*, S192–5.

Gardner, M. B. 1991. Simian and feline immunodeficiency viruses: animal lentivirus models for evaluation of AIDS vaccines and antiviral agents. *Antivir. Res. 15*, 267–86.

Gardner, M., Yamamoto, J., Marthas, M., Miller, C., Jennings, M., Rosenthal, A., Luciw, P., Planelles, V., Yilma, T., Giavedoni, L., Ahmed, S., Steimer, K., Haigwood, N., & Pedersen, N. 1992. SIV and FIV vaccine studies at UC Davis: 1991 update. *AIDS Res. Hum. Retroviruses 8*, 1495–8.

Garnham, P. C. C. 1977. The continuing mystery of relapses in malaria. *Protozool. Abst. 1*, 1–12.

Garnham, P. C. C. 1966. *Malaria parasites and other haemosporidia.* Oxford: Blackwell.

Gay, F. P. 1918. *Typhoid fever considered as a problem of scientific medicine.* New York: Macmillan.

Gayle, H. D., Gnaore, E., Adjorlolo, G., Ekpini, E., Coulibaly, R., Porter, A., Braun, M. M., Zabban, M. L. K., Andou, J., Timite, A., Assiadou, J., & Decock, K. M. 1992. HIV-1 and HIV-2 infection in children in Abidjan, Côte d'Ivoire. *J. Acquired Immune Defic. Syndr. 5*, 513–17.

Gazzard, B. G. 1992. When should asymptomatic patients with HIV infection be treated with zidovudine. *Br. Med. J. 304*, 456–7.

Gear, J., Monath, T. P., Bowen, G. S., & Kemp, G. E. 1987. Arboviruses of Africa. In *Textbook of pediatric infectious diseases*, 2nd edition, ed. R. D. Feigin & J. D. Cherry, pp. 1468– 89. Philadelphia: Saunders.

Geelen, J. L. M. C., & Goudsmit, J. 1991. Virus–host interactions in human immunodeficiency virus infection. *Prog. Med. Virol. 38*, 27–41.

Geldreich, E. E. 1972. Water-borne pathogens. In *Water pollution microbiology*, ed. R. Mitchell, pp. 207–41. London: Wiley.

Gellar, S. 1982. *Senegal. An African nation between Islam and the west.* Boulder, Colorado: Westview Press.

Gendelman, H. E., Ehrlich, G. D., Baca, L. M., Conley, S., Ribas, J., Kalter, D. C., Meltzer, M. S., Poiesz, B. J., & Nara, P. 1991. The inability of human immunodeficiency virus to infect chimpanzee monocytes can be overcome by serial viral passage *in vivo. J. Virol. 65*, 3853–63.

George, J. R., Ou, C. Y., Parekh, B., Brattegaard, K., Brown, V., Boateng, E., & Decock, K. M. 1992. Prevalence of HIV-1 and HIV-2 mixed infections in Côte d'Ivoire. *Lancet 340*, 337–9.

Gerding, D. N., Larson, T. A., Hughes, R. A., Weiler, M., Shanholtzer, C., & Peterson, L. R. 1991. Aminoglycoside resistance and aminoglycoside usage: Ten years of experience in one hospital. *Antimicrob. Agents Chemother. 35*, 1284–90.

Gershy-Damet, G. M., Koffi, K., Soro, B., Coulibaly, A., Koffi, D., Sangare, V., Josseran, R., Guelain, J., Aoussi, E., & Odehouri, K. 1991. Seroepidemiological survey of HIV-1 and HIV-2 infections in the five regions of Ivory Coast. *AIDS 5*, 462–3.

Gessain, A., Yanagihara, R., Franchini, G., Garruto, R. M., Jenkins, C. L., Ajdukiewicz, A. B., Gallo, R. C., & Gajdusek, D. C. 1991. Highly divergent molecular variants of human T-lymphotropic virus type I from isolated populations in Papua New Guinea and the Solomon Islands. *Proc. Natl. Acad. Sci. USA 88*, 7694–8.

Gezon, H. M., Schaberg, M. J., & Klein, J. O. 1973. Concurrent epidemics of *Staphylococcus aureus* and group A *streptococcus* disease in a newborn nursery—control with penicillin G and hexachlorophene bathing. *Pediatrics 51*, 383–90.

Ghosh, A. 1982. Deurbanization of the Harappan civilization. In *Harappan Civilization*, ed. G. Possehl, pp. 321–3. Warminster, U.K.: Aris & Phillips.

Ghosh, G., & Rao, A. V. 1965. Water supply in relation to cholera. *Ind. J. Med. Res. 53*, 659–68.

Gibbons, A. 1992. Researchers fret over neglect of 600 million patients. *Science 256*, 1135.

Gilks, C. 1991. AIDS, monkeys and malaria. *Nature 354*, 262.

Gill, D. E., & Mock, B. A. 1985. Ecological and evolutionary dynamics of parasites: The case of *Trypanosoma diemyctyli* in the red-spotted newt *Notophthalmus viridescens*. In *Ecology and genetics of host–parasite interaction*, ed. D. Rollinson & R. M. Anderson, pp. 157–83. London: Academic.

Gillies, R. R. 1968. Bacillary dysentery in Scotland: Some epidemiologic studies. *Arch. Immunol. Ther. Exp. (Warsaw) 16*, 410–20.

Gingeras, T. R., Prodanovich, P., Latimer, T., Guatelli, J. C., Richman, D. D., & Barringer, K. J. 1991. Use of self-sustained sequence replication amplification reaction to analyze and detect mutations in zidovudine-resistant human immunodeficiency virus. *J. Infect. Dis. 164*, 1066–74.

Gispen, R., & Garr, K. H. 1950. The antibacterial effect of riverwater on *Shigella shigae* in connection with the presence of corresonpding, antagonists and bacteriophages. *Antonie Leeuwenhoek J. Microbiol. Serol. 16*, 373–85.

Glass, R. I., Becker, S., & Huq, M. I. 1982. Endemic cholera in rural Bangladesh, 1966–1980. *Am. J. Epidemiol. 116*, 959–70.

Glass, R. I., Libel, M., & Brandling-Bennett, A. D. 1992. Epidemic cholera in the Americas. *Science 256*, 1524–5.

Gody, M., Ouattara, S. A., & De The, G. 1988. Clinical experience of AIDS in relation to HIV-1 and HIV-2 infection in a rural hospital in Ivory Coast, West Africa. *AIDS 2*, 433–6.

Goedert, J. J., Kessler, C. M., Aledort, L. M., Biggar, R. J., Andes, W. A., Gilbert, G. C., II, Drummond, J. E., Vaidya, K., Mann, D. L., Eyster, M. E., Ragni, M. V., Lederman, M. M., Cohen, A. R., Bray, G. L., Rosenberg, P. S., Friedman, R. M., Hilgartner, M. W., Blattner, W. A., Kroner, B., & Gail, M. H. 1989. A prospective study of human immunodeficiency virus type 1 infection and the development of AIDS in subjects with hemophilia. *N. Engl. J. Med. 321*, 1141–8.

Gokhale, B. G. 1959. *Ancient India*, 4th edition. New York: Asia Publishing House.

Goldenberg, M. M., Honkomp, L. J., & Castellion, A. W. 1975. The antidiarrheal action of bismuth subsalicylate. *Am. J. Dig. Dis. 20*, 955–60.

Gonzalez, J. P., Bouquety, J. C., Lesbordes, J. L., Madelon, M. C., Mathiot, C. C., Meunier, D. M. Y., & Georges, A. J. 1987. Rift Valley fever virus and haemorrhagic fever in the Central African Republic. *Ann. Inst. Past./Virol 138*, 385–90.

Goodenow, M., Huet, T., Saurin, W., Kwok, S., Sninsky, J., & Wain-Hobson, S. 1989. HIV-1 isolates are rapidly evolving quasispecies: Evidence for viral mixtures and preferred nucleotide substitutions. *J. Acquired Immune Defic. Syndr. 2*, 344–52.

Goodman, M. F., Creighton, S., Bloom, L. B., & Petruska, J. 1993. Biochemical basis of DNA replication fidelity. *Crit. Rev. Biochem. Mol. Biol. 28*, 83–126.

Gorbach, S. L., Banwell, J. G., Jacobs, B., Chatterjee, B. D., Mitra, R., Brigham, K. L., & Neogy, K. N. 1970. Intestinal microflora in Asiatic cholera. I. "Rice-water" stool. *J. Infect. Dis. 121*, 32.

Gore, S. M., Fontaine, O., & Pierce, N. F. 1992. Impact of rice based oral rehydration solution on stool output and duration of diarrhoea: meta-analysis of 13 clinical trials. *Br. Med. J. 304*, 287–91.

Gorman, A. E., & Wolman, A. 1939. Waterborne outbreaks in the United States and Canada and their significance. *J. Am. Water Works Assoc. 31*, 225–373.

Gorman, O. T., Bean, W. J., Kawaoka, Y., Donatelli, I., Guo, Y., & Webster, R. G. 1991. Evolution of influenza A virus nucleoprotein genes: Implications for the origins of H1N1 human and classical swine viruses. *J. Virol. 65*, 3704–14.

Gotzsche, P. C., Nielsen, C., Gerstoft, J., Nielsen, C. M., & Vestergaard, B. F. 1992. Trend towards decreased survival in patients infected with HIV resistant to zidovudine. *Scand. J. Infect. Dis. 24*, 563–5.

Goubau, P., Desmyter, J., Ghesquiere, J., & Kasereka, B. 1992. HTLV-II among pygmies. *Nature 359*, 201.

Goudsmit, J., Back, N. K. T., & Nara, P. L. 1991. Genomic diversity and antigenic variation of HIV-1: Links between pathogenesis, epidemiology and vaccine development. *FASEB J. 5*, 2427–36.

Gradon, J. D., Timpone, J. G., & Schnittman, S. M. 1992. Emergence of unusual opportunistic pathogens in AIDS: A review. *Clin. Infect. Dis. 15*, 134–57.

Graham, N. M. H., Gurrell, C. J., Douglas, R. M., Debelle, P., & Davies, L. 1990. Adverse-effects of aspirin, acetaminophen, and ibuprofen on immune function, viral shedding and clinical status in rhinovirus-infected volunteers. *J. Infect. Dis. 162*, 1277–82.

Graham, N. M. H., Zeger, S. L., Park, L. P., Phair, J. P., Detels, R., Vermund, S. H., Ho, M., Saah, A. J., & the Multicenter AIDS Cohort Study. 1991. Effect of zidovudine and *Pneumocystis carinii* pneumonia prophylaxis on progression of HIV-1 infection to AIDS. *Lancet 338*, 265–9.

Graham, N. M. H., Zeger, S. L., Park, L. P., Vermund, S. H., Detels, R., Rinaldo, C. R., & Phair, J. P. 1992. The effects on survival of early treatment of human immunodeficiency virus infection. *N. Engl. J. Med. 326*, 1037–42.

Grant, M. 1991. HIV and idiotypic T-cell regulation. *Immunol. Today 12*, 171–2.

Greaves, M. F., Verbi, W., Tilley, R., Lister, T. A., Habeshaw, J., Guo, H., Trainor, C. D., Robert-Guroff, M., Blattner, W., Reitz, M., & Gallo, R. C. 1984. Human T-cell leukaemia virus (HTLV) in the United Kingdom. *Int. J. Cancer 33*, 795–806.

Green, S. L., Nodell, C. C., & Porter, C. Q. 1978. The prevalence and persistence of group B streptococcal colonization among hospital personnel. *Int. J. Gynaecol. Obstet. 16*, 99–102.

Greenough, W. B., III & Bennett, R. G. 1990. Diarrhea in the elderly. In *Principles of geriatric medicine*, ed. W. R. Hazzard, R. Andres, E. L. Bierman, & J. P. Blass, pp. 1168–76. New York: McGraw Hill.

Grieger, T. A., & Kluger, M. J. 1978. Fever and survival: The role of serum iron. *J. Physiol. (Lond.) 279*, 187–96.

Griffith, R. S., & Black, H. R. 1976. Re: Increased virus shedding with aspirin treatment of rhinovirus infection. *JAMA 235*, 801–2.

Groopman, J. E. 1991. Straining credulity. *New Repub. 205 (18)*, 6.

Gross, P. A., Stein, M. R., Vanantwerpen, C., Demauro, P. J., Boscamp, J. R., Hess, W., & Wallenstein, S. 1991. Comparison of severity of illness indicators in an intensive care unit. *Arch. Intern. Med. 151*, 2201–5.

Gruters, R. A., Terpstra, F. G., Degoede, R. E. Y., Mulder, J. W., DeWolf, F., Schellekens, P. T. A., Vanlier, R. A. W., Tersmette, M., & Miedema, F. 1991. Immunological and virological markers in individuals progressing from seroconversion to AIDS. *AIDS 5*, 837–44.

Guiguet, M., Cohen, M., Flahault, A., Wells, J. A., & Valleron, A. J. 1991. French intravenous drug users: Knowledge and sexual behavior change. *Eur. J. Epidemiol. 7*, 423–6.

Gump, D. W., Nadeau, O. W., Hendricks, G. M., & Meyer, D. H. 1992. Evidence that bismuth salts reduce invasion of epithelial cells by enteroinvasive bacteria. *Med. Microbiol. Immunol. 181*, 131–43.

Gunn, R. A., Kimball, A. M., Mathew, P. P., Dutta, S. R., & Rifaat, A. H. M. 1981. Cholera in Bahrain: Epidemiological characteristics of an outbreak. *Bull. WHO 59*, 61–6.

Gust, I. D. 1991. AIDS vaccines. *Med. J. Austral. 155*, 403–6.

Hahn, B. H., & Shaw, G. M. 1990. Genetic variability in human immunodeficiency viruses. in *AIDS vaccine research and clinical trials*, ed. S. D. Putney & D. P. Bolognesi, pp. 121–35. New York: Marcel Dekker.

Hakenbeck, R., Briese, T., Chalkley, L., Ellerbrok, H., Kalliokoski, R., Latorre, C., Leinonen, M., & Martin, C. 1991. Antigenic variation of penicillin-binding proteins from penicillin-resistant clinical strains of *Streptococcus pneumoniae*. *J. Infect. Dis. 164*, 313–19.

Haldane, J. B. S. 1932. *The causes of evolution*. New York: Longmans, Green.

Haley, R. W., Culver, D. H., White, J. W., Morgan, W. M., & Emori, T. G. 1985a. The nationwide nosocomial infection rate: A new need for vital statistics. *Am. J. Epidemiol. 121*, 159–67.

Haley, R. W., Culver, D. H., White, J. W., Morgan, W. M., Emori, T. G., Munn, V. P., & Hooten, T. M. 1985b. The efficacy of infection surveillance and control programs in preventing nosocomial infections in US hospitals. *Am. J. Epidemiol. 121*, 182–205.

Hall, S. M., Plaster, P. A., Glasgow, J. F. T., & Hancock, P. 1988. Preadmission anti-pyretics in Reye's syndrome. *Arch. Dis. Child. 63*, 857–66.

Halsey, N. A., Coberly, J. S., Holt, E., Coreil, J., Kissinger, P., Moulton, L. H., Brutus, J. R., & Boulos, R. 1992. Sexual behavior, smoking, and HIV-1 infection in Haitian women. *JAMA 267*, 2062–66.

Halstead, S. 1981. Chikungunya. In *Handbook Series in Zoonoses, Section B. Viral Zoonoses*, ed. G. W. Beron, pp. 437–47. Boca Raton, Florida: CRC Press.

Halstead, S. B. 1980. Dengue haemorrhagic fever: A public health problem and a field for research. *Bull. WHO 58*, 1–21.

Hamilton, J. D., Hartigan, P. M., Simberkoff, M. S., Day, P. L., Diamond, G. R., Dickinson, G. M., Drusano, G. L., Egorin, M. J., George, W. L., Gordin, F. M., Hawkes, C. A., Jensen, P. C., Klimas, N. G., Labriola, A. M., Lahart, C. J., O'Brien, W. A., Oster, C. N., Weinhold, K. J., Wray, N. P., Zolla-Pazner, S. B. 1992. A controlled trial of early versus late treatment with zidovudine in symptomatic human immunodeficiency virus infection. *N. Engl. J. Med. 326*, 437–43.

Hamilton, W. D. 1963. The evolution of altruistic behavior. *Am. Nat. 97*, 354–6.

Hamilton, W. D. 1964. The genetical evolution of social behavior. *J. Theor. Biol 7*, 1–52.

Hamilton, W. D. 1966. On the moulding of senescence by natural selection. *J. Theor. Biol 12*, 12–45.

Hammes, S. R., Dixon, E. P., Malim, M. H., Cullen, B. R., & Greene, W. C. 1989. Nef protein of human immunodeficiency virus type 1: Evidence against its role as a transcriptional inhibitor. *Proc. Natl. Acad. Sci. USA 86*, 9549–53.

Hamon-Poupinel, V., Lecoutour, X., Vergnaud, M., & Malbruny, B. 1991. Experience of two intensive care units. *Presse Med. 20*, 1592–4.

Hamood, A. N., Sublett, R. D., & Parker, C. D. 1986. Plasmid-mediated changes in virulence of *Vibrio cholerae*. *Infect. Immun. 52*, 476–83.

Han, A. M., Oo, K. N., Aye, T., & Hlaing, T. 1991. Bacteriologic studies of food and water consumed by children in Myanmar: 2. Lack of association between diarrhoea and contamination of food and water. *J. Diar. Dis. Res. 9*, 91–3.

Hanley, K. A. 1989. Pathogenic threat and variation in febrile responses. Bachelor's honors thesis. Amherst College, Amherst, Mass.

Haq, J. A., & Szewczuk, M. R. 1991. Differential effect of aging on B-cell immune responses to cholera toxin in the inductive and effector sites of the mucosal immune system. *Infect. Immun. 59*, 3094–100.

Hardy, A. V. 1956. Diarrheal diseases of man: A historical review and global appraisal. *Ann. N.Y. Acad. Sci. 66*, 5–13.

Hardy, A. V., Watt, J., Kolodny, M. H., & De Capito, R. 1940. Studies of the acute diarrheal diseases. III. Infections due to the "Newcastle dysentery bacillus.". *Am. J. Public Hlth. 30*, 53–8.

Hardy, J. L., Houk, E. J., Kramer, L. D., & Reeves, W. C. 1983. Intrinsic factors affecting vector competence of mosquitoes for arboviruses. *Ann. Rev. Entomol. 28*, 229–62.

Harnisch, J. P., Tronca, E., Nolan, C. M., Turck, M., & Holmes, K. K. 1989. Diphtheria among alcoholic urban adults. *Ann. Intern. Med. 111*, 71–2.

Harrington, W. J., Sheremata, W., Hjelle, B., Dube, D. K., Bradshaw, P., Foung, S. K. H., Snodgrass, S., Toedter, G., Cabral, L., & Poiesz, B. 1993. Spastic ataxia associated with human T-cell lymphotropic virus type II infection. *Ann. Neurol. 33*, 411–14.

Harris, A. H., Yankauer, A., Greene, D. C., Coleman, M. B., & Phaneuf, M. Y. 1956. Control of epidemic diarrhea of the newborn in hospital nurseries and pediatric wards. *Ann. N.Y. Acad. Sci. 66*, 118–28.

Harris, R., & Paxman, J. 1982. *A higher form of killing: The secret story of chemical and biological warfare*. New York: Hill & Wang.

Harrison, L. H., da Silva, A. P. J., Gayle, H. D., Albino, P., George, R., Lee-Thomas, S., Rayfield, M. A., Del Castillo, F., & Heyward, W. L. 1991. Risk factors for HIV-2 infection in Guinea-Bissau. *J. Acquired Immune Defic. Syndr. 4*, 1155–60.

Hart, A. R., & Cloyd, M. W. 1990. Interference patterns of human immunodeficiency viruses HIV-1 and HIV-2. *Virology 177*, 1–10.

Hart, S. 1989. Baby bee odor lures cradle-robbing mites. *Sci. News 136*, 103.

Hartung, S., Boller, K., Cichutek, K., Norley, S. G., & Kurth, R. 1992. Quantitation of a lentivirus in its natural host: simian immunodeficiency virus in African green monkeys. *J. Virol. 66*, 2143–9.

Hasegawa, A., Tsujimoto, H., Maki, N., Ishikawa, K., Miura, T., Fukasawa, M., Miki, K., & Hayami, M. 1989. Genomic divergence of HIV-2 from Ghana. *AIDS Res. Hum. Retroviruses 5*, 593–604.

Haseltine, W. A. 1991. HIV research and *nef* alleles. *Science 253*, 366.

Hecht, M. F., Jewett, J., & Bateman, W. B. 1990. Management of HIV infection in the seropositive, asymptomatic patient. In *AIDS Dx/Rx*, ed. K. K. Holmes, L. Corey, A. C. Collier, & H. H. Handsfield, pp. 92–106. New York: McGraw-Hill.

Heckbert, S. R., Elarth, A., & Nolan, C. M. 1992. The impact of human immunodeficiency virus infection on tuberculosis in young men in Seattle-King County, Washington. *Chest 102*, 433–7.

Heeney, J. L., Devries, P., Dubbes, R., Koornstra, W., Niphuis, H., Tenhaaft, P., Boes, J., Dings, M. E. M., Morein, B., & Osterhaus, A. D. M. E. 1992. Comparison of protection from homologous cell-free vs. cell-associated SIV challenge afforded by inactivated whole SIV vaccines. *J. Med. Primatol. 21*, 126–30.

Heffernan, P. 1914. Asylum dysentery. *Indian Med. Gaz. 49*, 417– 24.

Heininger, U., Stehr, K., & Cherry, J. D. 1992. Serious pertussis overlooked in infants. *Eur. J. Pediatr. 151*, 342–3.

Hemming, V. G., Overall, J. C., & Britt, M. R. 1976. Nosocomial infections in a newborn intensive-care unit. *N. Engl. J. Med. 294*, 1310–16.

Hendrix, C. W., Volberding, P. A., & Chaisson, R. E. 1991. HIV antigen variability in ARC/AIDS. *J. Acquired Immune Defic. Syndr. 4*, 847–50.

Hentges, F., Hoffmann, A., De Araujo, F. O., & Hemmer, R. 1992. Prolonged clinically asymptomatic evolution after HIV-1 infection is marked by the absence of complement C4 null alleles at the MHC. *Clin. Exp. Immunol. 88*, 237–42.

Herbert, W. J., & Parratt, D. 1979. Virulence of trypansomes in the vertebrate host. In *Biology of the kinetoplastida*, ed. W. H. R. Lumsden & D. A. Evans, pp. 481–521. New York: Academic Press.

Herndier, B. G., Shiramizu, B. T., Jewett, N. E., Aldape, K. D., Reyes, G. R., & Mcgrath, M. S. 1992. Acquired immunodeficiency syndrome-associated T-cell lymphoma: evidence for human immunodeficiency virus type 1-associated T-cell transformation. *Blood 79*, 1768–73.

Herre, E. A. 1993. Population structure and the evolution of virulence in namatode parasites of fig wasps. *Science 259*, 1442– 5.

Hessol, N. A., Byers, R. H., Lifson, A. R., O'Malley, P. M., Cannon, L., Barnhart, J. L., Harrison, J. S., & Rutherford, G. W. 1990. Relationship between AIDS latency period and AIDS survival time in homosexual and bisexual men. *J. Acquired Immune Defic. Syndr. 3*, 1078–85.

Hewlett, E. L. 1990. *Bordetella* species. In *Principles and practice of infectious disease*, ed. G. L. Mandell, R. G. Douglas, & J. E. Bennett, pp. 1757–62. New York: Wiley.

Hewlett, I. K., Geyer, S. J., Hawthorne, C. A., Ruta, M., & Epstein, J. S. 1991. Kinetics of early HIV-1 gene expression in infected H9-cells assessed by PCR. *Oncogene 6*, 491–3.

Hill, A. R., Premkumar, S., Brustein, S., Vaidya, K., Powell, S., Li, P. W., & Suster, B. 1991. Disseminated tuberculosis in the acquired immunodeficiency syndrome era. *Am. Rev. Respir. Dis. 144*, 1164–70.

Hilleman, M. R. 1992. Past, present, and future of measles, mumps, and rubella virus vaccines. *Pediatrics 90*, 149–53.

Hinden, E. 1948. Etiological aspects of gastro-enteritis. *Arch. Dis. Child. 23*, 27–39.

Hino, S., Yamaguchi, K., Katamine, S., Amagasaki, T., Kinoshita, K., Yoshida, Y., Doi, H., Tsuji, Y., & Miyamoto, T. 1985. Mother-to-child transmission of human T-cell leukemia virus type I. *Jpn. J. Cancer Res. 76*, 474–80.

Hinton, N. A., Nelles, J. E., & Reed, G. B. 1953. The incidence of *E. coli* group 0111 in sporadic infantile gastroenteritis and the sensitivity to antibiotics of the strains isolated. *Can. J. Med. Sci. 1*, 431–6.

Hinuma, Y., Komoda, H., Chosa, T., Kondo, T., Kohakura, M., Takenaka, T., Kikuchi, M., Ichimaru, M., Yunoki, K., Sato, I., Matsuo, R., Takiuchi, Y., Uchino, H., & Hanaoka, M. 1982. Antibodies to adult T-cell leukemia-virus-associated antigen (ATLA) in sera from patients with ATL and controls in Japan: A nation-wide sero-epidemiologic study. *Int. J. Cancer 29*, 631.

Hirsch, I., Salaun, D., Brichacek, B., & Chermann, J. C. 1992. HIV-1 cytopathogenicity—genetic difference between direct cytotoxic and fusogenic effect. *Virology 186*, 647–54.

Hirschhorn, N., Greenough, W. B., III. 1991. Progress in oral rehydration therapy. *Sci. Am. 264 (5)*, 50–6.

Hizi, A., Tal, R., Shaharabany, M., & Loya, S. 1991. Catalytic properties of the reverse transcriptases of human immunodeficiency viruses type 1 and type 2. *J. Biol. Chem. 266*, 6230–9.

Hjelle, B., Appenzeller, O., Mills, R., Alexander, S., Torrez Martinez, N., Jahnke, R., & Ross, G. 1992. Chronic neurodegenerative disease associated with HTLV-II infection. *Lancet 339*, 645–6.

Ho, D. D., Moudgil, T., & Alam, M. 1989. Quantitation of human immunodeficiency virus type 1 in the blood of infected persons. *N. Engl. J. Med. 321*, 1621–5.

Ho, G. Y. F., Nomura, A. M. Y., Nelson, K., Lee, H., Polk, B. F., & Blattner, W. A. 1991. Declining seroprevalence and transmission of HTLV-I in Japanese families who immigrated to Hawaii. *Am. J. Epidemiol. 134*, 981–7.

Hoch, A. L., Pinheiro, F. P., Roberts, D. R., & Gomes, M. D. L. C. 1987. Laboratory transmission of oropouche virus by *Culex quinquefasciatus* Say. *Bol. Ofic. Sanit. Panam. 103*, 106–12.

Hoeprich, P. D. 1989. Host–parasite relationships and the pathogenesis of infectious disease. In *Infectious diseases*, 4th edition, ed. P. D. Hoeprich & M.C. Jordan, pp. 41–53. Philadelphia: J. B. Lippincott.

Hoffmann, G. W., Kion, T. A., & Grant, M. D. 1991. An idiotypic network model of AIDS immunopathogenesis. *Proc. Natl. Acad. Sci. USA 88*, 3060–4.

Hoffman, S. L., Nussenzweig, V., Sadoff, J. C., & Nussenzweig, R. S. 1991. Progress toward malaria preerythrocytic vaccines. *Science 252*, 520–1.

Holmes, J. C., & Bethel, W. M. 1972. Modification of intermediate host behaviour by parsites. In *Behavioural aspects of parasite transmission*, ed. E. U. Canning & C. A. Wright, pp. 123–49. London: Academic Press.

Holmgren, J. 1981. Actions of cholera toxin and the prevention and treatment of cholera. *Nature 292*, 413–17.

Holzman, R., Florman, A., & Lyman, M. 1980. Gentamicin resistant and sensitive strains of *S. aureus*. Factors affecting colonization and virulence for infants in a special care nursery. *Am. J. Epidemiol. 112*, 352–61.

Hood, M. A., Neww, G. E., & Rodrick, G. E. 1981. Isolation of *Vibrio cholerae* serotype 01 from the Eastern oyster *Crassostrea virginica*. *Appl. Environ. Microbiol. 41*, 559–60.

Hornick, R. B., Music, S. I., Wenzel, R., Cash, R., Libonati, J. P., Snyder, M. J., & Woodward, T. E. 1971. The Broad Street pump revisited: Responses of volunteers to ingested cholera vibrios. *Bull. N.Y. Acad. Med. 47*, 1181–91.

Horsburgh, C. R. 1992. Epidemiology of mycobacterial diseases in AIDS. *Res. Microbiol. 143*, 372–7.

House, J. A., Turell, M. J., & Mebus, C. A. 1992. Rift valley fever: present status and risk to the western hemisphere. *Ann. N.Y. Acad. Sci. 653*, 233–42.

Howard-Jones, N. 1972. Choleranomalies: The unhistory of medicine as exemplified by cholera. *Perspect. Biol. Med. 15*, 422–33.

Howell, R. M., Fitzgibbon, J. E., Noe, M., Ren, Z., Gocke, D. J., Schwartzer, T. A., & Dubin, D. T. 1991. *In vivo* sequence variation of the human immunodeficiency virus type 1 env gene: Evidence for recombination among variants found in a single individual. *AIDS Res. Hum. Retroviruses 7*, 869–76.

Hoxie, J. A., Brass, L. F., Pletcher, C. H., Haggarty, B. S., & Hahn, B. H. 1991. Cytopathic variants of an attenuated isolate of human immunodeficiency virus type-2 exhibit increased affinity for CD4. *J. Virol. 65*, 5096–101.

Hsia, K., & Spector, S. A. 1991. Human immunodeficiency virus DNA is present in a high percentage of CD4+ lymphocytes of seropositive individuals. *J. Infect. Dis. 164*, 470–5.

Hu, W., & Temin, H. M. 1990. Retroviral recombination and reverse transcription. *Science 250*, 1227–33.

Huet, T., Cheynier, A., Meyerhans, A., Roelants, G., & Wain-Hobson, S. 1990. Genetic organization of a chimpanzee lentivirus related to HIV-1. *Nature 345*, 356–9.

Huffman, S. L., & Combest, C. 1990. Role of breast feeding in the prevention and treatment of diarrhoea. *J. Diar. Dis. Res. 8*, 68– 81.

Hughes, A., & Corrah, T. 1990. Human immunodeficiency virus type 2 (HIV2). *Blood Rev. 4*, 158–64.

Hughes, A. L. 1992. Positive selection and interallelic recombination at the merozoite surface antigen-1 (MSA-1) locus of *Plasmodium falciparum. Mol. Biol. Evol. 9*, 381–93.

Humphery-Smith, I., Donker, G., Turzo, A., Chastel, C., & Schmidt-Mayerova, H. 1993. Evaluation of mechanical transmission of HIV by the African soft tick, *Ornithodoros moubata. AIDS 7*, 341–7.

Hunsmann, G., Schneider, J., Schmidt, L., & Yamamoto, N. 1983. Detection of serum antibodies to adult T cell leukemia virus in non-human primates and in peoples from Africa. *Int. J. Cancer 32*, 329–34.

Hunt, C. W. 1989. Migrant labor and sexually transmitted disease: AIDS in Africa. *J. Health Soc. Behav. 30*, 353–73.

Huq, M. I. 1979. *Investigation of an outbreak due to* Shigella sonnei. Dhaka, Bangladesh: International Center for Diarrheal Disease Research.

Huq, M. I., Sanyal, S. C., Samadi, A. R., & Monsur, K. A. 1983. Comparative behaviour of classical and el tor biotypes of *Vibrio cholerae* 01 isolated in Bangladesh during 1982. *J. Diar. Dis. Res. 1*, 5–9.

Hurst, A. F., & Knott, F. A. 1936. British dysenteric infections. *Lancet 231*, 1197–201.

Hutchinson, R. I. 1956. Some observations on the method of spread of Sonne dysentery. *Month. Bull. Min. Hlth. (Lond.) 15*, 110–18.

Hübner, A., Kruhoffer, M., Grosse, F., & Krauss, G. 1992. Fidelity of human immunodeficiency virus type I reverse transcriptase in copying natural RNA. *J. Mol. Biol 223*, 595–600.

Hwang, S. S., Boyle, T. J., Lyerly, H. K., & Cullen, B. R. 1992. Identification of envelope V3 loop as the major determinant of CD4 neutralization sensitivity of HIV-1. *Science 257*, 535–7.

Ijsselmuiden, C. B., Steinberg, M. H., Padayachee, G. N., Schoub, B. D., Strauss, S. A., Buch, E., Davies, J. C. A., De Beer, C., Gear, J. S. S., & Hurwitz, H. S. 1988. AIDS and South Africa—towards a comprehensive strategy. *S. Afr. Med. J. 73*, 465-7.

Imai, J., Terashi, S., Talonu, T., Komoda, H., Taufa, T., Nurse, G. T., Babona, D., Yamaguchi, K., Nakashima, H., Ishikawa, K., Kawamura, M., & Hayami, M. 1990. Geographic distribution of subjects seropositive for human T-cell leukemia virus type I in Papua New Guinea. *Jpn. J. Cancer Res. 81*, 1218-21.

Imberti, L., Sottini, A., Bettinardi, A., Puoti, M., & Primi, D. 1991. Selective depletion in HIV infection of T cells that bear specific T cell receptor Vß sequences. *Science 254*, 860-2.

Isaksson, B., Albert, J., Chiodi, F., Furucrona, A., Krook, A., & Putkonen, P. 1988. AIDS two months after primary human immunodeficiency virus infection. *J. Infect. Dis. 158*, 866-8.

Iseman, M. D. 1992. A leap of faith: What can we do to curtail intrainstitutional transmission of tuberculosis. *Ann. Intern. Med. 117*, 251-3.

Ivanoff, L. A., Looney, D. J., Mcdanal, C., Morris, J. F., Wongstaal, F., Langlois, A. J., Petteway, S. R., & Matthews, T. J. 1991. Alteration of HIV-1 infectivity and neutralization by a single amino acid replacement in the V3 loop domain. *AIDS Res. Hum. Retroviruses 7*, 595-603.

Jacobs, J. C. 1967. Sudden death in arthritic children receiving large doses of indomethacin. *JAMA 199*, 932-4.

Jacobs, S. I., Holzel, A., Wolman, B., Keen, J. H., Miller, V., Taylor, J., & Gross, R. J. 1970. Outbreak of infantile gastro-enteritis caused by *Escherichia coli* 0114. *Arch. Dis. Child. 45*, 656-63.

Jacoby, H. I., & Marshall, C. H. 1972. Antagonism of cholera enterotoxin by anti-inflammatory agents in the rat. *Nature 235*, 163-4.

Jaenike, J. 1993. Rapid evolution of host specificity in a parasitic nematode. *Evol. Ecol. 7*, 103-8.

Jameson, J. E., Mann, T. P., & Rothfield, N. J. 1954. Hospital gastro-enteritis: An epidemiological survey of infantile diarrhea and vomiting contracted in a children's hospital. *Lancet 267*, 459-65.

Japour, A. J., Chatis, P. A., Eigenrauch, H. A., & Crumpacker, C. S. 1991. Detection of human immunodeficiency virus type 1 clinical isolates with reduced sensitivity to zidovudine and dideoxyinosine by RNA–RNA hybridization. *Proc. Natl. Acad. Sci. USA 88*, 3092-6.

Ji, J. P., & Loeb, L. A. 1992. Fidelity of HIV-1 reverse transcriptase copying RNA *in vitro*. *Biochemistry 31*, 954-8.

Johnson, K. M. 1989. African hemorrhagic fevers caused by Marburg and Ebola viruses. In *Viral infections of humans: Epidemiology and control*, 3rd edition, ed. A. S. Evans, pp. 95-103. New York: Plenum.

Johnson, M. P., Coberly, J. S., Clermont, H. C., Chaisson, R. E., Davis, H. L., Losikoff, P., Ruff, A. J., Boulos, R., & Halsey, N. A. 1992. Tuberculin skin test reactivity among adults infected with human immunodeficiency virus. *J. Infect. Dis. 166*, 194-8.

Jones, J. 1776. *Plain concise practical remarks on the treatment of wounds and fractures*. Philadelphia: Robert Bell.

Jones, R. N. 1992. The current and future impact of antimicrobial resistance among nosocomial bacterial pathogens. *Diag. Microbiol. Infect. Dis. 15*, S3–10.

Juhlin, I., & Ericson, C. 1965. Hospital infections and hospital hygiene at Malmö General Hospital. *J. Hyg. 63*, 35–48.

Kajiyama, W., Kashiwagi, S., Hayashi, J., Nomura, H., Ikematsu, H., & Okochi, K. 1986. Intrafamilial clustering of anti-ATLA persons. *Am. J. Epidemiol. 124*, 800–6.

Kaliyugaperumal, V. 1978. Antimicrobial drug resistance and R-factors in *Shigella*. *Indian J. Med. Res. 68*, 220–4.

Kallick, C. A., Brooks, G. F., Dover, A. S., Brown, M. C., & Brolnitsky, O. 1970. A diphtheria outbreak in Chicago. *Ill. Med. J. 137*, 505–12.

Kalyanaraman, V. X., Sarngadharan, M. G., Robert-Guroff, M., Miyoshi, I., Blayney, D., Golde, D., & Gallo, R. C. 1982. A new subtype of human T-cell leukemia virus (HTLV-II) associated with a T-cell variant of hairy cell leukemia. *Science 218*, 571–3.

Kang, C. Y., Nara, P., Chamat, S., Caralli, V., Ryskamp, T., Haigwood, N., Newman, R., & Kohler, H. 1991. Evidence for non-V3-specific neutralizing antibodies that interfere with gp120/CD4 binding in human immunodeficiency virus 1-infected humans. *Proc. Natl. Acad. Sci. USA 88*, 6171–5.

Kangchuan, C., Chenshui, L., Qingxin, Q., Ningmei, Z., Guokui, Z., Gongli, C., Yijun, X., Yiejie, L., & Shifu, Z. 1991. The epidemiology of diarrhoeal diseases in southeastern China. *J. Diar. Dis. Res. 9*, 94–9.

Kanki, P. J. 1992. Virologic and biologic features of HIV-2. In *AIDS and other manifestations of HIV infection*, 2nd edition, ed. G. P. Wormser, pp. 85–93. New York: Raven Press.

Kanki, P., M'Boup, S., Marlink, R., Travers, K., Hsieh, C. C., Gueye, A., Boye, C., Sankalé, J. L., Donnelly, C., Leisenring, W., Siby, T., Thior, I., Dia, M., Gueye, E. H., N'Doye, I., & Essex, M. 1992. Prevalence and risk determinants of human immunodeficiency virus type 2 (HIV-2) and human immunodeficiency virus type 1 (HIV-1) in west African female prostitutes. *Am. J. Epidemiol. 136*, 895–907.

Kanki, P. J., Marlink, R. G., Siby, T., Essex, M., & M'Boup, S. 1990. Biology of HIV-2 infection in West Africa. In *Gene regulation and AIDS: Transcriptional activation, retroviruses, and pathogenesis. Advances in Applied Biotechnology Vol. 7*, ed. T. S. Papas, pp. 255–72. Houston: Gulf.

Kaper, J. B., Moseley, S. L., & Falkow, S. 1981. Molecular characterization of environmental and nontoxinogenic strains of *Vibrio cholerae*. *Infect. Immun. 32*, 661–7.

Kaplan, J. E., Lal, R. B., Davidson, M., Lanier, A. P., & Lairmore, M. D. 1993. HTLV-I in Alaska natives. *J. Acquired Immune Defic. Syndr. 6*, 327–8.

Kawamura, M., Katahira, J., Fukasawa, M., Sakuragi, J. I., Ishikawa, K. I., Nakai, M., Mingle, J. A. A., Oseikwasi, M., Netty, V. B. A., Akari, H., Hishida, O., Tomonaga, K., Miura, T., & Hayami, M. 1992. Isolation and characterization of a highly divergent HIV-2[GH-2]: Generation of an infectious molecular clone and functional analysis of its rev-responsive element in response to primate retrovirus transactivators (rev and rex). *Virology 188*, 850–3.

Kawamura, M., Yamazaki, S., Ishikawa, K., Kwofie, T. B., Tsujimoto, H., & Hayami, M. 1989. HIV-2 in west Africa in 1966. *Lancet i*, 385.

Kawaoka, Y., & Webster, R. G. 1988. Molecular mechanism of acquisition of virulence in influenza virus in nature. *Microb. Pathog.* 5, 311–18.

Kawase, K., Katamine, S., Moriuchi, R., Miyamoto, T., Kubota, K., Igarashi, H., Doi, H., Tsuji, Y., Yamabe, T., & Hino, S. 1992. Maternal transmission of HTLV-I other than through breast milk: discrepancy between the polymerase chain reaction positivity of cord blood samples for HTLV-I and the subsequent seropositivity of individuals. *Jpn. J. Cancer Res.* 83, 968–77.

Kazura, J. W., Saxinger, W. C., Wenger, J., Forsyth, K., Lederman, M. M., Gillespie, J. A., Carpenter, C. C. J., & Alpers, M. A. 1987. Epidemiology of human T-cell leukemia virus type I infection in East Sepik Province, Papua New Guinea. *J. Infect. Dis.* 155, 1100–7.

Keating, J. P. 1987. Reye syndrome. In *Textbook of pediatric infectious diseases*, 2nd edition, ed. R. D. Feigin & J. D. Cherry, pp. 1845–8. Philadelphia: W.B. Saunders.

Keet, I. P. M., Krijnen, P., Koot, M., Lange, J. M. A., Miedema, F., Goudsmit, J., & Coutinho, R. A. 1993. Predictors of rapid progression to AIDS in HIV-1 seroconverters. *AIDS* 7, 51–7.

Kellam, P., Boucher, C. A. B., & Larder, B. A. 1992. Fifth mutation in human immunodeficiency virus type 1 reverse transcriptase contributes to the development of high-level resistance to zidovudine. *Proc. Natl. Acad. Sci. USA* 89, 1934–8.

Kennedy, K. A. R. 1982. Skulls, aryans and flowing drains: The interface of archeology and skeletal biology in the study of the Harappan civilization. In *Harappan Civilization*, ed. G. Possehl, pp. 289–95. Warminster, U.K.: Aris & Phillips.

Kennedy, P. E., Moss, B., & Berger, E. A. 1993. Primary HIV-1 isolates refractory to neutralization by soluble CD4 are potently inhibited by CD4-*Pseudomonas* exotoxin. *Virology* 192, 375–9.

Kess, S., Bresolin, L., & Henning, J. 1991. HIV early care. AMA physician guidelines. Chicago: American Medical Association.

Kestler, H. W., Ringler, D. J., Mori, K., Panicall, D. L., Sehgal, P. K., Daniel M D, & Desrosiers, R. C. 1991. Importance of the *nef* gene for maintenance of high virus loads and for development of AIDS. *Cell* 65, 651–62.

Kettman, J. R., Robinson, R. A., Kuhn, L., & Lefkovits, I. 1991. Global analysis of lymphocyte gene expression: Perturbation of H-9 cells by infection with distinct isolates of human immunodeficiency virus: an exposition by multivariate analysis of a host–parasite interface. *Electrophoresis* 12, 554–69.

Khan, A. A., Srivastava, R., Sinha, V. B., & Srivastava, B. S. 1985. Regulation of toxin biosynthesis by plasmids in *Vibrio cholerae. J. Gen. Microbiol.* 131, 2653–7.

Khan, A. S., Galvin, T. A., Lowenstine, L. J., Jennings, M. B., Gardner, M. B., & Buckler, C. E. 1991. A highly divergent simian immunodeficiency virus (SIV$_{stm}$) recovered from stored stump-tailed macaque tissues. *J. Virol.* 65, 7061–5.

Khan, M., & Mosley, W. H. 1968. The significance of *Shigella* as a cause of diarrhea in a low economic urban community in Dacca. *East Pak. Med. J.* 12, 45–51.

Khan, M. U., Agrawal, S. K., Vrat, S., & Mehrotra, R. M. L. 1979. *Shigella* serotypes in recent infections at Lucknow. *Indian J. Med. Res.* 69, 393–8.

Khan, M. U., Roy, N. C., Islam, M. R., Huq, M. I., & Stoll, B. 1985. Fourteen years of shigellosis in Dhaka: An epidemiological analysis. *Int. J. Epidemiol.* 14, 607–13.

Khan, M. U., Samadi, A. R., Huq, M. I., Yunus, M., & Eusof, A. 1984a. Simultaneous classical and el tor cholera in Bangladesh. *J. Diar. Dis. Res. 2*, 13–18.

Khan, M., & Shahidullah, M. 1980. Cholera due to the el tor biotype equals the classical biotype in severity and attack rates. *J. Trop. Med. Hyg. 83*, 35-39.

Khan, M. U., Shahidullah, M., Haque, M. S., & Ahmed, W. U. 1984b. Presence of vibrios in surface water and their relation with cholera in a community. *Trop. Geogr. Med. 36*, 335–40.

Kielhofner, M., Atmar, R. L., Hamill, R. J., & Musher, D. M. 1992. Life-threatening *Pseudomonas aeruginosa* infections in patients with human immunodeficiency virus infection. *Clin. Infect. Dis. 14*, 403–11.

Kilbourne, E. D. 1979. Influenza. In *Cecil textbook of medicine*, ed. P. B. Beeson, W. McDermott, & J. B. Wyngaarden, pp. 240–6. Philadelphia: W. B. Saunders.

Kilbourne, E. D. 1990. New viral diseases: A real and potential problem without boundaries. *JAMA 264*, 68–70.

Kilbourne, E. D. 1991. New viruses and new disease: Mutation, evolution and ecology. *Curr. Opin. Immunol. 3*, 518–24.

Kim, S., Ikeuchi, K., Byrn, R., Groopman, J., & Baltimore, D. 1989. Lack of a negative influence on viral growth by the nef gene of human immunodeficiency virus type 1. *Proc. Natl. Acad. Sci. USA 86*, 9544–8.

Kingsley, L. A., Zhou, S. Y. J., Bacellar, H., Rinaldo, C. R., Chmiel, J., Detels, R., Saah, A., VanRaden, M., Ho, M., Munoz, A., & Multicenter AIDS Cohort Study Group. 1991. Temporal trends in human immunodeficiency virus type 1 seroconversion 1984–1989: A report from the Multicenter AIDS Cohort Study (MACS). *Am. J. Epidemiol. 134*, 331–9.

Kion, T. A., & Hoffmann, G. Q. 1991. Anti-HIV and anti-anti-MHC antibodies in alloimmune and autoimmune mice. *Science 253*, 1138– 40.

Kira, J., Koyanagi, Y., Yamada, T., Itoyama, Y., Goto, I., Yamamoto, N., Sasaki, H., & Sakaki, Y. 1991. Increased HTLV-I proviral DNA in HTLV-I-associated myelopathy: A quantitative polymerase chain reaction study. *Ann. Neurol. 29*, 194–201.

Kirby, A. C., Hall, E. G., & Coackley, W. 1950. Neonatal diarrhoea and vomiting, outbreaks in the same maternity unit. *Lancet 259*, 201–7.

Kirchhoff, F., & Hunsmann, G. 1992. The negative (?) factor of HIV and SIV. *Res. Virol. 143*, 66–9.

Kirkland, M. A., Frasca, J., & Bastian, I. 1991. Adult T-cell leukaemia lymphoma in an Aborigine. *Austral. New Zeal. J. Med 21*, 739–41.

Kitchen, S. F. 1949. Symptomatology: general considerations. in *Malariology*, ed. M. F. Boyd, pp. 966–94. Philadelphia: Saunders.

Klayman, D. L. 1989. Weeding out malaria. *Nat. Hist. 98(10)*, 18– 27.

Kluger, M. J. 1991. The adaptive value of fever. in *Fever: basic mechanisms and management*, ed. P. Mackowiak, pp. 105–24. New York: Raven Press.

Kluger, M. J., Ringler, D. J., & Anver, M. R. 1975. Fever and survival. *Science 188*, 166–8.

Kluger, M. J., & Rothenberg, B. A. 1979. Fever and reduced iron: Their interaction as a host defense response to bacterial infection. *Science 203*, 374–6.

Kluger, M. J., & Vaughn, L. K. 1978. Fever and survival in rabbits infected with *Pasteurella multocida. J. Physiol. 282*, 243–51.

Knittle, M. A., Eitzman, D. V., & Baer, H. 1975. Role of hand contamination of personnel in the epidemiology of gram-negative nosocomial infections. *J. Pediat. 86*, 433–7.

Ko, Y. C., Chen, M. J., & Yeh, S. M. 1992. The predisposing and protective factors against dengue virus transmission by mosquito vector. *Am. J. Epidemiol. 136*, 214–20.

Koblin, B. A., Morrison, J. M., Taylor, P. E., Stoneburner, R. L., & Stevens, C. E. 1992. Mortality trends in a cohort of homosexual men in New York City, 1978–1988. *Am. J. Epidemiol. 136*, 646–56.

Koffi, K., Gershy-Damet, G. M., Peeters, M., Soro, B., Rey, J. L., & Delaporte, E. 1992. Rapid spread of HIV infections in Abidjan, Ivory Coast, 1987–1990. *Eur. J. Clin. Microbiol. Infect. Dis. 11*, 271–3.

Kohler, P. F. 1964. Hospital salmonellosis. *JAMA 189*, 94–8.

Komurian-Pradel, F., Pelloquin, F., Sonoda, S., Osame, M., & de The, G. 1992. Geographical subtypes demonstrated by RFLP following PCR in the LTR region of HTLV-I. *AIDS Res. Hum. Retroviruses 8*, 429–34.

Komurian, F., Pelloquin, F., & De The, G. 1991. *In vivo* genomic variability of human T-cell leukemia virus type-I depends more upon geography than upon pathologies. *J. Virol. 65*, 3770–8.

Kondo, T., Kono, H., Miyamoto, N., Yoshida, R., Toki, H., Matsumoto, I., Hara, M., Inoue, H., Inatsuki, A., Funatsu, T., Yamano, N., Bando, F., Iwao, E., Miyoshi, I., Hinuma, Y., & Hanaoka, M. 1989. Age-and sex-specific cumulative rate and risk of ATLL for HTLV-I carriers. *Int. J. Cancer 43*, 1061–4.

Kong, L. I., Lee, S. W., Kappes, J. C., Parkin, J. S., Decker, D., Hoxie, J. A., Hahn, B. H., & Shaw, G. M. 1988. West African HIV-2-related human retrovirus with attenuated cytopathicity. *Science 240*, 1525–9.

Konings, E., Anderson, R. M., Morley, D., O'Riordan, T., & Meegan, M. 1989. Rates of sexual partner change among two pastoralist southern Nilotic groups in East Africa. *AIDS 3*, 245– 7.

Koopman, J. S., Prevots, D. R., Marin, M. A. V., Dantes, H. G., Aquino, M. L. Z., Longini, I. M., & Amor, J. S. 1991. Determinants and predictors of dengue infection in Mexico. *Am. J. Epidemiol. 133*, 1168–78.

Koot, M., Keet, I. P. M., Vos, A. H. V., Degoede, R. E. Y., Roos, M. T. L., Coutinho, R. A., Miedema, F., Schellekens, P. T. A., & Tersmette, M. 1993. Prognostic value of HIV-1 syncytium-inducing phenotype for rate of CD4+ cell depletion and progression to AIDS. *Ann. Intern. Med. 118*, 681–8.

Korneyeva, M., Stålhandske, P., & Åsjö, B. 1993. Jurkat-tat but not other tat-expressing cell lines support replication of slow/ low type HIV. *J. Acquired Immune Defic. Syndr. 6*, 231–6.

Kourany, M., & Vasquez, M. A. 1969. Enteropathogenic bacteria associated with diarrhea among infants in Panama. *Am. J. Hyg. 18*, 931–5.

Kourany, M., Vasquez, M. A., & Mata, L. 1971. Prevalence of pathogenic enteric bacteria in children of 31 Panamanian communities. *Am. J. Hyg. 20*, 608–15.

Kramer, J. M., Meunier, P. C., & Pollock, R. V. H. 1980. Canine parvovirus: Update. *Vet. Med. 75*, 1541–5.

Krämer, A., Goedert, J. J., Wachter, H., & Fuchs, D. 1992. Prognostic value of serum β_2 microglobulin in HIV infection. *Lancet 340*, 371.

Kreiss, J. K., Joech, D., Plummer, F. A., Holmes, K. K., Lightfoote, M., Piot, P., Ronald, A. R., Ndinya-Achola, J. O., D'Costa, L. J., Roberts, P., Ngugi, E. N., & Quinn, T. C. 1986. AIDS virus infection in Nairobi prostitutes: Spread of the epidemic to East Africa. *N. Engl. J. Med. 314*, 414–18.

Krieger, J. N., Coombs, R. W., Collier, A. C., Ross, S. O., Chaloupka, K., Cummings, D. K., Murphy, V. L., & Corey, L. 1990. Recovery of human immunodeficiency virus type 1 from semen: Minimal impact of stage of infection and current antiviral chemotherapy. *J. Infect. Dis. 163*, 386–8.

Kristiansen, B. E., Tveten, Y., Ask, E., Reiten, T., Knapskog, A. B., Steenjohnsen, J., & Hopen, G. 1992. Preventing secondary cases of meningococcal disease by identifying and eradicating disease-causing strains in close contacts of patients. *Scand. J. Infect. Dis. 24*, 165–73.

Krotoski, W. A. 1985. Discovery of the hypnozoite and a new theory of malarial relapse. *Roy. Soc. Trop. Med. Hyg. 79*, 1–11.

Kubota, R., Fujiyoshi, T., Izumo, S., Yashiki, S., Maruyama, I., Osame, M., & Sonoda, S. 1993. Fluctuation of HTLV-I proviral DNA in peripheral blood mononuclear cells of HTLV-I-associated myelopathy. *J. Neuroimmunol. 42*, 147–54.

Kuhls, T. L., Viering, T. P., Leach, C. T., Steele, M. I., Haglund, L. A., & Fine, D. P. 1992. Relapsing pneumococcal bacteremia in immunocompromised patients. *Clin. Infect. Dis. 14*, 1050–4.

Kumar, P., Hui, H., Kappes, J. C., Haggarty, B. S., Hoxie, J. A., Arya, S. K., Shaw, G. M., & Hahn, B. H. 1990. Molecular characterization of an attenuated human immunodeficiency virus type 2 isolate. *J. Virol. 64*, 890–901.

Kuo, J. M., Taylor, J. M. G., & Detels, R. 1991. Estimating the AIDS incubation period from a prevalent cohort. *Am. J. Epidemiol. 133*, 1050–7.

Kuroda, Y., Fujiyama, F., & Nagumo, F. 1991. Analysis of factors of relevance to rapid clinical progression in HTLV-I-associated myelopathy. *J. Neurol. Sci. 105*, 61–6.

Kurth, R., Binninger, D., Ennen, J., Denner, J., Hartung, S., & Norley, S. 1991. The quest for an AIDS vaccine: The state of the art and current challenges. *AIDS Res. Hum. Retroviruses 7*, 425– 33.

Kusuhara, K., Sonoda, S., Takahashi, K., Tokugawa, K., Fukushige, J., & Ueda, K. 1987. Mother-to-child transmission of human T-cell leukemia virus type I (HTLV-I): A fifteen-year follow-up study in Okinawa, Japan. *Int. J. Cancer 40*, 755–7.

Kyle, W. S. 1992. Simian retroviruses, poliovaccine, and origin of AIDS. *Lancet 339*, 600–1.

Lacey, S. F., Reardon, J. E., Furfine, E. S., Kunkel, T. A., Bebenek, K., Eckert, K. A., Kemp, S. D., & Larder, B. A. 1992. Biochemical studies on the reverse transcriptase and RNase H activities from human immunodeficiency virus strains resistant to 3'-azido-3'-deoxythymidine. *J. Biol. Chem. 267*, 15789–94.

Lal, R. B., & Griffis, K. P. 1991. Predictive B-and T-cell linear epitopes in structural proteins of HTLV-I, HTLV-II, and STLV-I. *AIDS Res. Hum. Retroviruses 7*, 663–70.

Land, S., Mcgavin, C., Lucas, R., & Birch, C. 1992. Incidence of zidovudine-resistant human immunodeficiency virus isolated from patients before, during, and after therapy. *J. Infect. Dis. 166*, 1139–42.

Land, S., McGavin, K., Birch, C., & Lucas, R. 1991. Reversion from zidovudine resistance to sensitivity on cessation of treatment. *Lancet 338*, 830–1.

Land, S., Treloar, G., McPhee, D., Birch, C., Doherty, R., Cooper, D., & Gust, I. 1990. Decreased *in vitro* susceptibility to zidovudine of HIV isolates obtained from patients with AIDS. *J. Infect. Dis. 161*, 326–9.

Lange, M., & Klein, E. B. 1991. Epidemic pneumocystis pneumonia in children before the AIDS era. *Lancet 338*, 1340–1.

Langhoff, E., Terwilliger, E. F., Bos, H. J., Kalland, K. H., Poznansky, M. C., Bacon, O. M. L., & Haseltine, W. A. 1991. Replication of human immunodeficiency virus type 1 in primary dendritic cell cultures. *Proc. Natl. Acad. Sci. USA 88*, 7998–8002.

Langmuir, A. D., & Schoenbaum, S. C. 1976. The epidemiology of influenza. *Hosp. Pract. 11*, 49–56.

Larder, B. A., Coates, K. E., & Kemp, S. D. 1991. Zidovudine-resistant human immunodeficiency virus selected by passage in cell culture. *J. Virol. 65*, 5232–6.

Larder, B. A., Darby, G., & Richman, D. D. 1989. HIV with reduced sensitivity to zidovudine (AZT) isolated during prolonged therapy. *Science 243*, 1731–4.

Larder, B. A., & Kemp, S. D. 1989. Multiple mutations in HIV-1 reverse transcriptase confer high-level resistance to zidovudine (AZT). *Science 246*, 1155–8.

Larson, A. 1989. Social context of HIV transmission in Africa: historical and cultural bases of east and central Africa sexual relations. *Rev. Infect. Dis. 11*, 716–31.

Larson, E. 1988. A causal link between handwashing and risk of infection? Examination of the evidence. *Infect. Control Hosp. Epidemiol. 9*, 28–36.

Larson, E. 1984. Effects of handwashing agent, handwashing frequency and clinical area on hand flora. *Am. J. Infect. Control 11*, 76.

Laurent, A. G., Hovanessain, A. G., Rivière, Y., Krust, B., Regnault, A., Montagnier, L., Findeli, A., Kieny, M. P., & Guy, B. 1990. Production of a nonfunctional *nef* protein in human immunodeficieny virus type-1-infected CEM cells. *J. Gen. Virol. 71*, 2273–81.

Layne, S. P., Merges, M. J., Spouge, J. L., Dembo, M., & Nara, P. L. 1991. Blocking of human immunodeficiency virus infection depends on cell density and viral stock age. *J. Virol. 65*, 3293–300.

Le Guenno, B., Pison, G., Enel, C., Lagarde, E., & Seck, C. 1992. HIV-2 infections in a rural Senegalese community. *J. Med. Virol. 38*, 67–70.

Lecatsas, G., & Alexander, J. J. 1992. Origins of HIV. *Lancet 339*, 1427.

Lee, C. A., Phillips A. N., Elford, J., Miller, E. J., Bofill, M., Griffiths, P. D., Kernoff, P. B. A. 1989. The natural history of human immunodeficiency virus infection in a haemophilic cohort. *Br. J. Haematol. 73*, 228–34.

Lee, C. A., Phillips, A. N., Elford, J., Janossy, G., Griffiths, P., & Kernoff, P. 1991. Progression of HIV disease in a haemophilic cohort followed for 11 years and the effect of treatment. *Br. Med. J. 303*, 1093–6.

Lee, H., Swanson, P., Shorty, V. S., Zack, J. A., Rosenblatt, J. D., & Chen, I. S. Y. 1989. High rate of HTLV-II infection in seropositive IV drug abusers in New Orleans. *Science 244*, 471–5.

Leedom, J. M. 1992. Pneumonia: Patient profiles, choice of empiric therapy, and the place of third-generation cephalosporins. *Diag. Microbiol. Infect. Dis. 15*, 57–65.

LeGrand, E. K. 1990. Endotoxin as an alarm signal of bacterial invasion: current evidence and implications. *J. Am. Vet. Med. Assoc. 197*, 454–6.

LeGrand, E. K. 1990. An evolutionary perspective of endotoxin: a signal for a well-adapted defense system. *Med. Hyp. 33*, 49–56.

Legrand, R., Vaslin, B., Vogt, G., Roques, P., Humbert, M., Dormont, D., & Aubertin, A. M. 1992. AIDS vaccine developments. *Nature 355*, 684.

LeGuenno, B. M., Barabe, P., Griffet, P. A., Guiraud, M., Morcillo, R. J., Peghini, M. E., Jean, P. A., M'Baye, P. S., Diallo, A., & Sarthou, J. L. 1991. HIV-2 and HIV-1 AIDS cases in Senegal: Clinical patterns and immunological perturbations. *J. Acquired Immune Defic. Syndr. 4*, 421–7.

Leiden, J. M., Wang, C. Y., Petryniak, B., Markovitz, D. M., Nabel, G. J., & Thompson, C. B. 1992. A novel ets-related transcription factor, elf-1, binds to human immunodeficiency virus type-2 regulatory elements that are required for inducible trans activation in T-cells. *J. Virol. 66*, 5890–7.

Lenahan, J. K., & Boreham, P. F. L. 1976. Effect of host movement on multiple feeding by *Aedes aegypti* (L.) (Diptera: Culicidae) in a laboratory experiment. *Bull. Entomol. Res. 66*, 681–4.

Lenihan, F. 1992. Thailand tries again to tackle AIDS. *Br. Med. J. 305*, 1385.

Lentino, J. R., Pachucki, C. T., Schaaff, D. M., Schaefer, M. R., Holzer, T. J., Heynen, C., Dawson, G., & Dorus, W. 1991. Seroprevalence of HTLV-I/II and HIV-1 infection among male intravenous drug abusers in Chicago. *J. Acquired Immune Defic. Syndr. 4*, 901–9.

Levin, B. R. 1992. Evolution and the future of AIDS. In *AIDS, the modern plague*, ed B. Wallace, pp. 101–11. Blacksburg, Virginia: Virginia Polytechnic Institute.

Levin, B. R., & Svanborg Edén, C. 1990. Selection and evolution of virulence in bacteria: an ecumenical excursion and modest suggestion. *Parasitology 100*, S103–15.

Levin, S. 1983. Some approaches to modelling of coevolutionary interactions. In *Coevolution*, ed. M. Nitecki, pp. 21–65. Chicago: The University of Chicago Press.

Levin, S., & Pimentel, D. 1981. Selection of intermediate rates of increase in parasite–host systems. *Am. Nat. 117*, 308–15.

Levine, P. H., Blattner, W. A., Clark, J., Tarone, R., Maloney, E. M., Murphy, E. M., Gallo, R. C., Robert-Guroff, M., & Saxinger, W. C. 1988. Geographic distribution of HTLV-I and identification of a new high-risk population. *Int. J. Cancer 42*, 7–12.

Levine, P. H., Reeves, W. C., Cuevas, M., Arosemena, J. R., Jaffe, E. S., Saxinger, W. C., Altafulla, M., De Bernal, J., Espino, H., Rios, B., Xatruch, H., Barnett, M., Drummond, J., Alexander, S., & Blattner, W. 1989. Human T-cell leukemia virus-I and hematologic malignancies in Panama. *Cancer 63*, 2186–91.

Levine, R. J., Khan, M. R., D'Souza, S., & Nalin, D. R. 1976. Cholera transmission near a cholera hospital. *Lancet ii*, 84–6.

Levy, J. A. 1991. HIV research and *nef* alleles. *Science 253*, 366.

Levy, J. A. 1989. Human immunodeficiency viruses and the pathogenesis of AIDS. *JAMA 261*, 2997–3006.

Li, W. H., Tanimura, M., & Sharp, P. M. 1988. Rates and dates of divergence between AIDS virus nucleotide sequences. *Mol. Biol. Evol. 5*, 313–30.

Lifson, A. R., Hessol, N. A., Buchbinder, S. P., O'Malley, P. M., Barnhart, L., Segal, M., Katz, M. H., & Holmberg, S. D. 1992a. Serum β_2 microglobulin and prediction of progression to AIDS in HIV infection. *Lancet 339*, 1436–40.

Lifson, A. R., Hessol, N. A., & Rutherford, G. W. 1992b. Progression and clinical outcome of infection due to human immunodeficiency virus. *Clin. Infect. Dis. 14*, 966–72.

Lindan, C., Allen, S., Carael, M., Nsengumuremyi, F., Vandeperre, P., Serufilira, A., Tice, J., Black, D., Coates, T., & Hulley, S. 1991. Knowledge, attitudes, and perceived risk of AIDS among urban Rwandan women: relationship to HIV infection and behavior change. *AIDS 5*, 993–1002.

Linneman, C. C., Shea, L., Kauffman, C. A., Schiff, G. M., Partin, J. C., & Schubert, W. K. 1974. Association of Reye's syndrome with viral infection. *Lancet ii*, 179–82.

Little, C. J. H., & Bornshin, W. 1930. The dysenteries of Mhow, central India and the central provinces. *Ind. J. Med. Res. 17*, 1015–36.

Lock, R. A., Hansman, D., & Paton, J. C. 1992. Comparative efficiency of autolysin and pneumolysin as immunogens protecting mice against infection by *Streptococcus pneumoniae*. *Microb. Pathog. 12*, 137–43.

Lockyer, M. J., March, D., & Newbold, C. I. 1989. Wild isolates of *Plasmodium falciparum* show extensive polymorphism in T-cell epitopes of the circumsporozoite protein. *Mol. Biochem. Parasit. 37*, 275–80.

Lorenz, K. 1964. *On aggression.* New York: Harcourt Brace.

Lorin, M. I. 1987. Fever: pathogenesis and treatment. In *Textbook of pediatric infectious diseases*, 2nd edition, ed. R. D. Feigin & J. D. Cherry, pp. 148–54. Philadelphia: W. B. Saunders.

Love, G. J., Gezon, H. M., Thompson, D. J., Rogers, K. D., & Hatch, T. F. 1963. Relation of intensity of staphylococcal infection in newborn infants to contamination of nurses' hands and surrounding environment. *Pediatrics 32*, 956–65.

Love, W. C., Gordon, A. M., Gross, R. J., & Rowe, B. 1972. Infantile gastroenteritis due to *Escherichia coli* 0142. *Lancet ii*, 355–7.

Lozano, F., Corzo, J. E., Nogales, C., & García-Bragado, F. 1992. Life-threatening *Pseudomonas aeruginosa* infections in patients with infection due to human immunodeficiency virus. *Clin. Infect. Dis. 15*, 751–2.

Luciw, P. A., Cheng-Mayer, C., & Levy, J. A. 1987. Mutational analysis of the human immunodeficiency virus: The orf-B region down-regulates virus replication. *Proc. Natl. Acad. Sci. USA 84*, 1434–8.

Lwoff, A. 1959. Factors influencing the evolution of viral diseases at the cellular level and in the organism. *Bacteriol. Rev. 23*, 109–24.

Lycke, N., Svennerholm, A. M., & Holmgren J. 1986. Strong biotype and serotype cross-protective antibacterial and antitoxic immunity in rabbits after cholera infection. *Microb. Pathog. 1*, 361–71.

Lynch, C., Ford, J. H., & Weed, F. W. 1925. *The medical department of the United States Army in the World War. Vol. VIII: Field operations.* Washington, D.C.: U. S. Government Printing Office.

Ma, X., Sakai, K., Sinangil, F., Golub, E., & Volsky, D. J. 1990. Interaction of a noncytopathic human immunodeficiency virus type 1 (HIV-1) with target cells: Efficient virus entry followed by delayed expression of its RNA and protein. *Virology 176*, 184–94.

Macaden, R., & Bhat, P. 1985. The changing pattern of resistance to ampicillin and co-trimoxazole in *Shigella* serotypes in Bangalore, Southern India. *J. Infect. Dis. 152*, 1348.

Macaden, R., & Bhat, P. 1986. Changing patterns of *Shigella* serotypes in a southern Indian population. *J. Diar. Dis. Res. 4*, 77–80.

Macaden, R., Gokul, B. N., Pereira, P., & Bhat, P. 1980. Bacillary dysentery due to multidrug resistant *Shigella dysenteriae* type 1. *Indian J. Med. Res. 71*, 178–85.

Macilwain, C. 1993. NIH plans to begin AIDS drug trials at earlier stage. *Nature 362*, 382.

Mackay, E. 1931. Architecture and masonry. in *Mohenjo-daro and the Indus civilization*, ed. J. Marshall, pp. 262–86. London: Probsthain.

Mackenzie, D. J. M. 1965. *Cholera and its control.* , Honolulu, Jan. 24–29, 1965. Pub. Hlth Serv. Publication No. 1328. Washington, D.C.: U.S. Govt. Printing Office.

Mackerras, I. M., & Mackerras, M. J. 1949. An epidemic of infantile gastro-enteritis in Queensland caused by *Salmonella bovis-morbificans* (Basenau). *J. Hyg. 47*, 166–81.

Mackowiak, P. A. 1983. Our microbial associates. *Nat. Hist. 92*, 80–7.

MacPherson, D. W., & Tonkin, M. 1992. Cholera vaccination: a decision analysis. *Can. Med. Assoc. J. 146*, 1947–52.

Maddox, J. 1993. The next step in AIDS treatment. *Nature 362*, 493.

Magura, S., Grossman, J. I., Lipton, D. S., Siddiqi, Q., Shapiro, J., Marion, I., & Amann, K. R. 1989. Determinants of needle sharing among intravenous drug users. *Am. J. Public Hlth. 79*, 459–61.

Maitra, R. K., Ahmad, N., Holland, S. M., & Venkatesan, S. 1991. Human immunodeficiency virus type 1 (HIV-1) provirus expression and LTR transcription are repressed in nef-expressing cell lines. *Virology 182*, 522–33.

Maloney, E. M., Biggar, R. J., Neel, J. V., Taylor, M. E., Hahn, B. H., Shaw, G. M., & Blattner, W. A. 1992. Endemic human T-cell lymphotropic virus type II infection among isolated Brazilian Amerindians. *J. Infect. Dis. 166*, 100–7.

Manifold, J. A. 1926. Important features in the correct diagnosis of dysentery in India. *J. Roy. Army Med. Corps 46*, 81–98.

Manos, J. P. 1982. Group B streptococcal infection in the neonate. *Ann. Clin. Lab. Sci. 12*, 239–43.

Manson-Bahr, P. 1944. *The dysentery disorders*, 2nd edition. London: Cassell.

Manson-Bahr, P. E. C., & Apted, F. I. C. 1982. *Manson's tropical diseases.* London: Bailliere Tindall.

Maramorosch, K. 1987. The curse of cadang-cadang. *Nat. Hist. 96*(7), 20–2.

Marcuzzi, A., Weinberger, J., & Weinberger, O. K. 1992. Transcellular activation of the human immunodeficiency virus type-1 long terminal repeat in cocultured lymphocytes. *J. Virol. 66*, 4228–32.

Marcy, S. M. 1976. Microorganisms responsible for neonatal diarrhea. in *Infectious diseases of the fetus and newborn infant*, ed. J. S. Remington & J. O. Klein, pp. 892–978. Philadelphia: W. B. Saunders.

Mariotto, A. B., Mariotti, S., Pezzotti, P., Rezza, G., & Verdecchia, A. 1992. Estimation of the acquired immunodeficiency syndrome incubation period in intravenous drug users: A comparison with male homosexuals. *Am. J. Epidemiol. 135*, 428–37.

Marshall, J. 1931. The buildings. In *Mohenjo-daro and the Indus civilization*, ed. J. Marshall, pp. 15–26. London: Prosthain.

Martin, P. M. V., Gresenguet, G., Massanga, M., Georges, A., & Testa, J. 1992. Association between HIV1 infection and sexually transmitted disease among men in central Africa. *Res. Virol. 143*, 205–9.

Mata, L. J., Catalan, M. A., & Gordon, J. E. 1966. Studies of diarrheal disease in Central America. IX. *Shigella* carriers among young children of a heavily seeded Guatemalan convalescent home. *Am. J. Trop. Med. Hyg. 15*, 632–8.

Mata, L., Gangarosa, E., Cáceras, A., Perera, D. R., & Mejicanos, M. L. 1970. Epidemic Shiga bacillus dysentery in Central America. I. *J. Infect. Dis. 122*, 170–80.

Mathez, D., Paul, D., De Belilovsky, C., Sultan, Y., Deleuze, J., Gorin, I., Saurin, W., Decker, R., & Liebowitch, J. 1990. Productive human immunodeficiency virus infection levels correlate with AIDS-related manifestations in the patient. *Proc. Natl. Acad. Sci. USA 87*, 7438–42.

Mavoungou, D. 1992. AIDS epicenter. *Science 257*, 598–9.

May, R. M., & Anderson, R. M. 1983. Epidemiology and genetics in the coevolution of parasites and hosts. *Proc. R. Soc. Lond. 219*, 281– 313.

Mayers, D. L., Mccutchan, F. E., Sanders-Buell, E. E., Merritt, L. I., Dilworth, S., Fowler, A. K., Marks, C. A., Ruiz, N. M., Richman, D. D., Roberts, C. R., & Burke, D. S. 1992. Characterization of HIV isolates arising after prolonged zidovudine therapy. *J. Acquired Immune Defic. Syndr. 5*, 749–59.

Maynard Smith, J. M. 1964. Group selection and kin selection. *Nature 201*, 1145–7.

McAllister, M. K., & Roitberg, B. D. 1987. Adaptive suicidal behaviour in pea aphids. *Nature 328*, 797–9.

McCandlish, I. A. P., Thompson, H., Fisher, E. W., Cornwell, H. J. C., Macartney, J., & Walton, I. A. 1981. Canine parvovirus infection. *In Practice 3*, 5–14.

McCusker, J., Stoddard, A. M., Zapka, J. G., Morrison, C. S., Zorn, M., & Lewis, B. F. 1992. AIDS education for drug abusers: Evaluation of short-term effectiveness. *Am. J. Public Hlth. 82*, 533–40.

McCutchan, F. E., Hegerich, P. A., Brennan, T. P., Phanuphak, P., Singharaj, P., Jugsudee, A., Berman, P. W., Gray, A. M., Fowler, A. K., & Burke, D. S. 1992. Genetic variants of HIV-1 in Thailand. *AIDS Res. Hum. Retroviruses 8*, 1887–95.

McLean, A. R., & Nowak, M. A. 1992. Competition between zidovudine-sensitive and zidovudine-resistant strains of HIV. *AIDS 6*, 71–9.

McLennon, J. L., & Darby, G. 1980. Herpes simplex virus latency: The cellular location of virus in dorsal root ganglia and the fate of the infected cells following virus activation. *J. Gen. Virol. 51*, 233–43.

McNearney, T., Hornickova, Z., Markham, R., Birdwell, A., Arens, M., Saah, A., & Ratner, L. 1992. Relationship of human immunodeficiency virus type 1 sequence heterogeneity to stage of disease. *Proc. Natl. Acad. Sci. USA 89* , 10247–51.

McNeill, W. H. 1976. *Plagues and peoples*. Garden City, New Jersey: Anchor.

McNicol, L. A., & Doetsch, R. N. 1983. A hypothesis accounting for the origin of pandemic cholera: a retrograde analysis. *Perspect. Biol. Med. 26*, 547–52.

Meiss, M. 1978. *Painting in Florence and Siena after the black death: The arts, religion, and society in the mid-fourteenth century*. Princeton, New Jersey: Princeton University Press.

Meitert, T., Pencu, E., Ciudin, L., & Tonciu, M. 1984. Vaccine strain *Sh. flexneri* T32-Istrati. Studies in animals and in volunteers. Antidysentery immunoprophylaxis and immunotherapy by live vaccine Vadizen (*Sh. flexneri* T-32-Istrati). *Arch. Roum. Pathol. Exp. Microbiol. 43*, 251–78.

Mekalanos, J. J., Moseley, S. L., Murphy, J. R., & Falkow, S. 1982. Isolation of enterotoxin structural gene deletion mutations in *Vibrio cholerae* induced by two mutagenic vibriophages. *Proc. Natl. Acad. Sci. USA 79*, 151–5.

Melish, M. E., & Glasgow, L. A. 1970. The staphyolococcal scalded-skin syndrome: Development of an experimental model. *N. Engl. J. Med. 282*, 1114–19.

Mellors, J. W., Dutschman, G. E., Im, G. J., Tramontano, E., Winkler, S. R., & Cheng, Y. C. 1992. *In vitro* selection and molecular characterization of human immunodeficiency virus-1 resistant to non-nucleoside inhibitors of reverse transcriptase. *Mol. Pharmacol. 41*, 446–51.

Mercereau-Puijalon, O., Fandeur, T., Guillotte, M., & Bonnefoy, S. 1991. Parasite features impeding malaria immunity: antigenic diversity, antigenic variation and poor immunogenicity. *Res. Immunol. 142*, 690-7.

Mercereau-Puijalon, O., Fandeur, T., Bonnefoy, S., Jacquemot, C., & Sarthou, J. L. 1991. A study of the genomic diversity of *Plasmodium falciparum* in Senegal. 2. Typing by the use of the polymerase chain reaction. *Acta Trop. 49*, 293-304.

Merino, F., Robert-Guroff, M., Clark, J., Biondo-Bracho, M., Blattner, W. A., & Gallo, R. C. 1984. Natural antibodies to human T-cell leukemia/lymphoma virus in healthy Venezuelan populations. *Int. J. Cancer 44*, 419-23.

Mermin, J. H., Holodniy, M., Katzenstein, D. A., & Merigan, T. C. 1991. Detection of human immunodeficiency virus DNA and RNA in semen by the polymerase chain reaction. *J. Infect. Dis. 164*, 769–72.

Metler, R., Conway, G. A., & Stehr-Green, J. 1991. AIDS surveillance among American Indians and Alaska natives. *Am. J. Public Hlth. 81*, 1469-71.

Meunier, P. C., Blickman, L. T., Appel, M. J. G., & Shin, S. J. 1981. Canine parvovirus in a commercial kennel: epidemiologic and pathologic findings. *Cornell Vet. 71*, 96-110.

Meyerhans, A., Cheynier, R., Albert, J., Seth, M., Kwok, S., Sninsky, J., Morfeldt-Manson, L., Åsjö, B., & Wain-Hobson, S. 1989. Temporal fluctuations in HIV quasispecies *in vivo* are not reflected by sequential HIV isolations. *Cell 58*, 901-10.

Mhalu, F. S., Mmari, P. W., & Ijumba, J. 1979. Rapid emergence of el tor *Vibrio cholerae* resistant to antimicrobial agents during first 6 months of 4th cholera epidemic in Tanzania. *Lancet i*, 345-7.

Michael, N. L., Vahey, M., Burke, D. S., & Redfield, R. R. 1992. Viral DNA and messenger RNA expression correlate with the stage of human immunodeficiency virus (HIV) type 1 infection in humans: evidence for viral replication in all stages of HIV disease. *J. Virol. 66*, 310-16.

Miller, B. R., & Mitchell, C. J. 1991. Genetic selection of a flavivirus-refractory strain of the yellow fever mosquito *Aedes aegypti*. *Am. J. Trop. Med. Hyg. 45*, 399-407.

Miller, C. J., Alexander, N. J., Gettie, A., Hendricks, A. G., & Marx, P. A. 1992. The effect of contraceptives containing nonoxynol-9 on the genital transmission of simian immunodeficiency virus in rhesus macaques. *Fertil. Steril. 57*, 1126-8.

Miller, C. J., Feachem, R. G., & Drasar, B. S. 1985. Cholera epidemiology in developed and developing countries: New thoughts on transmission, seasonality, and control. *Lancet i*, 261-3.

Miller, D., Yoshikawa, T., Castle, S. C., & Norman, D. 1991. Effect of age on fever response to a recombinant tumor necrosis factor alpha. *J. Gerontol. 46*, M176-9.

Miller, J. A. 1989. Diseases for our future: Global ecology and emerging viruses. *Bioscience 39*, 509-17.

Miller, J. F., Melakanos, J. J., & Falkow, S. 1989. Coordinate regulation and sensory transduction in the control of bacterial virulence. *Science 243*, 916-22.

Miller, L. W., Older, J. J., Drake, J., & Zimmerman, S. 1972. Diphtheria immunization. Effect upon carriers and the control of outbreaks. *Am. J. Dis Child 123*, 197-9.

Miller, V., & Mekalanos, J. J. 1984. Synthesis of cholera toxin is positively regulated at the transcriptional level by toxR. *Proc. Natl. Acad. Sci. USA 81*, 3471-5.

Minami, A., Hashimoto, S., Abe, H., Arita, M., Taniguchi, T., Honda, T., Miwatani, T., & Nishibuchi, M. 1991. Cholera enterotoxin production in *Vibrio cholerae*-O1 strains isolated from the environment and from humans in Japan. *Appl. Environ. Microbiol. 57*, 2152-7.

Mitchell, C. J., Niebylski, M. L., Smith, G. C., Karabatsos, N., Martin, D., Mutebi, J. P., Craig, G. B., & Mahler, M. J. 1992. Isolation of eastern equine encephalitis virus from *Aedes albopictus* in Florida. *Science 257*, 526-7.

Mitscherlich, E., & Marth, E. H. 1984. *Microbial survival in the environment*. Berlin: Springer-Verlag.

Mitsuya, H., Yarchoan, R., & Broder, S. 1990. Molecular targets for AIDS therapy. *Science 249*, 1533-44.

Mitsuya, H., Yarchoan, R., Kageyama, S., & Broder, S. 1991. Targeted therapy of human immunodeficiency virus-related disease. *FASEB J. 5*, 2369-81.

Miura, T., Sakuragi, J. I., Kawamura, M., Fukasawa, M., Moriyami, E. N., Gojobori, T., Ishikawa, K. I., Mingle, J. A. A., Nettey, V. B. A., Akari, H., Enami, M., Tsujimoto, H., & Hayami, M. 1990. Establishment of a phylogenetic survey system for AIDS-related lentiviruses and demonstration of a new HIV-2 subgroup. *AIDS 4*, 1257-61.

Miyamoto, K., Kamiya, T., Minowada, J., Tomita, N., & Kitajima, K. 1991. Transformation of CD8+ T-cells producing a strong cytopathic effect on CD4+ T-cells through syncytium formation by HTLV II. *Jpn. J. Cancer Res. 82*, 1178-83.

Mogabgab, W. J., & Pollack, B. 1976. Re: increased virus shedding with aspirin treatment of rhinovirus infection. *JAMA 235*, 801.

Mohri, H., Singh, M. K., Ching, W. T. W., & Ho, D. D. 1993. Quantitation of zidovudine-resistant human immunodeficiency virus type 1 in the blood of treated and untreated patients. *Proc. Natl. Acad. Sci. USA 90*, 25-9.

Molavi, A., & LeFrock, J. L. 1984. *Enterobacteriaceae, Pseudomonas aeruginosa* and *Acinetobacter*. In *The pneumonias. Clinical approaches to infectious diseases of the lower respiratory tract*, ed. M. E. Levison, pp. 309-33. Boston: John Wright/PSG.

Molineaux, L., & Gramiccia, G. 1980. *The Garki project*. Geneva: World Health Organization.

Molla, A. M., & Bari, A. 1992. Role of cereal-based oral rehydration therapy in persistent diarrhoea in children. *Acta Paediatr. Scand. 81*, 104-7.

Monath, T. P. 1991. Yellow fever—Victor, Victoria?—Conqueror, Conquest? Epidemics and research in the last 40 years and prospects for the future. *Am. J. Trop. Med. Hyg. 45*, 1-43.

Monk, R. J., Malik, F. G., Stokesberry, D., & Evans, L. H. 1992. Direct determination of the point mutation rate of a murine retrovirus. *J. Virol. 66*, 3683-9.

Monsur, K. A. 1983. How this happened? *J. Diar. Dis. Res. 1*, 3–4.

Montagnier, L. 1988. Origin and evolution of HIVs and their role in AIDS pathogenesis. *J. Acquired Immune Defic. Syndr. 1*, 517– 20.

Montaner, J. S. G., Singer, J., Schechter, M. T., Raboud, J. M., Tsoukas, C., O'Shaughnessy, M., Ruedy, J., Nagai, K., Salomon, H., Spira, B., & Wainberg, M. A. 1993. Clinical correlates of *in vitro* HIV-1 resistance to zidovudine: results of the multicentre Canadian AZT trial. *AIDS 7*, 189–96.

Montgomery, S. B., & Joseph, J. G. 1989. Behavioral change in homosexual men at risk for AIDS: Intervention and policy implications. In *The AIDS epidemic: Private rights and the public interest*, ed. P. O'Malley, pp. 323–33. Boston: Beacon Press.

Moon, H., Orskov, F., Rowe, B., & Sack, R. B. 1980. *Escherichia coli* diarrhea. *Bull. WHO 58*, 23–36.

Moore, H. A., de la Cruz, E., & Vargas-Mendez, O. 1965. Diarrheal disease studies in Costa Rica IV. *Am. J. Epidemiol. 82*, 162–84.

Moore, H. A., de la Cruz, E., & Vargas-Mendez, O. 1966. Diarrheal disease studies in Costa Rica. II. *Am. J. Public Hlth. 59*, 442– 51.

Moore, J. P., McKeating, J. A., Huang, Y. X., Ashkenazi, A., & Ho, D. D. 1992. Virions of primary human immunodeficiency virus type 1 isolates resistant to soluble CD4 (sCD4) neutralization differ in sCD4 binding and glycoprotein gp120 retention from sCD4-sensitive isolates. *J. Virol. 66*, 235–43.

Moore, R. D., Creagh-Kirk, T., Keruly, J., Link, G., Wang, M. C., Richman, D., & Chaisson, R. E. 1991a. Long-term safety and efficacy of zidovudine in patients with advanced human immunodeficiency virus disease. *Arch. Intern. Med. 151*, 981–6.

Moore, R. D., Hidalgo, J., Sugland, B. W., & Chaisson, R. E. 1991b. Zidovudine and the natural history of the acquired immunodeficiency syndrome. *N. Engl. J. Med. 324*, 1412–16.

Morens, D. M., Marchette, N. J., Chu, M. C., & Halstead, S. B. 1991. Growth of dengue type-2 virus isolates in human peripheral blood leukocytes correlates with severe and mild dengue disease. *Am. J. Trop. Med. Hyg. 45*, 644–51.

Morozov, V. A., Lagaye, S., Saal, F., Bazarbachi, A., Gout, O., Lyoncaen, O., & Peries, J. 1992. High level of HTLV-I specific protein expression in a patient with adult T-cell leukemia, chronic progressive myelopathy and Kaposi's sarcoma. *Leukemia 6*, 746–50.

Morrey, J. D., Okleberry, K. M., & Sidwell, R. W. 1991. Early-initiated zidovudine therapy prevents disease but not low levels of persistent retrovirus in mice. *J. Acquired Immune Defic. Syndr. 4*, 506–12.

Morrison, A. J., & Wenzel, R. P. 1984. Epidemiology of infections due to *Pseudomonas aeruginosa*. *Rev. Infect. Dis. 6 (Suppl 3)*, S627–42.

Morrison, N. K., McCarthy, K., & Hart, C. A. 1991. Growth of human immunodeficiency virus 1 in cultured cells in the absence of the CD4 antigen. *J. Med. Virol. 35*, 187–91.

Morse, R. A., & Nowogrodzki, R. 1990. Introduction. In *Honey bee pests, predators, and diseases*, 2nd edition, ed. R. A. Morse & R. Nowogrodzki, pp. 1–11. Ithaca: Cornell University Press.

Morse, S. S. 1991. Emerging viruses: Defining the rules for viral traffic. *Perspect. Biol. Med. 34*, 387–409.

Mortimer, E. A., Lipsitz, P. J., Wolinsky, E., Bonzaga, A. J., & Rammelkamp, D. H. 1962. Transmission of staphylococci between newborns. *Am. J. Dis. Child. 104*, 289–95.

Moseley, S. L., & Falkow, S. 1980. Nucleotide sequence homology between the heat-labile enterotoxin gene of *Escherichia coli* and *Vibrio cholerae* DNA. *J. Bacteriol. 144*, 444–6.

Moses, S., Plummer, F. A., Ngugi, E. N., Nagelkerke, N. J. D., Anzala, A. O., & Ndinya-Achola, J. O. 1991. Controlling HIV in Africa: Effectiveness and cost of an intervention in a high-frequency STD transmitter core group. *AIDS 5*, 407–11.

Mosley, W. H., & Khan, M. 1979. Cholera epidemiology—some environmental aspects. *Prog. Wat. Tech. 11*, 309–16.

Muckenthaler, M., Gunkel, N., Levantis, P., Broadhurst, K., Goh, B., Colvin, B., Forster, G., Jackson, G. G., & Oxford, J. S. 1992. Sequence analysis of an HIV-1 isolate which displays unusually high-level AZT resistance *in vitro. J. Med. Virol. 36*, 79–83.

Mufson, M. A., Mocega, H. E., & Drause, H. E. 1973. Acquisition of parainfluenza 3 virus infection by hospitalized children. I. Frequencies, rates and temporal data. *J. Infect. Dis. 138*, 141–7.

Mukhopadhyay, A., Sarnaik, A. P., & Deshmukh, D. R. 1992. Interactions of ibuprofen with influenza infection and hyperammonemia in an animal model of Reye's syndrome. *Pediatr. Res. 31*, 258–60.

Mulder, J. W., De Wolf, F., Goudsmit, J., Cload, P. A., Coutinho, R. A., Fiddian, A. P., Schellekens, P. T., Van Der Noordaa, J., & Lange, J. M. A. 1990. Long-term zidovudine treatment of asymptomatic HIV-1-infected subjects. *Antivir. Res. 13*, 127–38.

Mulder, J., & Masurel, N. 1960. The epidemiology of pandemic A2 influenza in the Netherlands, 1957–1958. *Bull. WHO 22*, 399–407.

Mulligan, M. J., Yamshchikov, G. V., Ritter, G. D., Gao, F., Jin, M. J., Nail, C. D., Spies, C. P., Hahn, B. H., & Compans, R. W. 1992. Cytoplasmic domain truncation enhances fusion activity by the exterior glycoprotein complex of human immunodeficiency virus type 2 in selected cell types. *J. Virol. 66*, 3971–5.

Muñoz, R., Musser, J. M., Crain, M., Briles, D. E., Marton, A., Parkinson, A. J., Sorensen, U., & Tomasz, A. 1992. Geographic distribution of penicillin-resistant clones of *Streptococcus pneumoniae*: Characterization by penicillin-binding protein profile, surface protein-A typing, and multilocus enzyme analysis. *Clin. Infect. Dis. 15*, 112–18.

Murphey-Corb, M., Montelaro, R. C., Miller, M. A., West, M., Martin, L. N., Davisonfairburn, B., Ohkawa, S., Baskin, G. B., Zhang, J. Y., Miller, G. B., Putney, S. D., Allison, A. C., & Eppstein, D. A. 1991. Efficacy of SIV/deltaB670 glycoprotein-enriched and glycoprotein-depleted subunit vaccines in protecting against infection and disease in rhesus monkeys. *AIDS 5*, 655–62.

Murphy, E. L., & Blattner, W. 1988. HTLV-I associated leukemia: A model for chronic retroviral diseases. *Ann. Neurol. 23 (Suppl.)*, S174–80.

Murphy, E. L., Figueroa, J. P., Gibbs, W. N., Holdingcobham, M., Cranston, B., Malley, K., Bodner, A. J., Alexander, S. S., & Blattner, W. A. 1991. Human T-lymphotropic virus type-I (HTLV-I) seroprevalence in Jamaica. 1. Demographic determinants. *Am. J. Epidemiol. 133*, 1114–24.

Murphy, E. L., Figueroa, J. P., Gibbs, W. N., Brathwaite, A., Holding-Cobham, M., Waters, D., Cranston, B., Hanchard, B., & Blattner, W. A. 1989. Sexual transmission of human T-lymphotropic virus type I (HTLV I). *Ann. Intern. Med. 111,* 555–60.

Mushin, R. 1948. An outbreak of gastro-enteritis due to *Salmonella derby. J. Hyg. 46,* 151–7.

Myers, G., MacInnes, K., & Korber, B. 1992. The emergence of simian/human immunodeficiency viruses. *AIDS Res. Hum. Retroviruses 8,* 373–86.

Myers, W. F., & Wisseman, C. L. 1980. Genetic relatedness among the typhus group of rickettsiae. *Int. J. Syst. Bacteriol. 30,* 143–50.

Nagamine, M., Nakashima, Y., Uemura, S., Takei, H., Toda, T., Maehama, T., Nakachi, H., & Nakayama, M. 1991. DNA amplification of human T Lymphotropic virus type I (HTLV-I) proviral DNA in breast milk of HTLV-I carriers. *J. Infect. Dis. 164,* 1024–5.

Nagelkerke, N. J. D., Plummer, F. A., Holton, D., Anzala, A. O., Manji, F., Ngugi, E. N., & Moses, S. 1990. Transition dynamics of HIV disease in a cohort of African prostitutes: A Markov model approach. *AIDS 4,* 743–8.

Nahmias, A. J., Weiss, J., Yao, Z., Lee, F., Kodsi, R., Schandfield, M., Matthews, T., Bolognesi, D., Durack, D., Motulsky, A., Kanki, P., & Essex, M. 1986. Evidence for human infection with an HTLV-III/LAV-like virus in central Africa, 1959. *Lancet i,* 1279–80.

Nair, G. B., Oku, Y., Takeda, Y., Ghosh, A., Ghosh, R. K., Chattopadhyay, S., Pal, S. C., Kaper, J. B., & Takeda, T. 1988. Toxin profiles of *Vibrio cholerae* non-01 from environmental sources in Calcutta, India. *Appl. Environ. Microbiol. 54,* 3180–3.

Nara, P. L., Garrity, R. R., & Goudsmit, J. 1991. Neutralization of HIV-1: A paradox of humoral proportions. *FASEB J. 5,* 2437–55.

National Academy of Sciences 1969. *An evaluation of the* Salmonella *problem.* Publ. No. 1683. Washington, D.C.: National Academy of Sciences.

National Institute of Allergy and Infectious Diseases. 1990. State-of-the-art conference on azidothymidine therapy for early HIV infection. *Am. J. Med. 89,* 335–44.

Natoli, C., Dianzani, F., Mazzotta, F., Balocchini, E., Pierotti, P., Antonelli, G., & Iacobelli, S. 1993. 90K protein: A new predictor marker of disease progression in human immunodeficiency virus infection. *J. Acquired Immune Defic. Syndr. 6,* 370–5.

Nauclér A, Andreasson P-Å, Costa C M, Thorstensson R, & Biberfeld G. 1989. HIV-2 associated AIDS and HIV-2 seroprevalence in Bissau, Guinea-Bissau. *J. Acquired Immune Defic. Syndr. 2,* 88–93.

Nauclér, A., Albino, P., Da Silva, A. P., Andreasson, P. A., Andersson, S., & Biberfeld, G. 1991. HIV-2 infection in hospitalized patients in Bissau, Guinea-Bissau. *AIDS 5,* 301-4.

Neequaye, A. R., Neequaye, J. E., & Biggar, R. J. 1991. Factors that could influence the spread of AIDS in Ghana, west Africa: knowledge of AIDS, sexual behavior, prostitution, and traditional medical practices. *J. Acquired Immune Defic. Syndr. 4,* 914-19.

Nesbitt, J. A. A., & Minuk, G. Y. 1988. Adult Reye's syndrome. *Ann. Emerg. Med. 17,* 155-8.

Neter, E., Korns, R. F., & Trussell, R. E. 1953. Association of *Escherichia coli* serogroup 0111 with two hospital outbreaks of epidemic diarrhea of the newborn infant in New York State during 1947. *Pediatrics 12,* 377-83.

Neu, H. C. 1992. The crisis in antibiotic resistance. *Science 257*, 1064-73.

Neustadt, R. E., & Fineberg, H. 1983. *The epidemic that never was: Policy-making and the swine flu affair*. New York: Random House.

Niederman, T. M. J., Garcia, J. V., Hastings, W. R., Luria, S., & Ratner, L. 1992. Human immunodeficiency virus type 1 nef protein inhibits NF-κab induction in human T cells. *J. Virol. 66*, 6213-19.

Niederman, T. M. J., Thielan, B. J., & Ratner, L. 1989. Human immunodeficiency virus type 1 negative factor is a transcriptional silencer. *Proc. Natl. Acad. Sci. USA 86*, 1128-32.

Niklasson, B., Liljestrand, J., Berstrom, S., & Peters, C. J. 1987. Rift Valley fever a sero-epidemiological survey among pregnant women in Mozambique. *Epidemiol. Infect. 99*, 517-22.

Norden, C. W., & Ruben, F. L. 1981. Staphylococcal infections. In *Communicable and infectious diseases*, 9th edition, ed. P. F. Wehrle & F. H. Top, pp. 589-605. St. Louis: C. V. Mosby.

Novembre, F. J., Hirsch, V. M., Mcclure, H. M., Fultz, P. N., & Johnson, P. R. 1992. SIV from stump-tailed macaques: Molecular characterization of a highly transmissible primate lentivirus. *Virology 186*, 783-7.

Nowak, M. A., Anderson, R. M., McLean, A. R., Wolfs, T. F. W., Goudsmit, J., & May, R. M. 1991. Antigenic diversity thresholds and the development of AIDS. *Science 254*, 963-9.

Nowak, M. A., May, R. M., & Anderson, R. M. 1990. The evolutionary dynamics of HIV-1 quasispecies and the development of immunodeficiency disease. *AIDS 4*, 1095-103.

Nuland, S. B. 1981. The enigma of Semmelweis—an interpretation. In *The etiology, the concept and the prophylaxis of childbed fever, by Ignac Fulop Semmelweis*, ed. S. B. Nuland & F. A. Gyorgyey, pp. xiii-xlii. Birmingham: Gryphon.

Nzila, N., Laga, M., Thiam, M. A., Mayimona, K., Edidi, B., Vandyck, E., Behets, F., Hassig, S., Nelson, A., Mokwa, K., Ashley, R. L., Piot, P., & Ryder, R. W. 1991. HIV and other sexually transmitted diseases among female prostitutes in Kinshasa. *AIDS 5*, 715-21.

Nzilambi, N., De Cock, K. M., Forthal, D. N., Francis, H., Ryder, R. W., Malebe, I., Gretchell, J., Laga, M., Piot, P., & McCormick, J. B. 1988. The prevalence of infection with human immunodeficiency virus over a 10-year period in rural Zaire. *N. Engl. J. Med. 318*, 276–9.

Odehouri, K., De Cock, K. M., Krebs, J. W., Moreau, J., Rayfield, M., McCormick, J. B., Schochetman, G., Bretton, R., Bretton, G., Ouattara, D., Heroin, P., Kanga J-M, Beda, B., Niamkey, E., Kadio, A., Gariepe, E., & Heyward, W. L. 1989. HIV-1 and HIV-2 infection associated with AIDS in Abidjan, Côte d'Ivoire. *AIDS 3*, 509–12.

Oduola, A. M. J., Sowunmi, A., Milhous, W. K., Kyle, D. E., Martin, R. K., Walker, O., & Salako, L. A. 1992. Innate resistance to new antimalarial drugs in *Plasmodium falciparum* from Nigeria. *Trans. Roy. Soc. Trop. Med. Hyg. 86*, 123–6.

Oka, S., Urayama, K., Hirabayashi, Y., Ohnishi, K., Goto, H., Mitamura, K., Kimura, S., & Shimada, K. 1991. Quantitative estimation of human immunodeficiency virus type-1 provirus in CD4+ lymphocytes-T using the polymerase chain reaction. *Mol. Cell. Probes 5*, 137–42.

O'Keefe, E., Kaplan, E., & Khoshnood, K. 1991. *City of New Haven needle exchange program: Preliminary report*. New Haven, Conn.: New Haven Health Department.

Olson, W. W. 1974. *Animal parasites: Their life cycles and ecology*. Baltimore, Md.: University Park Press.

Ong, E. L. C., & Mandal, B. K. 1991. Tuberculosis in patients infected with the human immunodeficiency virus. *Q. J. Med. 80*, 613–17.

Oo, K. N., Han, M., Hlaing, T., & Aye, T. 1991. Bacteriologic studies of food and water consumed by children in Myanmar: 1. *J. Diar. Dis. Res. 9*, 87–90.

O'Reilly, D. R., & Miller, L. K. 1989. A baculovirus blocks molting by producing an ecdysteroid UDP-glucosyl transferase. *Science 245*, 1110–12.

O'Reilly, T., & Zak, O. 1992. Elevated body temperature restricts growth of *Haemophilus influenzae* type b during experimental meningitis. *Infect. Immun. 60*, 3448–51.

Osek, J., Svennerholm, A. M., & Holmgren, J. 1992. Protection against *Vibrio cholerae* el tor infection by specific antibodies against mannose-binding hemagglutinin pili. *Infect. Immun. 60*, 4961–4.

O'Shea, S., Rostron, T., Hamblin, A. S., Palmer, S. J., & Banatvala, J. E. 1991. Quantitation of HIV: Correlation with clinical, virological, and immunological status. *J. Med. Virol. 35*, 65–9.

Osmond, D. H., Shiboski, S., Bacchetti, P., Winger, E. E., & Moss, A. R. 1991. Immune activation markers and AIDS prognosis. *AIDS 5*, 505–11.

Osoba, A. O. 1981. Sexually transmitted diseases in tropical africa. *Br. J. Ven. Dis 57*, 89–94.

Ouattara, S. A., Meite, M., Cot, M. C., & de-The, G. 1989. Compared prevalence of infections by HIV-1 and HIV-2 during a 2-year period in suburban and rural areas of Ivory Coast. *J. Acquir Immune Defic Diseases 2*, 94–9.

Owens, D. K., & Nease, R. F. 1992. Occupational exposure to human immunodeficiency virus and hepatitis-B virus: A comparative analysis of risk. *Am. J. Med. 92*, 503–12.

Padian, N., Marquis, L., Francis, D. P., Anderson, R. E., Rutherford, G. W., O'Malley, P. M., & Winkelstein, W. 1987. Male-to-female transmission of human immunodeficiency virus. *JAMA 258*, 788–90.

Padian, N. S., Shiboski, S. C., & Jewell, N. P. 1991. Female-to-male transmission of human immunodeficiency virus. *JAMA 266*, 1664–7.

Pal, A., Ramamurthy, T., Bhadra, R. K., Takeda, T., Shimada, T., Takeda, Y., Nair, G. B., Pal, S. C., & Chakrabarti, S. 1992. Reassessment of the prevalence of heat-stable enterotoxin (NAG-ST) among environmental *Vibrio cholerae* non-01 strains isolated from Calcutta, India, by Using a NAG-ST DNA probe. *Appl. Environ. Microbiol. 58*, 2485–9.

Palmieri, J. R. 1982. Be fair to parasites. *Nature 298*, 220.

Panda, G. K., & Gupta, S. P. 1964. *Shigella* serotypes in Uttar Pradesh. *Indian J. Med. Res. 52*, 235–40.

Paniker, C. K. J., Vimala, K. N., Bhat, P., & Stephen, S. 1978. Drug resistant shigellosis in South India. *Indian J. Med. Res. 68*, 413–17.

Pantaleo, G., Graziosi, C., Demarest, J. F., Butini, L., Montroni, M., Fox, C. H., Orenstein, J. M., Kotler, D. P., & Fauci, A. S. 1993. HIV infection is active and progressive in lymphoid tissue during the clinically latent stage of disease. *Nature 362*, 355–8.

Pappenheimer, A. M. 1977. Diphtheria toxin. *Annu. Rev. Biochem. 46*, 69–94.

Pappenheimer, A. M. 1982. Diphtheria: Studies on the biology of an infectious disease. *Harvey Lect. 76*, 45–73.

Pappenheimer, A. M., & Gill, D. M. 1973. Diphtheria. *Science 182*, 353–8.

Pappenheimer, A. M., & Murphy, J. R. 1983. Studies on the molecular epidemiology of diphtheria. *Lancet ii*, 923–6.

Parker, E. R., & Horne, W. T. 1932. The transmission of avocado sun-blotch. *Calif. Avocado Assoc. Yearbook* 50–6.

Patterson, J. E., Vecchio, J., Pantelick, E. L., Farrel, P., Mazon, D., Zervos, M. J., & Hierholzer, W. J. 1991. Association of contaminated gloves with transmission of *Acinetobacter calcoaceticus* var. *anitratus* in an intensive care unit. *Am. J. Med. 91*, 479–83.

Pavillard, R., Harvey, K., Douglas, D., Hewstone, A., Andrew, J., Collopy, B., Asche, V., Carson, P., Davidson, A., Gilbert, G., Spicer, J., & Tosolini, F. 1982. Epidemic of hospital-acquired infection due to methicillin-resistant *Staphylococcus aureus* in major Victorian hospitals. *Med. J. Austral. 1*, 451–4.

Pavlakis, G. N., Felber, B. K., Ciminale, V., Unge, T., Solomin, L., & Harrison, J. E. 1992. Structure, regulation and oncogenic mechanisms of HTLV-I and HTLV-II. *Leukemia 6*, S176–80.

Pearson, M. L., Jereb, J. A., Frieden, T. R., Crawford, J. T., Davis, B. J., Dooley, S. W., & Jarvis, W. R. 1992. Nosocomial transmission of multidrug-resistant *Mycobacterium tuberculosis*: A risk to patients and health care workers. *Ann. Intern. Med. 117*, 191–6.

Pedersen, C., Nielsen, J., Dickmeis, E., & Sordal, R. 1989. Early progression to AIDS following primary HIV infections. *AIDS 158*, 866–8.

Peeters, M., Fransen, K., Delaporte, E., Van den Haesevelde, M., Gershy-Damet, G. M., Kestens, L., van der Groen, G., & Piot, P. 1992. Isolation and characterization of a new chimpanzee lentivirus (simian immunodeficiency virus isolate cpz-ant) from a wild-captured chimpanzee. *AIDS 6*, 447–51.

Peeters, M., Honore, C., Huet, T., Bedjabaga, L., Ossari, S., Bussi, P., Cooper, R. W., & Delaporte, E. 1989. Isolation and partial characterization of an HIV-related virus occurring naturally in chimpanzees in Gabon. *AIDS 3*, 625–30.

Pela, A. O., & Platt, J. J. 1989. AIDS in Africa: Emerging trends. *Soc. Sci. Med. 28*, 1–8.

Pepin, J., Morgan, G., Dunn, D., Gevao, S., Mendy, M., Gaye, I., Scollen, N., Tedder, R., & Whittle, H. 1991. HIV-2-induced immunosuppression among asymptomatic West African prostitutes: evidence that HIV-2 is pathogenic, but less so than HIV-1. *AIDS 5*, 1165–72.

Perkins, H. A., Smaon, S., Garner, J., Echenberg, D., Allen, J. R., Cowan, M., & Levy, J. A. 1987. Risk of AIDS for recipients of blood components from donors who subsequently developed AIDS. *Blood 70*, 1604–10.

Pesola, G. R., & Charles, A. 1992. Pneumococcal bacteremia with pneumonia: Mortality in acquired immunodeficiency syndrome. *Chest 101*, 150–5.

Peterman, T. A., Jaffe, H. W., Friedmankien, A. E., & Weiss, R. A. 1991. The aetiology of Kaposi's sarcoma. *Cancer Surv. 10*, 23– 37.

Peters, B. S., Beck, E. J., Coleman, D. G., Wadsworth, M. J. H., McGuinness, O., Harris, J. R. W., & Pinching, A. J. 1991. Changing disease patterns in patients with AIDS in a referral centre in the United Kingdom: The changing face of AIDS. *Br. Med. J. 302*, 203–7.

Peters, W. 1987. *Chemotherapy and drug resistance in malaria*. London and New York: Academic Press.

Petersen, J. W., Ibsen, P. H., Bentzon, M. W., Capiau, C., & Heron, I. 1991. The cell mediated and humoral immune response to vaccination with acellular and whole cell pertussis vaccine in adult humans. *FEMS Microbiol. Immunol. 76*, 279–87.

Petersen, J. W., & Ochoa, L. G. 1989. Role of prostaglandin and cAMP in the secretory effects of cholera toxin. *Science 245*, 857– 9.

Petritsch, W., Eherer, A. J., Holzer-Petsche, U., Hinterleitner, T., Beubler, E., & Krejs, G. J. 1992. Effect of cholera toxin on the human jejunum. *Gut 33*, 1174–8.

Pfützner, A., Dietrich, U., Voneichel, U., Vonbriesen, H., Brede, H. D., Maniar, J. K., & Rübsamen-Waigmann, H. 1992. HIV-1 and HIV-2 infections in a high-risk population in Bombay, India: evidence for the spread of HIV-2 and presence of a divergent HIV-1 subtype. *J. Acquired Immune Defic. Syndr. 5*, 972–7.

Phair, J., Jacobson, L., Detels, R., Rinaldo, C., Saah, A., Schrager, L., & Muñoz, A. 1992. Acquired immune deficiency syndrome occurring within 5 years of infection with human immunodeficiency virus type-1: the multicenter AIDS cohort study. *J. Acquired Immune Defic. Syndr. 5*, 490–6.

Phillips, R. E., Rowland Jones, S., Nixon, D. F., Gotch, F. M., Edwards, J. P., Ogunlesi, A. O., Elvin, J. G., & Rothbard, J. A. 1991. Human immunodeficiency virus genetic variation that can escape cytotoxic T-cell recognition. *Nature 354*, 453–9.

Piatak, M., Saag, M. S., Yang, L. C., Clark, S. J., Kappes, J. C., Luk, K. C., Hahn, B. H., Shaw, G. M., & Lifson, J. D. 1993. High levels of HIV-1 in plasma during all stages of infection determined by competitive PCR. *Science 259*, 1749–54.

Pichichero, M. E., Francis, A. B., Blatter, M. M., Reisinger, K. S., Green, J. L., Marsocci, S. M., & Disney, F. A. 1992. Acellular pertussis vaccination of 2-month-old infants in the United States. *Pediatrics 89*, 882–7.

Pinheiro, F. P., Travassos da Rosa, A. P. A., Travassos da Rosa, J. F., & Bensabath, G. 1976. An outbreak of oropouche virus disease in the vicinity of Santarem Para Brazil. *Tropenmed. Parasitol. 27*, 213– 23.

Piot, P., Laga, M., Ryder, R., Perriens, J., Temmerman, M., Heyward, W., & Curran, J. W. 1990. The global epidemiology of HIV infection: Continuity, heterogeneity, and change. *J. Acquired Immune Defic. Syndr. 3*, 403–12.

Pison, G., Le Guenno, B., Lagarde, E., Enel, C., & Seck, C. 1993. Seasonal migration: A risk factor for HIV infection in rural Senegal. *J. Acquired Immune Defic. Syndr. 6*, 196–200.

Pluda, J. M., Yarchoan, R., Jaffe, E. S., Feuerstein, I. M., Solomon, D., Steinberg, S. M., Wyvill, K. M., Raubitschek, A., Katz, D., & Broder, S. 1990. Development of non-Hodgkin lymphoma in a cohort of patients with severe human immunodeficiency virus (HIV) infection on long-term antiretroviral therapy. *Ann. Intern. Med. 113*, 276–82.

Podda, A., Nencioni, L., Marsili, I., Peppoloni, S., Volpini, G., Donati, D., Ditommaso, A., Demagistris, M. T., & Rappuoli, R. 1991. Phase-I clinical trial of an acellular pertussis vaccine composed of genetically detoxified pertussis toxin combined with FHA and 69-kDa. *Vaccine 9*, 741–5.

Poiesz, B., Ruscetti, F. W., Gazdar, A. F., Bunn, P. A., Minna, J. D., & Gallo, R. C. 1980. Detection and isolation of type C retrovirus particles from fresh and cultured lymphocytes of a patient with cutaneous T-cell lymphoma. *Proc. Natl. Acad. Sci. USA* 77, 7415–19.

Pokrovsky, V. V. 1989. Nosocomial outbreak of HIV infection in Elista, USSR, Abstract W.A.0.5. In *Proceedings of the 5th International Conference on AIDS, Montreal, Quebec* 63.

Pokrovsky, V. V., Eramova, I. Y., Deulina, M. A., Lipetinov, V. V., Yashkutov, K. B., Slyusareva, L. A., Chemizova, N. M., & Savchenko, S. P. 1990. Outbreak of hospital infection caused by human immunodeficiency virus (HIV) in Elista. *Z. Mikrobiol. Epidemiol. Immunobiol. (April)*, 17–23.

Pollitzer, K. 1959. *Cholera*. Geneva: World Health Organization.

Polsky, B., Gold, J. W. M., Whimbey, E., Dryjanski, J., Brown, A. E., Schiffman, G., & Armstrong, D. 1986. Bacterial pneumonia in patients with the acquired immune deficiency syndrome. *Ann. Intern. Med. 104*, 38–41.

Pomerantz, R. J., Bagasra, O., & Baltimore, D. 1992. Cellular latency of human immunodeficiency virus type-1. *Curr. Opin. Immunol. 4*, 475–80.

Poulsen, A., Kvinesdal, B., Aaby, P., Molbak, K., Frederiksen, K., Dias, F., & Lauritzen, E. 1989. Prevalence of and mortality from human immunodeficiency virus type 2 in Bissau, west Africa. *Lancet i*, 827–30.

Prasad, V. R., Lowy, I., Delossantos, T., Chiang, L., & Goff, S. P. 1991. Isolation and characterization of a dideoxyguanosine triphosphate-resistant mutant of human immunodeficiency virus reverse transcriptase. *Proc. Natl. Acad. Sci. USA 88*, 11363–7.

Prescott, S. C., & Horwood, M. P. 1935. *Sedgwick's principles of sanitary science and public health*. New York: Macmillan.

Preston, B. D., Poiesz, B. J., & Loeb, L. A. 1988. Fidelity of HIV-I reverse transcriptase. *Science 242*, 1168.

Price, P. W. 1980. *Evolutionary biology of parasites*. Princeton: Princeton University Press.

Prince, H. E., Jensen, E. R., & York, J. 1992. Lymphocyte subsets in HTLV-II-infected former blood donors: relationship to spontaneous lymphocyte proliferation. *Clin. Immunol. Immunopathol. 65*, 201–6.

Profet, M. 1988. The evolution of pregnancy sickness as protection to the embryo against Pleistocene teratogens. *Evol. Theory 8*, 177–90.

Profet, M. 1991. The function of allergy: Immunological defense against toxins. *Q. Rev. Biol. 66*, 23–62.

Profet, M. 1992. Pregnancy sickness as adaptation: A deterrent to maternal ingestion of teratogens. In *The adapted mind: Evolutionary psychology and the generation of culture*, ed. J. Barkow, L. Cosmides, & J. Tooby, pp. 327–65. New York: Oxford University Press.

Puel, J., Lheritier, D., Guyader, M., Izopet, J., Briant, L., Tricoire, J., & Berrebi, A. 1992. Viral load and mother-to-infant HIV transmission. *Lancet 340*, 859.

Puffer, R. R., & Serrano, C. V. 1973. *Patterns of mortality in childhood*. Washington, DC: Pan Am Health Organization.

Putkonen, P., Thorstensson, R., Albert, J., Hild, K., Norrby, E., Biberfeld, P., & Biberfeld, G. 1990. Infection of cynomolgus monkeys with HIV-2 protects against pathogenic consequences of a subsequent simian immunodeficiency virus infection. *AIDS 4*, 783-9.

Rademaker, C. M. A., Wolfhagen, M. J. H. M., Jansze, M., Oteman, M., Fluit, A. C., Glerum, J. H., & Verhoef, J. 1992. Digoxigenin labelled DNA probes for rapid detection of enterotoxigenic, enteropathogenic and Vero cytotoxin producing *Escherichia coli* in faecal samples. *J. Microbiol. Methods 15*, 121–7.

Rahman, A. S. M. M., Bari, A., & Molla, A. M. 1991. Rice-ORS shortens the duration of watery diarrhoeas: Observation from rural Bangladesh. *Trop. Geogr. Med. 43*, 23–7.

Rajasekaran, P., Dutt, P. R., & Pisharoti, K. A. 1977. Impact of water supply on the incidence of diarrhea and shigellosis among children in rural communities in Madurai. *Indian J. Med. Res. 66*, 189–99.

Raju, T. N. K., & Kobler, C. 1991. Improving handwashing habits in the newborn nurseries. *Am. J. Med. Sci. 302*, 355–8.

Ramamurthy, T., Garg, S., Sharma, R., Bhattacharya, S. K., Nair, G. B., Shimada, T., Takeda, T., Karasawa, T., Kurazano, H., Pal, A., & Takeda, Y. 1993. Emergence of novel strain of *Vibrio cholerae* with epidemic potential in southern and eastern India. *Lancet 341*, 703–4.

Ranford-Cartwright, L. C., Balfe, P., Carter, R., & Walliker, D. 1991. Genetic hybrids of *Plasmodium falciparum* identified by amplification of genomic DNA from single oocysts. *Mol. Biochem. Parasitol. 49*, 239–44.

Rao, S. R. 1973. *Lothal and the Indus civilization*. New York: Asia Publishing House.

Rapoport, F. H. 1919. The complement fixation test in influenzal pneumonia. *JAMA 72*, 633–6.

Rappuoli, R., Pizza, M., DeMagistris, M. T., Podda, A., Bugnoli, M., Manetti, R., & Nencioni, L. 1992. Development and clinical testing of an acellular pertussis vaccine containing genetically detoxified pertussis toxin. *Immunobiology 184*, 230–9.

Rather, L. J. 1962. Introduction to *Disease, life, and man*, by Rudolf Virchow. New York: Collier.

Reddy, M. M., McKinley, G., Euglard, A., & Grieco, M. H. 1989. Effect of azidothymidine (AZT) on p24 antigen levels in patients with AIDS-related complex and AIDS. *J. Clin. Lab. Analysis 3*, 199–201.

Reddy, M. M., McKinley, G. F., & Grieco, M. H. 1991. Evaluation of HIV P24 antigen, β_2 microglobulin, neopterin, soluble CD4, soluble CD8, and soluble interleukin-2 receptor levels in patients with AIDS or AIDS-related complex treated with 2´, 3´-dideoxyinosine (ddI). *J. Clin. Lab. Analysis 5*, 396–8.

Reddy, M. M., Winger, E. E., Hargrove, D., McHugh, T., McKinley, G. F., & Grieco, M. H. 1992. An improved method for monitoring efficacy of anti-retroviral therapy in HIV-infected individuals: a highly sensitive HIV p24 antigen assay. *J. Clin. Lab. Analysis 6*, 125–9.

Reeves, W. C., Levine, P. H., Cuevas, M., Quiroz, E., Maloney, E., & Saxinger, W. C. 1990. Seroepidemiology of human T-cell lymphotropic virus type I in the Republic of Panama. *Am. J. Trop. Med. Hyg. 42*, 374–9.

Reeves, W. C., Saxinger, C., Brenes, M. M., Quiroz, E., Clark, J. W., Hoh, M. W., & Blattner, W. A. 1988. Human T-cell lymphotropic virus type I (HTLV-I) seroepidemiology and risk factors in metropolitan Panama. *Am. J. Epidemiol. 127*, 532–9.

Regan, J. A., San Giovani, T., Greenberg, E., & Konowitz, L. 1987. Nosocomial transmission of group B streptococci (GBS) in a well baby nursery: 1986 update. *Pediatr. Res. 21*, 420.

Samadi, A. R., Huq, M. I., Shahid, N., Khan, M. U., Eusof, A., Rahaman, A. S. M. M., Yunus, M., & Faruque, A. S. G. 1983. Classical *Vibrio cholerae* biotype displaces el tor in Bangladesh. *Lancet i*, 805–7.

Samuel, M. C., Guydish, J., Ekstrand, M., Coates, T. J., & Winkelstein, W. 1991. Changes in sexual practices over five years of follow-up among heterosexual men in San Francisco. *J. Acquired Immune Defic. Syndr. 4*, 896–900.

Sanchez-Lanier, M., Davis, L. E., Blisard, K. S., Woodfin, B. M., Wallace, J. M., & Caskey, L. S. 1991. Influenza A virus in the mouse: Hepatic and cerebral lesions in a Reye's syndrome-like illness. *Int. J. Exp. Pathol. 72*, 489–500.

Santhanakrishnan, B. R., Ganga, N., & Lakshminarayana, C. S. 1987. Shigellosis in children. *Indian J. Pediatr. 54*, 739–42.

Saracco, A., Musicco, M., Nicolosi, A., Angarano, G., Arici, C., Gavazzeni, G., Costigliola, P., Gafa, S., Gervasoni, C., Luzzati, R., Piccinino, F., Puppo, F., Salassa, B., Sinicco, A., Stellini, R., Tirelli, U., Turbessi, G., Vigevani, G. M., Visco, G., Zerboni, R., & Lazzarin, A. 1993. Man-to-woman sexual transmission of HIV: longitudinal study of 343 steady partners of infected men. *J. Acquired Immune Defic. Syndr. 6*, 497–502.

Sarver, N., Black, R. J., Bridges, S., & Chrisey, L. 1992. Frontiers in HIV-1 therapy: Fourth conference of the NIAID National Cooperative Drug Discovery Groups-HIV. *AIDS Res. Hum. Retroviruses 8*, 659–67.

Sato, H., Orenstein, J., Dimitrov, D., & Martin, M. 1992. Cell-to-cell spread of HIV-1 occurs within minutes and may not involve the participation of virus particles. *Virology 186*, 712–24.

Sawada, M., Suzumura, A., Kondo, N., & Marunouchi, T. 1992. Induction of cytokines in glial cells by transactivator of human T cell lymphotropic virus type I. *FEBS Let. 313*, 47–50.

Saxon, A. J., Calsyn, D. A., Whittaker, S., & Freeman, G. 1991. Sexual behaviors of intravenous drug users in treatment. *J. Acquired Immune Defic. Syndr. 4*, 938–44.

Scarlatti, G., Lombardi, V., Plebani, A., Principi, N., Vegni, C., Ferraris, G., Bucceri, A., Fenyo, E. M., Wigzell, H., Rossi, P., & Albert, J. 1991. Polymerase chain reaction, virus isolation and antigen assay in HIV-1-antibody-positive mothers and their children. *AIDS 5*, 1173–8.

Schaberg, D. R., Alford, R. H., Anderson, R., Farmer, J. J., Melly, M. A., & Schaffner, W. 1976. An outbreak of nosocomial infection due to a multiply resistant *Serratia marcescens*: Evidence of interhospital spread. *J. Infect. Dis. 134*, 181–8.

Schaberg, D. R., Rubens, C. E., Alford, R. H., Farrar, W. E., Schaffner, W., & McGee, Z. A. 1981. Evolution of antimicrobial resistance and nosocomial infection: Lessons from the Vanderbilt experience. *Am. J. Med. 70*, 445–8.

Schall, J. J. 1990. Virulence of lizard malaria: The evolutionary ecology of an ancient parasite-host association. *Parasitology 100*, S35–52.

Schatzl, H., Yakovleva, L., Lapin, B., Rose, D., Inzhiia, L., Gaedigknitschko, K., Deinhardt, F., & Vonderhelm, K. 1992. Detection and characterization of T-cell leukemia virus-like proviral sequences in PBL and tissues of baboons by PCR. *Leukemia 6*, S158–60.

Schechter, M. T., Marion, S. A., Elmslie, K. D., Ricketts, M. N., Nault, P., & Archibald, C. P. 1991a. Geographic and birth cohort associations of Kaposi's sarcoma among homosexual men in Canada. *Am. J. Epidemiol. 134*, 485–8.

Schechter, M. T., Neumann, P. W., Weaver, M. S., Montaner, J. S. G., Cassol, S. A., Le, T. N., Craib, K. J. P., & O'Shaughnessy, M. V. 1991b. Low HIV-1 proviral DNA burden detected by negative polymerase chain reaction in seropositive individuals correlates with slower disease progression. *AIDS 5*, 373–9.

Schellekens, P. T. A., Tersmette, M., Roos, M. T. L., Keet, R. P., Dewolf, F., Coutinho, R. A., & Miedema, F. 1992. Biphasic rate of CD4+ cell count decline during progression to AIDS correlates with HIV-1 phenotype. *AIDS 6*, 665–9.

Schmitt, M. P., & Holmes, R. K. 1991. Characterization of a defective diphtheria toxin repressor (dtxR) allele and analysis of dtxR transcription in wild-type and mutant strains of *Corynebacterium diphtheriae*. *Infect. Immun. 59*, 3903–8.

Schmitt, M. P., Twiddy, E. M., & Holmes, R. K. 1992. Purification and characterization of the diphtheria toxin repressor. *Proc. Natl. Acad. Sci. USA 89*, 7576–80.

Schneiderman, L. J., & Kaplan, R. M. 1992. Fear of dying and HIV infection vs hepatitis-B infection. *Am. J. Public Hlth. 82*, 584– 6.

Schneweis K E, Kleim J-P, Bailly E, Niese D, Wagner N, & Brackmann H H. 1990. Graded cytopathogenicity of the human immunodeficiency virus (HIV) in the course of HIV infection. *Med. Microbiol. Immunol. 179*, 193–203.

Schnittman, S. M., Greenhouse, J. J., Lane, H. C., Pierce, P. F., & Fauci, A. S. 1991. Frequent detection of HIV-1-specific mRNAs in infected individuals suggests ongoing active viral expression in all stages of disease. *AIDS Res. Hum. Retroviruses 7*, 361–7.

Schoepf, B. G. 1988. Women, AIDS, and the economic crisis in central Africa. *Can. J. Afric. Stud. 22*, 625–44.

Schrijvers, D., Delaporte, E., Peeters, M., Dupont, A., & Meheus, A. 1991. Seroprevalence of retroviral infection in women with different fertility statuses in Gabon western Equatorial Africa. *J. Acquired Immune Defic. Syndr. 4*, 468–70.

Schulman, K. A., Lynn, L. A., Glick, H. A., & Eisenberg, J. M. 1991. Cost effectiveness of low-dose zidovudine therapy for asymptomatic patients with human immunodeficiency virus (HIV) infection. *Ann. Intern. Med. 114*, 798–802.

Schulz, T. F. 1992. Origin of AIDS. *Lancet 339*, 867.

Schwartz, B., Schuchat, A., Oxtoby, M. J., Cochi, S. L., Hightower, A., & Broome, C. V. 1991. Invasive group B streptococcal disease in adults: A population-based study in metropolitan Atlanta. *JAMA 266*, 1112–14.

Schwartz, J. B., Akin, J. S., Guilkey, D. K., & Paqueo, V. 1989. The effect of contraceptive prices on method choice in the Philippines, Jamaica, and Thailand. In *Choosing a contraceptive. Method choice in Asia and the United States*, ed. R. A. Bulatao, J. A. Palmore, & S. E. Ward, pp. 78–102. Boulder, Colorado: Westview Press.

Seal, S. C., & Banerjea, R. K. 1949. Incidence of gastrointestinal disorders in relation to the drinking-water sources in a rural area in Bengal. *J. Indian Med. Assoc. 18*, 319–26.

Selwyn, P. A., Alcabes, P., Hartel, D., Buono, D., Schoenbaum, E. E., Klein, R. S., Davenny, K., & Friedland, G. H. 1992. Clinical manifestations and predictors of disease progression in drug users with human immunodeficiency virus infection. *N. Engl. J. Med. 327*, 1697–1703.

Semmelweis, I. P. 1861/1981. *The cause, concept, and prophylaxis of childbed fever.* Birmingham: Classics of Medicine Library. [Translation of 1861 text].

Semple, M., Loveday, C., Weller, I., & Tedder, R. 1991. Direct measurement of viraemia in patients infected with HIV-1 and its relationship to disease progression and zidovudine therapy. *J. Med. Virol. 35*, 38–45.

Seshamma, T., Bagasra, O., Trono, D., Baltimore, D., & Pomerantz, R. J. 1992. Blocked early-stage latency in the peripheral blood cells of certain individuals infected with human immunodeficiency virus type 1. *Proc. Natl. Acad. Sci. USA 89*, 10663–7.

Shanks, R. A., & Studzinski, L. P. 1952. *Bact. coli* in infantile diarrhoea. *Br. Med. J. i*, 119–23.

Sharma, A. K., Majumdar, S. K., & Chakrabarty, A. N. 1967. Bacteriological findings of dysenteric disorders in Calcutta. *Indian J. Med. Res. 55*, 1181–3.

Shearer, G. M., & Clerici, M. 1991. Early T-helper cell defects in HIV infection. *AIDS 5*, 245–53.

Sheppard, H. W., Ascher, M. S., McRae, B., Anderson, R. E., Lang, W., & Allain, J. P. 1991. The initial immune response to HIV and immune system activation determine the outcome of HIV disease. *J. Acquired Immune Defic. Syndr. 4*, 704–12.

Sherman, M. P., Saksena, N. K., Dube, D. K., Yanagihara, R., & Poiesz, B. J. 1992. Evolutionary insights on the origin of human T-Cell lymphoma/leukemia virus type I (HTLV-I) derived from sequence analysis of a new HTLV-I variant from Papua New Guinea. *J. Virol. 66*, 2556–63.

Shiga, K. 1936. The trend of prevention, therapy and epidemiology of dysentery since the discovery of its causitive organism. *N. Engl. J. Med. 215*, 1205–11.

Shimanuki, H. 1990. Bacteria. In *Honey bee pests, predators, and diseases*, 2nd edition, ed. R. A. Morse & R. Nowogrodzki, pp. 27–47. Ithaca, N.Y.: Cornell University Press.

Shimoyama, M. 1991. Diagnostic criteria and classification of clinical subtypes of adult T-cell leukaemia-lymphoma: A report from the Lymphoma Study Group (1984–7). *Br. Med. Haematol. 79*, 428–37.

Shinefield, H. R. 1976. Staphylococcal infections. in *Infectious diseases of the fetus and newborn infant*, ed. J. S. Remington & J. O. Klein, pp. 979–1019. Philadelphia: W. B. Saunders.

Shu-Cheng, D. 1983. Shigellosis in children in China. In *Shigellosis, a continuing global problem*, ed. M. Rahaman, W. B. Greenough, N. R. Novack, & S. Rahman, pp. 14–25. Dhaka: International Center for Diarrheal Disease Research, Bangladesh.

Shute, P. G., Lupascu, G. H., Branzei, P., Maryon, M., Constantinescu, P., Bruce-Chwatt, L. J., Draper, C. C., Killick-Kendrick, R., & Garnham, P. C. C. 1976. A strain of *Plasmodium vivax* characterized by prolonged incubation: The effect of numbers of sporozoites on the length of the prepatent period. *Trans. Roy. Soc. Trop. Med. Hyg. 70*, 474–81.

Siddique, A. K., Baqui, A. H., Eusof, A., Haider, K., Hossain, M. A., Bashir, I., & Zaman, K. 1991. Survival of classic cholera in Bangladesh. *Lancet 337*, 1125–7.

Siegmund, O. H., & Fraser, C H. (eds.) 1973. *The Merck veterinary manual*, 4th edition, Rahway, New Jersey: Merck.

Sigel, S. P., Lanier, S., Baselski, V. S., & Parker, C. D. 1980. *In vivo* evaluation of pathogenicity of clinical and environmental isolates of *Vibrio cholerae. Infect. Immun.* *28*, 681–7.

Sigerist, H. E. 1943. *Civilization and disease.* Ithaca, N.Y.: Cornell University Press.

Silva, M. L. M., & Giampaglia, C. M. S. 1992. Colostrum and human milk inhibit localized adherence of enteropathogenic *Escherichia coli* to HeLa cells. *Acta Paediatr. Scand. 81*, 266–7.

Silver, D. R., Cohen, I. L., & Weinberg, P. F. 1992. Recurrent *Pseudomonas aeruginosa* pneumonia in an intensive care unit. *Chest 101*, 194–8.

Simon, H. J. 1960. *Attenuated infection: The germ theory in contemporary perspective.* Philadelphia: J. B. Lippincott.

Sinden, R. E. 1991. Asexual blood stages of malaria modulate gametocyte infectivity to the mosquito vector—possible implications for control strategies. *Parasitology 103*, 191–6.

Singh, R. P. 1983. Viroids and their potential danger to potatoes in hot climates. *Can. Plant. Dis. Surv. 63*, 13–18.

Sittitrai, W., Brown, T., & Sterns, J. 1990. Opportunities for overcoming the continuing restraints to behavior change and HIV risk reduction. *AIDS 4 (Suppl. 1)*, S269–76.

Sivinski, J. 1984. The behavioral ecology of vermin. *Florida Entomol. 67*, 57–67.

Skidmore, C. A., Robertson, J. R., Robertson, A. A., & Elton, R. A. 1990. After the epidemic: Follow up study of HIV seroprevalence and changing patterns of drug use. *Br. Med. J. 300*, 219–23.

Slater, I. H. 1965. Strychnine, picrotoxin, pentylenetetrazol, and miscellaneous drugs. *Drill's pharmacology in medicine*, 3rd edition, ed. J. R. DiPalma, pp. 379–93. New York: Blakiston/ McGraw-Hill.

Smart, C. 1888. *The medical and surgical history of the war of the rebellion, Part III, Vol. I: Medical history.* Washington, D.C.: U.S. Government Printing Office.

Smith, D. T. 1972. The typhus group of rickettsioses. In *Zinsser microbiology*, 15th edition, ed. W. K. Joklik & D. T. Smith, pp. 677–84. New York: Appleton-Century-Crofts.

Smith, I. M. 1979. *Staphylococcus aureus.* In *Principles and practice of infectious disease*, 3rd edition, ed. G. L. Mandell, R. G. Douglas, & J. E. Bennett, pp. 1530–52. New York: Wiley.

Smith, K. M. 1957. *A textbook of plant virus diseases*, 2nd edition. Boston: Little, Brown.

Smith, T. 1934. *Parasitism and disease.* Princeton: Princeton University Press.

Snewin, V. A., Longacre, S., & David, P. H. 1991. *Plasmodium vivax*: Older and wiser? *Res. Immunol. 142*, 631–6.

Snow, J. 1855/1966. *On the mode of communication of cholera*, 2nd edition, London: Churchill.

Snyder, J. C. 1965. Typhus fever rickettsiae. In *Viral and rickettsial disease of man*, ed. F. L. Horsfall & Tam I, pp. 1059– 94. Philadelphia: J. P. Lippencott.

Snyder, J. D., & Merson, M. H. 1982. The magnitude of the global health problem of acute diarrhoeal disease: A review of active surveillance data. *Bull. WHO 60*, 605–13.

Somasundaran, M., & Robinson, H. L. 1988. Unexpectedly high levels of HIV-1 RNA and protein synthesis in a cytocidal infection. *Science 242*, 1554–7.

South, M. A. 1971. Enteropathogenic Escherichia coli disease: New developments and perspectives. *J. Pediat. 79*, 1–11.

Southwood, T. R. E. 1987. The natural environment and disease: An evolutionary perspective. *Br. Med. J. 294*, 1086–9.

Spear, J. B., Benson, C. A., Pottage, J. C., Paul, D. A., Landay, A. L., & Kessler, H. A. 1988. Rapid rebound of serum human immunodeficiency virus antigen after discontinuing zidovudine therapy. *J. Infect. Dis. 158*, 1132–3.

Spiegel, H., Herbst, H., Niedobitek, G., Foss, H. D., & Stein, H. 1992. Follicular dendritic cells are a major reservoir for human immunodeficiency virus type 1 in lymphoid tissues facilitating infection of CD4+ T-helper cells. *Am. J. Pathol. 140*, 15–22.

Sprunt, K., & Redman, W. 1968. Evidence suggesting importance of role of interbacterial inhibition in maintaining balance of normal flora. *Ann. Intern. Med. 68*, 579–90.

Srugo, I., Brunell, P. A., Chelyapov, N. V., Ho, D. D., Alam, M., & Israele, V. 1991. Virus burden in human immunodeficiency virus type 1-infected children: Relationship to disease status and effect of antiviral therapy. *Pediatrics 87*, 921–5.

St. Clair, M. H., Martin, J. L., Tudor-Williams, G., Bach, M. C., Vavro, C. L., King, D. M., Kellam, P., Kemp, S. D., & Larder, B. A. 1991. Resistance to ddI and sensitivity to AZT induced by a mutation in HIV-1 reverse transcriptase. *Science 253*, 1557–9.

Stahmer, I., Zimmer, J. P., Ernst, M., Fenner, T., Finnern, R., Schmitz, H., Flad, H. D., & Gerdes, J. 1991. Isolation of normal human follicular dendritic cells and CD4-independent *in vitro* infection by human immunodeficiency virus (HIV-1). *Eur. J. Immunol. 21*, 1873–8.

Stall, R. D., Coates, T. J., & Hoff, C. 1988. Behavioral risk reduction of HIV infection among gay and bisexual men: A review of results from the United States. *Am. Psychol. 43*, 878–85.

Stanley, E. D., Jackson, G. G., Panusam, C., Rubenis, M., & Dirda, V. 1975. Increased virus shedding with aspirin treatment of rhinovirus infection. *JAMA 231*, 1248–51.

Stanley, E. D., Jackson, G. G., Dirda, V., & Rubenis, M. 1976. Re: Increased virus shedding with aspirin treatment of rhinovirus infection. *JAMA 235*, 802–3.

Stead, W. W., Lofgren, J. P., Warren, E., & Thomas, C. 1985. Tuberculosis as an epidemic and nosocomial infection among the elderly in nursing homes. *N. Engl. J. Med. 312*, 1483–7.

Stead, W. W., & Lofgren, J. P. 1991. Tuberculosis and HIV infection. *N. Engl. J. Med. 325*, 1882.

Stebbins, E. L. 1940. Recent studies of epidemic diarrhea and dysentery. *South. Med. J. 33*, 197–203.

Steiner, P. E. 1968. *Disease in the civil war: Natural biological warfare in 1861–1865.* Springfield, Ill.: C. C. Thomas.

Sternberg, S. 1992. HIV comes in five family groups. *Science 256*, 966.

Stevenson, J. S. 1952. Further observations on the occurrence of *Bact. coli* D 433 in adult faeces. *Br. Med. J. ii*, 123–4.

Stevens, K. M. 1981. The pathophysiology of influenzal pneumonia in 1918. *Perspect. Biol. Med. 25*, 115–25.

Stevenson, M., Stanwick, T. L., Dempsey, M. P., & Lamonica, C. A. 1990. HIV-1 replication is controlled at the level of T cell activation and proviral integration. *EMBO J. 9*, 1551–60.

Stoll, B. J., Glass, R. I., Huq, M. I., Khan, M. U., Banu, H., & Holt, J. 1982. Epidemiologic and clinical features of patients infected with *Shigella* who attended a diarrheal disease hospital in Bangladesh. *J. Infect. Dis. 146*, 177–83.

Storsaeter, J. 1991. *Studies on the protective efficacy of two acellular pertussis vaccines: The importance of appropriate diagnostic methods and case definitions.* Stockholm: Kongl Carolinska Medico Chirurgiska Institutet.

Studdert, M. J., Oda, C., Riegl, C. A., & Roston, R. P. 1983. Aspects of the diagnosis, pathogenesis and epidemiology of canine parvovirus. *Austral. Vet. J. 60*, 197–200.

Stulberg, C. S., & Zuelzer, W. W. 1956. Infantile diarrhea due to *Escherichia coli. Ann. N.Y. Acad. Sci. 66*, 90–9.

Sudre, P., ten Dam, G., & Kochi, A. 1992. Tuberculosis—A global overview of the situation today. *Bull. WHO 70*, 149–59.

Sugiyama, H., Doi, H., Yamaguchi, K., Tsuji, Y., Miyamoto, T., & Hino, S. 1986. Significance of post-natal mother-to-child transmission of human T-lymphotropic virus type-I on the development of adult T-cell leukemia/lymphoma. *J. Med. Virol. 20*, 253–60.

Súarez, P., Valcarcel, J., & Ortin, J. 1992. Heterogeneity of the mutation rates of influenza A viruses: Isolation of mutator mutants. *J. Virol. 66*, 2491–4.

Swanson, C. E., & Cooper, D. A. 1990. Factors influencing outcome of treatment with zidovudine of patients with AIDS in Australia. *AIDS 4*, 749–57.

Swart, A. M., Weller, I., & Darbyshire, J. H. 1990. Early HIV infection: To treat or not to treat? *Br. Med. J. 301*, 825–6.

Swellengrebel, N. H. 1940. The efficient parasite. In *Proceedings of the Third International Congress of Microbiology* pp. 119–27. Baltimore: Waverly.

Szturm-Rubenstein, S. 1968. Determination of biotype, phage type and colicinogenic character of *Shigella sonnei*, and its epidemiologic importance. *Arch. Immunol. Ther. Exp. (Warsaw) 16*, 421–28.

Tachibana, N., Okayama, A., Ishihara, S., Shioiri, S., Murai, K., Tsuda, K., Goya, N., Matsuo, Y., Essex, M., Stuver, S., & Mueller, N. 1992. High HTLV-I proviral DNA level associated with abnormal lymphocytes in peripheral blood from asymptomatic carriers. *Int. J. Cancer 51*, 593–5.

Tacket, C. O., Shahid, N., Huq, M. I., Alim, A. R. M. A., & Cohen, M. L. 1984. Usefulness of plasmid profiles for differentiation of *Shigella* isolates in Bangladesh. *J. Clin. Microbiol. 20*, 300–1.

Tajima, K. 1988. The T-and B-cell malignancy study group. The third nation-wide study on adult T-cell leukemia/lymphoma (ATL) in Japan: Characteristic patterns of HLA antigen and HTLV-I infection in ATL patients and their relatives. *Int. J. Cancer 41*, 505–12.

Tajima, K., & Ito, S. 1990. Prospective studies of HTLV-I and associated diseases in Japan. In *Human retrovirology: HTLV*, ed. W. A. Blattner, pp. 267–79. New York: Raven Press.

Tajima, K., Tominaga, S., Suchi, T., Kawagoe, T., Komoda, H., Hinuma, Y., Oda, T., & Fujita, K. 1982. Epidemiological analysis of the distribution of antibody to adult T-cell leukemia virus associated antigen (ATLA): Possible horizontal transmission of adult T-cell leukemia virus. *Gann 73*, 893–901.

Takeda, Y. 1983. Shigellosis in Japan. In *Shigellosis: A continuing global problem*, ed. M. Rahaman, W. B. Greenough, N. R. Novack, & S. Rahman, pp. 48-58. Dhaka: International Center for Diarrheal Disease Research, Bangladesh.

Takeuchi, Y., Nagumo, T., & Hoshino, H. 1988. Low fidelity of cell-free DNA synthesis by reverse transcriptase of human immunodeficiency virus. *J. Virol. 62*, 3900–2.

Taylor, J. 1966. Host–parasite relations of *Escherichia coli* in man. *J. Appl. Bacteriol 29*, 1–12.

Tedder, R. S., O'Connor, T., Hughes, A., N'jie, H., Corrah, T., & Whittle, H. 1988. Envelope cross-reactivity in western blot for HIV-1 and HIV-2 may not indicate dual infection. *Lancet ii*, 927– 30.

Temin, H. M. 1989a. Is HIV unique or merely different? *J. Acqured Immune Defic. Syndr. 2*, 1–9.

Temin, H. M. 1989b. Retrovirus variation and evolution. *Genome 31*, 17–22.

Tersmette, M., Gruters, R. A., de Wolf, F., de Goede, R. E. Y., Lange, J. M. A., Schellekens, P. T. A., Goudsmit, J. A. A. P., Huisman, H. G., & Miedema, F. 1989. Evidence for a role of virulent human immunodeficiency virus (HIV) variants in the pathogenesis of acquired immunodeficiency syndrome: Studies on sequential HIV isolates. *J. Virol. 63*, 2118–25.

Tersmette, M., & Miedema, F. 1990. Interactions between HIV and the host immune system in the pathogenesis of AIDS. *AIDS 4 (Suppl. 1)*, S57–66.

Terwilliger, E. F., Langhoff, E., & Haseltine, W. A. 1991. The nef gene of HIV-1. A review of recent results. In *Genetic structure and regulation of HIV*, ed. W. A. Haseltine & F. Wongstaal, pp. 457–71. New York: Raven Press.

Tesh, R. B. 1980. Experimental studies on the transovarial transmission of Kunjin and San Angelo viruses in mosquitoes. *J. Trop. Med. Hyg. 29*, 657–66.

Tesh, R. B., & Shroyer, D. A. 1980. The mechanism of arbovirus transovarial transmission in mosquitoes: San Angelo virus in *Aedes albopictus*. *Am. J. Trop. Med. Hyg. 29*, 1394–1404.

Thomas, L. 1972. Notes of a biology-watcher: Germs. *N. Engl. J. Med. 247*, 553–5.

Thompson, R. L., Cabezudo, I., & Wenzel, R. P. 1982. Epidemiology of nosocomial infections caused by methicillin-resistant *Staphylococcus aureus*. *Ann. Intern. Med. 97*, 309–17.

Thomson, S. 1955. The numbers of pathogenic bacilli in faeces in intestinal diseases. *J. Hyg. 53*, 217–24.

Tilton, J. 1813. *Economic observations on military hospitals and the prevention of diseases incident to an army*. Wilmington, Del.: Wilson.

Tiollais, P., & Buendia, M. A. 1991. Hepatitis B virus. *Sci. Am. 264(4)*, 116–23.

Tjøtta, E., Hungnes, O., & Grinde, B. 1991. Survival of HIV-1 activity after disinfection, temperature and pH changes, or drying. *J. Med. Virol. 35*, 223–7.

Tokudome, S. 1991. Possible environmental factors related with transmission of HTLV-I among children. *Eur. J. Epidemiol. 7*, 437– 8.

Tomonaga, K., Katahira, J., Fukasawa, M., Hassan, M. A., Kawamura, M., Akari, H., Miura, T., Goto, T., Nakai, M., Suleman, M., Isahakia, M., & Hayami, M. 1993. Isolation and characterization of simian immunodeficiency virus from African white-crowned mangabey monkeys (*Cercocebus torquatus lunulatus*). *Arch. Virol. 129*, 77–92.

Trager, J. 1982. *Letters from Sachiko*. New York: Atheneum.

Tremblay M, & Wainberg M A. 1990. Neutralization of multiple HIV-1 isolates from a single subject by autologous sequential sera. *J. Infect. Dis. 162*, 735–7.

Trujillo, J. M., Concha, M., Muñoz, A., Bergonzoli, G., Mora, C., Borrero, I., Gibbs, C. J., & Arango, C. 1992. Seroprevalence and cofactors of HTLV-I infection in Tumaco, Colombia. *AIDS Res. Hum. Retroviruses 8*, 651–7.

Tsujimoto, H., Hasegawa, A., Maki, N., Fukasawa, M., Miura, T., Speidel, S., Cooper, R. W., Moriyama, E. N., Gojobori, T., & Hayami, M. 1989. Sequence of a novel simian immunodeficiency virus from a wild-caught African mandrill. *Nature 341*, 539–41.

Tudor-Williams, G., St. Clair, M. H., Mckinney, R. E., Maha, M., Walter, E., Santacroce, S., Mintz, M., O'Donnell, K., Rudoll, T., Vavro, C. L., Connor, E. M., & Wilfert, C. M. 1992. HIV-1 sensitivity to zidovudine and clinical outcome in children. *Lancet 339*, 15–19.

Turnbull, P. C. B., Lee, J. V., Miliotis, M. D., Still, C. S., Isaacson, M., & Ahmad, Q. S. 1985. *In vitro* and *in vivo* cholera toxin production by classical and el tor isolates of *Vibrio cholerae*. *J. Clin. Microbiol. 21*, 884–90.

Turner, B. J., & Ball, J. K. 1992. Variations in inpatient mortality for AIDS in a national sample of hospitals. *J. Acquired Immune Defic. Syndr. 5*, 978–87.

Turner-Lowe, S. 1991. New strategies needed to combat malaria. *News Report, U.S. National Research Council 41(8)*, 5–8.

Uchida, T., Gill, D. M., & Pappenheimer, A. M. 1971. Mutation in the structural gene for diphtheria toxin carried by temperate phage ß. *Nature New Biol. 233*, 8–11.

Ueda, K., Tokugawa, K., & Kusuhara, K. 1992. Perinatal viral infections. *Early Hum. Dev. 29*, 131–6.

Uherová, P., Schmidtmayerova, H., & Mayer, V. 1991. Failure of azidothymidine to inhibit human immunodeficiency virus (HIV) replication in a promonocytic cell line (U937). *Acta Virol 35*, 357–64.

U.S. Department of State 1986. *Gabon: Post report*. Washington, D.C.: U.S. Government Printing Office.

van Beneden, P. J. 1885. *Animal parasites and messmates*. New York: Appleton.

van den Hoek, J. A. R., Al, E. J. M., Huisman, J. G., Goudsmit, J., & Coutinho, R. A. 1991. Low prevalence of human T-cell leukaemia virus-I and -II infection among drug users in Amsterdam, the Netherlands. *J. Med. Virol. 34*, 100–3.

van den Hoek, J. A. R., van Haastrecht, H. J. A., & Coutinho, R. A. 1992. Little change in sexual behavior in injecting drug users in Amsterdam. *J. Acquired Immune Defic. Syndr. 5*, 518–22.

van den Hoek, J. A. R., van Haastrech, H. J. A., & Coutinho, R. A. 1989. Risk reduction among intravenous drug users in Amsterdam under the influence of AIDS. *Am. J. Public Hlth. 79*, 1355–7.

van der Werf, T. S., Das, P. K., van Soolingen, D., Yong, S., van der Mark, T. W., & van den Akker, R. 1992. Sero-diagnosis of tuberculosis with A60 antigen enzyme-linked immunosorbent assay: Failure in HIV-infected individuals in Ghana. *Med. Microbiol. Immunol. 181*, 71–6.

van Griensven, G. J. P., De Vroome, E. M. M., Goudsmit, J., & Coutinho, R. A. 1989. Changes in sexual behavior and the fall in incidence of HIV among homosexual men. *Br. Med. J. 298*, 218–21.

van Griensven, G. J. P., de Vroome, E. M. M., de Wolf, F., Goudsmit, J., Roos, M., & Coutinho, R. A. 1990. Risk factors for progression of human immunodeficiency virus (HIV) infection among seroconverted and seropositive homosexual men. *Am. J. Epidemiol. 182*, 203–10.

van Loon, F. P. L., Rabbani, G. H., Bukhave, K., & Rask-Madsen, J. 1992. Indomethacin decreases jejunal fluid secretion in addition to luminal release of prostaglandin-E2 in patients with acute cholera. *Gut 33*, 643–5.

van Oye, E., Pfeifer, I., & Krüger, W. 1968. The epidemiology of shigellosis in Belgium with special reference to the phage-types of *Shigella sonnei*. *Arch. Immunol. Ther. Exp. (Warsaw) 16*, 452–8.

Varavithya, W., Sunthornkachit, R., & Eampokalap, B. 1991. Oral rehydration therapy for invasive diarrhea. *Rev. Infect. Dis. 13*, S325–31.

Varela-Echavarria, A., Garvey, N., Preston, B. D., & Dougherty, J. P. 1992. Comparison of moloney murine leukemia virus mutation rate with the fidelity of its reverse transcriptase *in vitro*. *J. Biol. Chem. 267*, 24681–8.

Vasquez, P., Sanchez, G., Volante, C., Vera, L., Ramirez, E., Soto, G., & Lee, H. 1991. Human T-lymphotropic virus type I (HTLV-I): New risk for Chilean population. *Blood 78*, 850–1.

Venkatesan, S. 1992. Virological and cellular physiological roles of HIV nef protein. *Res. Virol. 143*, 38–42.

Verghese, A., Mireault, K., & Arbeit, R. C. 1986. Group B streptococcal bacteremia in men. *Rev. Infect. Dis. 8*, 912–17.

Veyssier-Belot, C. 1990. Kaposi's sarcoma and HTLV-I infection. *Lancet 336*, 575.

Victoria, C. G., Smith, P. G., Vaughan, J. P., Nobre, L. C., Lombardi, C., Teixeira, A. M. B., Fuchs, S. M. C., Moreira, L. B., Gigante, L. P., & Barros, F. C. 1987. Evidence for protection by breast-feeding against infant deaths from infectious diseases in Brazil. *Lancet ii*, 319–22.

Virchow, R. 1877/1962. *Disease, life, and man*. New York: Collier.

Volberding, P. A., Lagakos, S. W., Koch, M. A., Pettinelli, C., Myers, M. W., Booth, D. K., Balfour, H. H., Reichman, R. C., Bartlett, J. A., Hirsch, M. S., Murphy, R. L., Hardy, W. D., Soeiro, R., Fischl, M. A., Bartlett, J. G., Merigan, T. C., Hyslop, N. E., Richman, D. D., Valentine, F. T., & Corey, L. 1990. Zidovudine in asymptomatic human immunodeficiency virus infection: A controlled trial in persons with fewer than 500 CD4-positive cells per cubic millimeter. *N. Engl. J. Med. 322*, 941–9.

Waage, J. K., & Nondo, J. 1982. Host behaviour and mosquito feeding success: an experimental study. *Trans. Roy. Soc. Trop. Med. Hyg. 76*, 119–22.

Wade, A. W., Green-Johnson, J., & Szewczuk, M. R. 1988. Functional changes in systemic and mucosal lymphocyte repertoires with age: An update review. *Aging: Immunol. Infect. Dis. 1*, 65– 97.

Wahman, A., Melnick, S. L., Rhame, F. S., & Potter, J. D. 1991. The epidemiology of classic, African, and immunosuppressed Kaposi's sarcoma. *Epidemiol. Rev. 13*, 178–99.

Wainberg, M. A., Tremblay, M., Rooke, R., Fanning, M., Tsoukas, C., Montaner, J. S. G., O'Shaughnessy, M., & Ruedy, J. 1992. Characterization of zidovudine resistant variants of HIV-1 isolated from patients on prolonged therapy. *Drugs Exptl. Clin. Res. 18*, 283–90.

Wallace, B. 1972. *Disease, sex, communication, behavior: Essays in social biology, Vol III.* Englewood Cliffs, New Jersey: Prentice-Hall.

Wallace, B. 1989. Can "stepping stones" form stairways. *Am. Nat. 133*, 578–9.

Wallace, J. M. 1950. Prevention of sunblotch disease of avocados in new plantings. *Calif. Avocado Assoc. Yearbook 1950*, 97–100.

Wallace, J. M., & Drake, R. J. 1962. A high rate of seed transmission of avocado sun-blotch virus from symptomless trees and the origin of such trees. *Phytopathology 52*, 237–41.

Wallace, J. M., & Drake, R. J. 1953. Seed transmission of the avocado sunblotch virus. *Citr. Leaves 33*, 18–20.

Walliker, D., Quakyi, I. A., Wellems, T. E., McCutchan, T. F., Szarfman, A., London, W. T., Corcoran, L. M., Burkot, T. R., & Carter, R. 1987. Genetic analysis of the human malaria parasite *Plasmodium falciparum. Science 236*, 1661–6.

Walsh, J., & Warren, K. 1979. Selective primary health care: An interim strategy for disease control in developing countries. *N. Engl. J. Med. 301*, 967–74.

Wang, B. 1984. Study on the effect of oral immunization of T32-Istrati strain against bacillary dysentery in field trials. *Arch. Roum. Pathol. Exp. Microbiol. 43*, 285–9.

Ward, J. W., Bush, T. J., Perkins, H. A., Lieb, L. E., Allen, J. R., Goldfinger, D., Samson, S. M., Pepkowitz, S. H., Fernando, L. P., Holland, P. V., Kleinman, S. H., Grindon, A. J., Garner, J. L., Rutherford, G. W., & Holmberg, S. D. 1989. The natural history of transfusion-associated infection with human immunodeficiency virus. Factors influencing the rate of progression to disease. *N. Engl. J. Med. 321*, 947–52.

Warren, J. T., & Dolatshahi, M. 1992. Worldwide survey of AIDS vaccine challenge studies in nonhuman primates: Vaccines associated with active and passive immune protection from live virus challenge. *J. Med. Primatol. 21*, 139–86.

Watanabe, M., Ringler, D. J., Fultz, P. N., Mackey, J. J., Boyson, J. E., Levine, C. G., & Letvin, N. L. 1991. A chimpanzee-passaged human immunodeficiency virus isolate is cytopathic for chimpanzee cells but does not induce disease. *J. Virol. 65*, 3344–8.

Watanakunakorn, C., & Jura, J. 1991. *Klebsiella* bacteremia: A review of 196 episodes during a decade (1980–1989). *Scand. J. Infect. Dis. 23*, 399–405.

Waters, A. P., Higgins, D. G., & McCutchan, T. F. 1991. *Plasmodium falciparum* appears to have arisen as a result of lateral transfer between avian and human hosts. *Proc. Natl. Acad. Sci. USA 88*, 3140–4.

Wats, R. C., Loganadan, A. D., & Conquest, C. N. 1928. Dysentery in Secunderabad. *Indian Med. Gaz. 63*, 13–16.

Wattel, E., Mariotti, M., Agis, F., Gordien, E., Le Coeur, F. F., Prin, L., Rouger, P., Chen, I. S. Y., Wain-Hobson, S., & Lefrere, J. J. 1992. Quantification of HTLV-I proviral copy number in peripheral blood of symptomless carriers from the French West Indies. *J. Acquired Immune Defic. Syndr. 5*, 943–6.

Weber, D. J., Becherer, P. R., Rutala, W. A., Samsa, G. P., Wilson, M. B., & White, G. C. 1991. Nosocomial infection rate as a function of human immunodeficiency virus type 1 status in hemophiliacs. *Am. J. Med. 91*, S206–12.

Weintraub, Z., Regev, R., Iancu, T., Ferne, M., & Rabinowitz, B. 1983. Perinatal group B streptococcal infections in Israel. *Israel J. Med. Sci. 19*, 900–2.

Weiss, P. J., Brodine, S. K., Goforth, R. R., Kennedy, C. A., Wallace, M. R., Olson, P. E., Garland, F. C., Hall, F. W., Ito, S. I., & Oldfield, E. C. 1992. Initial low CD4 lymphocyte counts in recent human immunodeficiency virus infection and lack of association with identified coinfections. *J. Infect. Dis. 166*, 1149–53.

Weiss, R. 1989a. The viral advantage. *Sci. News 136*, 200–3.

Weiss, R. 1989b. Allergy-triggering receptor made *en masse. Sci. News 135*, 246.

Weiss, R. 1991. Brain killer stable in soil. *Sci. News 139*, 84.

Weiss, R. 1992. Measles battle loses potent weapon. *Science 258*, 546–47.

Weiss, R. 1990. The swat team. *Sci. News 137*, 72–4.

Weissman, J. B., Murton, K. I., Lewis, J. N., Friedemann, C. H. T., & Gangarosa, E. J. 1974. Impact in the U.S. of the Shiga dysentery pandemic of Central America and Mexico: A review of surveillance data through 1972. *J. Infect. Dis. 129*, 218–23.

West, A. P. 1991. Drug abuse treatment as a strategy to prevent human immunodeficiency virus infection among intravenous drug users: How can we maximize prevention of infection? *Arch. Intern. Med. 151*, 1493–96.

Wheeler, M. 1966. *Civilizations of the Indus Valley and beyond.* London: Thames & Hudson.

Wheeler, M. 1968. *The Indus civilization.* Cambridge: Cambridge University Press.

Wheeler, W. E., & Wainerman, B. 1954. The treatment and prevention of epidemic infantile diarrhea due to *E. coli* 0-111 by the use of chloramphenicol and neomycin. *Pediatrics 14*, 357–63.

Whitley, R. J. 1990. Herpes simplex viruses. In *Virology*, 2nd edition, ed. B. N. Fields, D. M. Knipe, R. M. Chanock, M. S. Hirsch, J. L. Melnick, T. P. Monath, & B. Roizman, pp. 1843–87. New York: Raven Press.

Whittle, H., Egboga, A., Todd, J., Corrah, T., Wilkins, A., Demba, E., Morgan, G., Rolfe, M., Berry, N., & Tedder, R. 1992. Clinical and laboratory predictors of survival in Gambian patients with symptomatic HIV-1 or HIV-2 infection. *AIDS 6*, 685–9.

Wignall, F. S., Hyams, K. C., Phillips, I. A., Escamilla, J., Tejada, A., Li, O., Lopez, F., Chauca, G., Sanchez, S., & Roberts, C. R. 1992. Sexual transmission of human T-lymphotropic virus type I in Peruvian prostitutes. *J. Med. Virol. 38*, 44–8.

Wilbur, C. K. 1980. *Revolutionary medicine 1700–1800.* Chester, Conn.: Globe Pequot.

Williams, G. 1959. *Virus hunters.* New York: Knopf.

Williams, G. C. 1966. *Adaptation and natural selection.* Princeton, New Jersey: Princeton University Press.

Williams, G. C. 1957. Pleiotropy, natural selection and the evolution of senescence. *Evolution 11*, 398–411.

Williams, G. C., & Nesse, R. M. 1991. The dawn of Darwinian medicine. *Q. Rev. Biol. 66*, 1–22.

Wilson, C. M., Serrano, A. E., Wasley, A., Bogenshutz, M. P., Shankar, A. J., & Wirth, D. F. 1989. Amplification of a gene related to mammalian *mdr* genes in drug-resistant *Plasmodium falciparum. Science 244*, 1184–86.

Wilson, D. S. 1980. *The natural selection of populations and communitites.* Menlo Park, Cal.: Benjamin/Cummings.

Winkelstein, W., Wiley, J. A., Padian, N. S., Samuel, M., Shiboski, S., Ascher, M. S., & Levy, J. A. 1988. The San Francisco Men's Health Study: Continued decline in HIV seroconversion rates among homosexual/bisexual men. *Am. J. Public Hlth. 78*, 1472–74.

Winther, B., Gwaltney, J. M., & Hendley, J. O. 1990. Respiratory virus infection of monolayer culture of human nasal epithelial cells. *Am. Rev. Respir. Dis. 141*, 839–45.

Wolff, H. L., & Croon, J. J. A. B. 1968. The survival of smallpox virus (*Variola minor*) in natural circumstances. *Bull. WHO 38*, 492–93.

Wolfs, T. F. W., de Jong, J. J., van den Berg, H., Tijnagel, J. M. G. H., Krone, W. J. A., & Goudsmit, J. 1990. Evolution of sequences encoding the principal neutralization epitope of human immunodeficiency virus 1 is host dependent, rapid and continuous. *Proc. Natl. Acad. Sci. USA 87*, 9938–42.

Wolfs, T. F. W., Zwart, G., Bakker, M., & Goudsmit, J. 1992. HIV-1 genomic RNA diversification following sexual and parenteral virus transmission. *Virology 189*, 103–10.

Wolfs, T. F. W., Zwart, G., Bakker, M., Valk, M., Kuiken, C. L., & Goudsmit, J. 1991. Naturally occurring mutations within HIV-1 V3 genomic RNA lead to antigenic variation dependent on a single amino acid substitution. *Virology 185*, 195–205.

Wolinsky, E. 1992. Mycobacterial diseases other than tuberculosis. *Clin. Infect. Dis. 15*, 1–12.

Wolinsky, E., Lipsitz, P. J., Mortimer, E. A., & Rammelkamp, C. H. 1960. Acquisition of staphylococci by newborns. Direct versus indirect transmission. *Lancet ii*, 620–22.

Wolinsky, S. M., Wike, C. M., Korber, B. T. M., Hutto, C., Parks, W. P., Rosenblum, L. L., Kunstman, K. J., Furtado, M. R., & Muñoz, J. L. 1992. Selective transmission of human immunodeficiency virus type-1 variants from mothers to infants. *Science 255*, 1134-37.

Wolman, A., & Gorman, A. E. 1931. *The significance of waterborne typhoid fever outbreaks, 1920–1930.* Baltimore: Williams and Wilkins.

Wood, R., Dong, H. L., Katzenstein, D. A., & Merigan, T. C. 1993. Quantification and comparison of HIV-1 proviral load in peripheral blood mononuclear cells and isolated CD4+ T cells. *J. Acquired Immune Defic. Syndr. 6*, 237–40.

Woodcock, H. M. 1909. Hemoflagellates and allied forms. In *A treatise on zoology* Part 1, pp. 193–273. London: Adam & Charles Black.

Woodward, J. J. 1870. *The medical and surgical history of the war of the rebellion (1861–65), Part I, Vol. I: Medical history.* Washington, D.C.: U.S. Gov. Printing Office.

Woodward, J. J. 1879. *The medical and surgical history of the war of the rebellion (1861–1865), Part II, Vol. I: Medical history.* Washington, D.C.: U.S. Gov. Printing Office.

World Health Organization. 1992. Tuberculosis control and research strategies for the 1990s—memorandum from a WHO meeting. *Bull. WHO 70*, 17–21.

Wormser, G. P., Forseter, G., Joline, C., Tupper, B., & O'Brien, T. A. 1991. Hepatitis C in HIV-infected intravenous drug users and homosexual men in suburban New York City. *JAMA 265*, 2958.

Wynne-Edwards, V. C. 1962. *Animal dispersion in relation to social behaviour.* Edinburgh: Oliver & Boyd.

Yahi, N., Fantini, J., & Chermann, J. C. 1992. Infection of HIV-1 and HIV-2 through the luminal and serosal sides of polarized human intestinal epithelial cells. *AIDS 6*, 335–6.

Yamaguchi, K., Kiyokawa, T., Nakada, K., Yul, L. S., Asou, N., Ishii, T., Sanada, I., Seiki, M., Yoshida, M., Matutes, E., Catovsky, D., & Takatsuki, K. 1988. Polyclonal integration of HTLV-I proviral DNA in lymphocytes from HTLV-I seropositive individuals: An intermediate state between the healthy carrier state and smouldering ATL. *Br. J. Haematol. 68*, 169–74.

Yamaguchi, K., Nishimura, H., & Takatsuki, K. 1983. Clinical features of malignant lymphoma and adult T-cell leukemia in Kumamoto. *Rinsho Ketsekui 24*, 1271–76.

Yamaoka, S., Tobe, T., & Hatanaka, M. 1992. Tax protein of human T-cell leukemia virus type I is required for maintenance of the transformed phenotype. *Oncogene 7*, 433–37.

Yanagihara, R., Ajdukiewicz, A. B., Garruto, R. M., Sharlow, E. R., Wu, X., Alemaena, O., Sale, H., Alexander, S. S., & Gajdusek, D. C. 1991a. Human T lymphotropic virus type I infection in the Solomon Islands. *Am. J. Trop. Med. Hyg. 44*, 122–30.

Yanagihara, R., Jenkins, C. L., Alexander, S. S., Mora, C. A., & Garruto, R. M. 1990. Human T lymphotropic virus type I infection in Papua New Guinea: High prevalence among the Hagahai confirmed by western analysis. *J. Infect. Dis. 162*, 649–54.

Yanagihara, R., Nerurkar, V. R., Garruto, R. M., Miller, M. A., Leon-Monzon, M. E., Jenkins, C. L., Sanders, R. C., Liberski, P. P., Alpers, M. P., & Gajdusek, D. C. 1991b. Characterization of a variant of human T lymphotropic virus type I isolated from a member of a remote, recently contacted group in Papua New Guinea. *Proc. Natl. Acad. Sci. USA 88*, 1446–50.

Yoshida, M., Osame, M., Kawai, H., Toita, M., Kuwasaki, N., Nishida, Y., Hiraki, Y., Takahashi, K., Nomura, K., Sonoda, S., Eiraku, N., Ijichi, S., & Usuku, K. 1989. Increased replication of HTLV-I in HTLV-I-associated myelopathy. *Ann. Neurol. 26*, 331–35.

Yu, F., Itoyama, Y., Fujihara, K., & Goto, I. 1991. Natural killer (NK) cells in HTLV-I-associated myelopathy/tropical spastic paraparesis—decrease in NK cell subset populations and activity in HTLV-I seropositive individuals. *J. Neuroimmunol. 33*, 121–28.

Zack, J. A., Haislip, A. M., Krogstad, P., & Chen, I. S. Y. 1992. Incompletely reverse-transcribed human immunodeficiency virus type 1 genomes in quiescent cells can function as intermediates in the retroviral life cycle. *J. Virol. 66*, 1717–25.

Zanetti, A. R., & Galli, C. 1992. Seroprevalence of HTLV-I and HTLV-II. *N. Engl. J. Med. 326*, 1783.

Zazopoulos, E., & Haseltine, W. A. 1993. Effect of *nef* alleles on replication of human immunodeficiency virus type 1. *Virology 194*, 20–7.

Zazopoulos, E., & Haseltine, W. A. 1992. Mutational analysis of the human immunodeficiency virus type-1 Eli nef function. *Proc. Natl. Acad. Sci. USA 89*, 6634–38.

Zervos, M. J., Dembinski, S., Mikesell, T., & Schaberg, D. R. 1986a. High-level resistance to gentamicin in *Streptococcus faecalis*: Risk factors and evidence for exogenous acquisition of infection. *J. Infect. Dis. 153*, 1075–83.

Zervos, M. J., Kauffman, C. A., Therasse, P. M., Bergman, A. G., Mikesell, T. S., & Schaberg, D. R. 1987. Nosocomial infection by gentamicin-resistant *Streptococcus faecalis*: An epidemiologic study. *Ann. Intern. Med. 106*, 687–91.

Zervos, M. J., Mikesell, T. S., & Schaberg, D. R. 1986b. Heterogeneity of plasmids determining high-level resistance to gentamicin in clinical isolates of *Streptococcus faecalis. Antimicrob. Agents Chemother. 30*, 78–81.

Zhang, L. Q., Simmonds, P., Ludlam, C. A., & Leigh-Brown, A. J. 1991. Detection, quantification and sequencing of HIV-1 from the plasma of seropositive individuals and from factor VIII concentrates. *AIDS 5*, 675–81.

Zinsser, H. 1935. *Rats, lice and history.* Boston: Little Brown.

Zuber, P. L. F., Gruner, E., Altwegg, M., & Vongraevenitz, A. 1992. Invasive infection with non-toxigenic *Corynebacterium diphtheriae* among drug users. *Lancet 339*, 1359.

Zucker-Franklin, D., Hooper, W. C., & Evatt, B. L. 1992. Human lymphotropic retroviruses associated with mycosis fungoides: evidence that human T-cell lymphotropic virus type II (HTLV-II) as well as HTLV-I may play a role in the disease. *Blood 80*, 1537–45.

Zweig, M., Samuel, K. P., Showalter, S. D., Bladen, S. V., DuBois, G. C., Lautenberger, J. A., & Papas, T. S. 1990. Enhanced production of HIV-1 nef protein in high-passage cultures of infected cells. In *Gene regulation and AIDS: Transcriptional activation, retroviruses, and pathogenesis*, ed. T. S. Papas, pp. 193–204. Houston: Gulf.

Index